Molecular Mechanisms and Biological Procedures of Biomaterials in Medical Applications

Molecular Mechanisms and Biological Procedures of Biomaterials in Medical Applications

Guest Editor

Yi Zhang

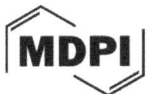

Basel • Beijing • Wuhan • Barcelona • Belgrade • Novi Sad • Cluj • Manchester

Guest Editor
Yi Zhang
Department of Minerals
Processing and
Bioengineering
Central South University
Changsha
China

Editorial Office
MDPI AG
Grosspeteranlage 5
4052 Basel, Switzerland

This is a reprint of the Special Issue, published open access by the journal *Journal of Functional Biomaterials* (ISSN 2079-4983), freely accessible at: https://www.mdpi.com/journal/jfb/special_issues/07992YW6Q0.

For citation purposes, cite each article independently as indicated on the article page online and as indicated below:

Lastname, A.A.; Lastname, B.B. Article Title. *Journal Name* **Year**, *Volume Number*, Page Range.

ISBN 978-3-7258-4157-8 (Hbk)
ISBN 978-3-7258-4158-5 (PDF)
https://doi.org/10.3390/books978-3-7258-4158-5

© 2025 by the authors. Articles in this book are Open Access and distributed under the Creative Commons Attribution (CC BY) license. The book as a whole is distributed by MDPI under the terms and conditions of the Creative Commons Attribution-NonCommercial-NoDerivs (CC BY-NC-ND) license (https://creativecommons.org/licenses/by-nc-nd/4.0/).

Contents

About the Editor vii

Seânia Santos Leal, Gustavo Oliveira de Meira Gusmão, Valdiléia Teixeira Uchôa, José Figueiredo-Silva, Lucielma Salmito Soares Pinto, Carla R. Tim, et al.
Evaluation of How Methacrylate Gelatin Hydrogel Loaded with *Ximenia americana* L. Extract (Steam Bark) Effects Bone Repair Activity Using Rats as Models
Reprinted from: *J. Funct. Biomater.* **2023**, *14*, 438, https://doi.org/10.3390/jfb14090438 1

Aneta Fraczek-Szczypta, Natalia Kondracka, Marcel Zambrzycki, Maciej Gubernat, Pawel Czaja, Miroslawa Pawlyta, et al.
Exploring CVD Method for Synthesizing Carbon–Carbon Composites as Materials to Contact with Nerve Tissue
Reprinted from: *J. Funct. Biomater.* **2023**, *14*, 443, https://doi.org/10.3390/jfb14090443 18

Renata de Lima Barbosa, Emanuelle Stellet Lourenço, Julya Vittoria de Azevedo dos Santos, Neilane Rodrigues Santiago Rocha, Carlos Fernando Mourão and Gutemberg Gomes Alves
The Effects of Platelet-Rich Fibrin in the Behavior of Mineralizing Cells Related to Bone Tissue Regeneration—A Scoping Review of In Vitro Evidence
Reprinted from: *J. Funct. Biomater.* **2023**, *14*, 503, https://doi.org/10.3390/jfb14100503 45

Ishita Allu, Ajay Kumar Sahi, Meghana Koppadi, Shravanya Gundu and Alina Sionkowska
Decellularization Techniques for Tissue Engineering: Towards Replicating Native Extracellular Matrix Architecture in Liver Regeneration
Reprinted from: *J. Funct. Biomater.* **2023**, *14*, 518, https://doi.org/10.3390/jfb14100518 80

Carmen Grierosu, Gabriela Calin, Daniela Damir, Constantin Marcu, Radu Cernei, Georgeta Zegan, et al.
Development and Functionalization of a Novel Chitosan-Based Nanosystem for Enhanced Drug Delivery
Reprinted from: *J. Funct. Biomater.* **2023**, *14*, 538, https://doi.org/10.3390/jfb14110538 106

Yibei Jiang, Zhou Wang, Ke Cao, Lu Xia, Dongqing Wei and Yi Zhang
Montmorillonite-Sodium Alginate Oral Colon-Targeting Microcapsule Design for WGX-50 Encapsulation and Controlled Release in Gastro-Intestinal Tract
Reprinted from: *J. Funct. Biomater.* **2024**, *15*, 3, https://doi.org/10.3390/jfb15010003 119

Elisa Restivo, Emanuela Peluso, Nora Bloise, Giovanni Lo Bello, Giovanna Bruni, Marialaura Giannaccari, et al.
Surface Properties of a Biocompatible Thermoplastic Polyurethane and Its Anti-Adhesive Effect against *E. coli* and *S. aureus*
Reprinted from: *J. Funct. Biomater.* **2024**, *15*, 24, https://doi.org/10.3390/jfb15010024 130

Zhou Wang, Yibei Jiang, Guangjian Tian, Chuyu Zhu and Yi Zhang
Toxicological Evaluation toward Refined Montmorillonite with Human Colon Associated Cells and Human Skin Associated Cells
Reprinted from: *J. Funct. Biomater.* **2024**, *15*, 75, https://doi.org/10.3390/jfb15030075 145

About the Editor

Yi Zhang

Prof. Dr. Yi Zhang is currently a full-time employee at Sch. Miner. Process. Bioeng., Cent. South Univ., whom has long engaged in clay mineral nanoprocessing and their applications in controlling drug release and tissue regeneration. He has also contributed one edited book, one edited book chapter, and more than 40 journal publications (including *Nature Communications*, *Science Advances*, *Advanced Functional Materials*, *Science China Materials*, *Applied Clay Science*, etc.). He has succeeded in winning 2 National Natural Science Foundation of China, and 2 Natural Science Foundation of Hunan Province. He also won some prestigious Fellowships/awards including China Building Materials Science and Technology Award (2018 and 2016), China Non-Ferrous Metals Industry Science and Technology Award (2013) and Ministry of Education's Academic Youth Award for Doctoral Candidate (2012). He has been invited as board members of the Chinese Ceramic Society's Mineral Materials Division, International Journal of Materials, Mechanics and Manufacturing, and Standardization Committee of Chinese Society for Testing and Materials (Inorganic Nonmetallic Material Field).

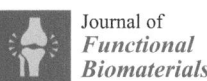

Article

Evaluation of How Methacrylate Gelatin Hydrogel Loaded with *Ximenia americana* L. Extract (Steam Bark) Effects Bone Repair Activity Using Rats as Models

Seânia Santos Leal [1,2], Gustavo Oliveira de Meira Gusmão [3], Valdiléia Teixeira Uchôa [4], José Figueiredo-Silva [2], Lucielma Salmito Soares Pinto [2], Carla R. Tim [1], Lívia Assis [1], Antonio Luiz Martins Maia-Filho [2], Rauirys Alencar de Oliveira [5], Anderson Oliveira Lobo [6,*] and Adriana Pavinatto [1,*]

1. Scientific and Technological Institute, Brazil University, São Paulo 08230-030, Brazil; seaniasantos@gmail.com (S.S.L.); carla.tim@universidadebrasil.edu.br (C.R.T.); livia.assis@universidadebrasil.edu.br (L.A.)
2. Biotechnology and Biodiversity Research Center, State University of Piauí, Teresina 64002-150, Brazil; figueredo_silva@hotmail.com (J.F.-S.); lucielmasalmito@ccs.uespi.br (L.S.S.P.); almmaiaf@ccs.uespi.br (A.L.M.M.-F.)
3. GrEEnTeC-PPGQ, State University of Piauí—UESPI, 2231 João Cabral Street, P.O. Box 381, Teresina 64002-150, Brazil; gomgusmao@ccn.uespi.br
4. PPGQ-GERATEC-CD, State University of Piauí, Teresina 64002-150, Brazil; valdileiateeira@ccn.uespi.br
5. School of Health Sciences, State University of Piauí, Teresina 64002-150, Brazil; rauirysalencar@ccs.uespi.br
6. Interdisciplinary Laboratory for Advanced Materials (LIMAV), Materials Science & Engineering Graduate Program (PPGCM), Federal University of Piauí (UFPI), Teresina 64049-550, Brazil
* Correspondence: lobo@ufpi.edu.br (A.O.L.); adriana.pavinatto@universidadebrasil.edu.br (A.P.)

Abstract: The use of bioactive materials, such as *Ximenia americana* L., to stimulate the bone repair process has already been studied; however, the synergistic effects of its association with light emitting diode (LED) have not been reported. The present work aims to evaluate the effect of its stem bark extract incorporated into methacrylate gelatin hydrogel (GelMA) on the bone repair process using pure hydrogel and hydrogel associated with LED therapy. For this purpose, the GelMA hydrogel loaded with *Ximenia americana* L. extract (steam bark) was produced, characterized and applied in animal experiments. The tests were performed using 50 male Wistar rats (divided into 5 groups) submitted to an induced tibia diaphyseal fracture. The therapy effects were verified for a period of 15 and 30 days of treatment using histological analysis and Raman spectroscopy. After 15 days of induced lesion/treatment, the new bone formation was significantly higher in the GXG (GelMA + *X. americana* L.) group compared to the control group ($p < 0.0001$). After 30 days, a statistically significant difference was observed when comparing the GXLEDG (GelMA + *X. americana* L. + LED) and the control group ($p < 0.0001$), the GXG and the control group ($p < 0.001$), and when comparing the GG, GXG ($p < 0.005$) and GXLEDG ($p < 0.001$) groups. The results shows that the *Ximenia americana* L. stem extract incorporated into GelMA hydrogel associated with LED therapy is a potentiator for animal bone repair.

Keywords: biomaterials; plant extract; hydrogel; bone repair; photobiomodulation

1. Introduction

Bone repair is a natural process that involves a series of complex biological events aimed at restoring bone integrity and function. Some factors that can affect bone repair include age, nutrition, blood supply, stability, diabetes, smoking and certain medications [1]. In cases of severe fractures or complications, bone grafts or growth factors can be used to stimulate bone repair. Although bone grafts can be effective in promoting bone regeneration, there are several challenges and limitations associated with this approach, such as limited availability, healing time, graft resorption, non-union and late union, risk of infection, immune response, rejection and nonviable cost [2,3]. Given the challenges associated with conventional approaches, researchers and healthcare professionals are continually exploring alternative treatments for bone repair. Some promising options include tissue engineering, including structures, growth factors and stem cells [3–6]; bone morphogenetic proteins (BMPs) [7]; mesenchymal stem cell therapy [6]; 3D printing [4,5,8]; and gene therapy [7,9].

Photo-crosslinkable hydrogels with exceptional biocompatibility and biodegradability possess the capacity to substantially enhance cell migration, proliferation and differentiation, making them extensively employed in the field of tissue engineering [8,10]. Methacryloyl gelatin (GelMA) is a flexible hydrogel derived from gelatin and modified with methacrylamide and methacrylate groups, allowing it to crosslink when exposed to light irradiation. This versatile hydrogel can be fabricated using diverse methodologies, including microforming, photomasking, bioprinting and microfluidic techniques. It is characterized by high flexibility, porosity and hydrophilicity, leading to minimal inflammatory responses when used in the body. In addition, they exhibit promising osteoinductive properties that are beneficial for bone repair [11–13]. Their structure closely resembles the cell matrix, making them well suited for cell culture both in vitro and in vivo [14].

In the same context, natural compounds derived from medicinal plant extracts, such as *Davallina orientalis, Lepidium sativum* L., Cimicifuga racemose (Actaea), *Piper sarmentosum, Ormocarpum cochinchinense, Peperomia pellucida, Symphytum officinale,* Chenopodium ambroisioides L., *Epimedium sagittatum, Nigella sativa, Aloe vera, Sambucus williamsii, Ulmus davidiana, Spinacia oleracea, Dalbergia sissoo, Marantodes pumilum, Cassia occidentalis* L. [15], Astragalus membranaceus [16], Anredera cordifolia [17], Cissus quadrangularis, Withania somnifera and Tinospora cordifolia [18], are widely used to promote bone repair. Among the most studied herbal medicines, *Ximenia americana* L., which is a plant that is found in various regions of the world, possesses medicinal properties that are utilized and recognized [19]. The pulverized stem of *Ximenia americana* L. has been recommended for the repair and control of the inflammatory process, and proven results in research carried out through experimental models showed that this extract can be used to promote tissue repair [20]. The aqueous crude extract derived from various parts of the plant, including the leaves, roots, stem and stem bark, contains a range of secondary metabolites. These include tannins, flavonoids, saponins, steroids and triterpenes [21–23].

Phytochemical investigations of *Ximenia americana* L. steam bark reported by Santana et al. [19] and Almeida et al. [24] have revealed the presence of several bioactive compounds in different extracts, including aqueous, ethanolic and hydroalcoholic extracts. These compounds include condensed tannins, hydrolysable tannins, saponins, glycosides, polyphenols, flavonoids and terpenoids [23]. Flavonoids play a crucial role in various physiological processes within the body. They aid in the absorption of iron and vitamins and exhibit several beneficial properties, including antioxidant, antimicrobial, immunomodulatory, anti-inflammatory, and antinociceptive effects [25]. In addition, flavonoids possess analgesic properties and contribute to the regeneration of cartilage [26] and bones [27–30]. They also promote vasodilation and tissue healing in incisional wounds. In the context of bone repair, flavonoids exhibit anti-osteoclastic and anti-inflammatory effects by inhibiting the expression of osteoclastic markers, reducing reactive oxygen species and pro-inflammatory cytokine levels, as well as matrix metalloproteinases. Additionally, flavonoids enhance the osteogenic potential of pre-osteoblastic cells and stimulate the overexpression of osteogenic markers [29,31]. The flavonoids found in *Ximenia americana* L. are catechin, rutin, myricetin and (-)-epicatechin, the latter being found in greater amounts in the stem and root extracts [32–34].

The application of photobiomodulation LED therapy (light emitting diode therapy) has been widely studied in the treatment of different bone conditions [35–38]. The results of these studies have shown that the LED therapy in the near-infrared (invisible) wavelength spectrum has a positive effect on bone tissue metabolism and on fracture consolidation [39–42], as it stimulates mitochondrial metabolism, resulting in increased differentiation and proliferation of osteogenic cells and subsequent higher bone matrix deposition [43,44]. This evidence emphasizes the ability of LED therapy to stimulate bone formation and optimize bone repair.

Recent research demonstrates the association of poly (β-aminoester) (PBAE) hydrogel with total flavonoids with osteogenic properties [45]. Given this perspective, the interest in the subject is justified by the scarcity of studies that investigate the incorporation of *Ximenia americana* L. extract into GelMA hydrogel, as well as the association of the components (GelMA and GelMA/extract of *Ximenia americana* hydrogel) with LED (photobiomodulation) in bone repair. Therefore, in the present study, the synergistic effect from pure GelMA hydrogel loaded with aqueous extract from *Ximenia americana* L. stem-bark, and the effect of the hydrogel combined with LED therapy was evaluated.

2. Materials and Methods

2.1. Ximenia americana L. Extract

A sample of *Ximenia americana* L. was collected in Domingos Mourão (4°09′14.8″ S and 41°18′28.3″ W), a city in Piauí, Brazil, in January 2018. The different parts of the plant, including the stem, leaves, flowers and fruits, were identified and documented. A voucher specimen was preserved under the accession number HAF 03541 at the Herbarium Afrânio Gomes Fernandes (UESPI).

Following the methodology proposed by Carvalho et al. in 2020 [33], the bark of the *Ximenia americana* L. stem (300 g) was washed with water and placed in a beaker containing 2 L of distilled water. The beaker was then stored at 4 °C for 5 days. After this period, the liquid was filtered, and the aqueous extract was obtained. A portion of the extract was lyophilized, and both the aqueous and lyophilized samples were kept frozen until further use.

2.2. Incorporation of Ximenia americana L. in GelMA Hydrogel

The photopolymerizable methacrylate gelatin (GelMA) was obtained following the procedure described by Nichol et al. [46]. Briefly, 10 g of Type A gelatin (from pork skin, Sigma-Aldrich, Sao Paulo, Brazil), were dissolved in 100 mL of phosphate buffer solution (pH 7.4, Sigma-Aldrich), mixed and stirred for 1 h at 50 °C. Next, 3 mL of methacrylate anhydride 3-(trimethoxysilyl) propyl methacrylate (Sigma-Aldrich) was slowly dropped and stirred into the system for 3 h at 50 °C. Separately, 400 mL of PBS was pre-warmed to 50 °C and then mixed into the initial solution (reaching a volume of 500 mL). Next, the solution was then dialyzed using deionized (DI) water (12–14 KDa dialysis membranes, Sigma-Aldrich) for 7 days at 40 °C. The deionized water was changed twice a day. Finally, the solution was transferred to Falcon tubes, frozen at −80 °C and lyophilized, and the GelMA was obtained.

The GelMA/*Ximenia americana* L. hydrogel was obtained by adding *Ximenia americana* L. aqueous extract at a concentration of 5% in GelMA solution before the photoinitiator agent Irgacure insertion at a concentration of 0.5% 2-hydroxy-4′-(2-hydroxyethoxy)-2-methylpropiophenone (from Irgacure 2959, Sigma-Aldrich) to a 10% gelatin solution. Eppendorf tubes (used as a template) were taken to UV photocrosslinking (360–480 nm) for 5 min.

2.3. Hydrogel Characterization

The spectra were obtained from KBr pellets (spectroscopic grade), at a ratio of 1:100 sample/KBr. Before analyses, all samples (*Ximenia americana* L., GelMA and GelMA/*Ximenia americana* L.) and KBr were dried at 50 °C for 40 min. Next, the tablets were prepared using a press. The analyses were carried out using a Thermo Nicolet Nexus 470 equipment with Fourier transform infrared spectroscopy (FTIR) while using a transmittance module with an accumulation of 48 scans from 4000 to 500 cm^{-1}, observing a resolution of 2 cm^{-1}.

Thermogravimetric analysis curves (TGA) were obtained on a SDT Q600 analyzer model (TA Instruments, São Paulo, Brazil). TGA curves were obtained using alumina sample support, and approximately 8 ± 0.1 mg of sample was used. The analyses were performed with a heating rate of 10 °C min^{-1} in an atmosphere composed of air and N2, using a flow rate of 40 mL min^{-1}.

Differential scanning calorimetry (DSC) curves were obtained in a DSC Q20 calorimeter model (TA Instruments), using an aluminum pan containing 2 ± 10 mg of sample in a nitrogen atmosphere under a flow rate of 20 mL min^{-1}. All results were obtained using the temperature ranging from 20 to 800 °C at a heating rate of 10 °C min^{-1}. All data analyses were performed using the TA Instruments Universal Analysis 2000 software, version 4.7A.

X-ray diffraction measurements were performed on the GelMA hydrogel samples, including those containing *Ximenia americana* L. and those without it. The samples were ground, the spectra acquisition time increased, and the scan was performed from 10° to 70°, with a step of 0.0200/s and speed of 0.5°/min for a total of 2 h of analyses for each sample. X-ray diffraction analyses were performed in a Rigaku X-ray unit, last model IV 2Theta/Theta, 40 kV voltage and 30 mA current, and a sealed Cu tube was used.

2.4. Controlled Release Test of Epicatechin—Main Compound of Ximenia americana L.

UV-Vis (Shimadzu UV-160A, Barueri, Brazil) absorption spectra were performed from 200 to 700 nm to identify the absorbance band of epicatechin, the main compound of the *Ximenia americana* L. sample. An analytical curve, observing the λ max. = 278 nm, was obtained from the *Ximenia americana* L. stock solution (1 mg/mL) in concentrations ranging from 50 to 250 µg/mL. All curves were performed in triplicate (n = 3).

The analytical curve constructed was then used to determine the concentration of epicatechin release through an in vitro release assay of the GelMA epicatechin. For this purpose, the experiment was carried out using the GelMA + *Ximenia americana* L. 5% hydrogel (m = 0.0005 g) was inserted in 10 mL of PBS (pH 7.4 ± 0.1) and incubated at 37 °C under 100 rpm of stirring. In the periods fixed at 15 min, 30 min, 1 h, 2 h, 24 h and for 30 days (maximum experimental time in the in vivo tests for the hydrogel), 3.0 mL of solution was removed from these mediums, and the amount of the epicatechin was detected using UV-Vis spectroscopy. Each experiment was performed in triplicate.

2.5. In Vivo Study

2.5.1. Ethical and Legal Aspects, and Experimental Animals

The present study was approved by the Animal Ethics Committee of the State University of Piaui (protocol 00089.007021/2021-66). Fifty male Wistar rats (Rattus norvegicus albinus), 8 weeks old and weighting 250–300 g, were kept at the Animal Hospital located at the State University of Piaui. The animals were housed in standard polyethylene cages under controlled conditions, including a temperature of 24 ± 1 °C, humidity of 60% and a 12/12 h light/dark cycle. They were provided with unrestricted access to suitable food and water.

The animals were divided into five groups (n = 10), with 5 rats from each group euthanized at the experimental times of 15 and 30 days. The groups were submitted to the following:

- Control Group (CG): induced fracture and no treatment;
- GelMA Group (GG): induced fracture and GelMA as treatment;
- GelMA + LED Group (GLEDG): induced fracture and GelMA + LED as treatment;
- GelMA/*Ximenia americana* L. Group (GXG): induced fractures and GelMA/*Ximenia americana* L. as treatment;
- GelMA/*Ximenia americana* L. + LED Group (GXLEDG): induced fractures and GelMA/*Ximenia americana* L. + LED as treatment.

2.5.2. Surgical Procedure

A pre-treatment using atropine provided by Alergan® (Guarulhos, Brazil) was administrated to the animals (0.04 mL/100 g of animal weight). After 15 min, they were anesthetized intramuscularly using 10% ketamine hydrochloride and 2% xylazine hydrochloride provided by Syntec® (0.1 mL/100 g of animal weight) [47,48]. Next, the animals were submitted to depilation and asepsis in the right tibia region with topical polvidone (Bioquímica®, Belo Horizonte, Brazil).

The procedures for fracture and implantation of the biomaterial were performed using the protocol adapted by Kido 2015 et al. [49]. Briefly, the critical bone defect was induced after a longitudinal incision in the skin, and the separation of the subcutaneous connective tissue was performed with a surgical micromotor (3 mm in diameter), followed by insertion of the biomaterial at the injury site, according to the treated groups. To obtain this cavity, a constant torque of 45 N was stipulated at a speed of 45,000 rpm and abundant irrigation with saline solution for the viability of bone regeneration.

At the end of the procedure, the animals received subcutaneous tramadol hydrochloride analgesic (12.5 mg/Kg), administered every 6 h. Periodic assessments (every 2 h), were also performed to identify pain by facial expression and behavior. The euthanasia of the animals was proceeded in the period of 15 and 30 days after induction of injury by overdose administrating 150 mg/kg of sodium thionembutal [50,51]. Samples of bone tissue from the groups were removed and kept in liquid nitrogen. The collected samples were sent for Raman spectroscopy analysis and histopathological analysis.

2.5.3. LED Therapy

To stimulate bone repair, 1 LED light device (Endophoton, KLD, Biosistemas, Amparo, Brazil) was used, which emitted in the near infrared electromagnetic spectrum of 858 ± 20 nm. The intervention of the LED group was performed after the surgical procedure, which corresponds to the period from the beginning of the inflammatory phase of bone repair for several days after the postoperative period until euthanasia. The application was performed on the right tibia using the punctual technique (one point on the fracture), with the equipment pen positioned perpendicularly to the bone tissue for 120 s using 6 J of energy, 12 J/cm^2 of energy density and 0.1 W/cm^2 of potency.

2.5.4. Histological Analysis

Buffered formalin was used for 48 h to fix each sample, and after fixation, the samples were decalcified with EDTA (ethylendiaminetetra acetic acid, 10% w/v, pH 7.2) for four weeks. After decalcification, the samples were immersed in alcoholic solutions (gradually increasing concentrations) for dehydration and treated with xylene in an automatized tissue processor (PT05 TS Luptec, Sao Carlos, Brazil). After being embedded in paraffin, a rotating microtome (MRP09 Luptec, Sao Carlos, Brazil) was used to obtain serial histopathological sections (with a thickness of 5 µm and a distance between 2 and 3 µm,), and the samples were colored using hematoxylin and eosin (H.E.) at two sections/blade.

The samples were studied using a trinocular light microscope (model Olympus CX31, Tokyo, Japan), and photographic images were made in triplicate using a digital camera (Moticam WiFi X, MoticMicroscopes, Richmond, VA, USA) with connection to a computer. The histopathological semiquantitative analysis of new bone formation was performed according to the aspects described in the literature [52,53]. All images were enlarged using a micrometric ruler as a parameter of magnitude of amplification, which was inserted into all images collected using 4× and 10× magnification objectives. The processed specimens were evaluated through comparative descriptive analysis.

2.5.5. Dispersive Raman Spectroscopy

To perform the Raman spectroscopy, the samples were kept at room temperature (removed from the nitrogen). The spectra were obtained in a Raman spectrometer (model Senterra II, Bruker, Fällanden, Switzerland), using $\lambda = 785$ nm laser for excitation. The laser parameters used are 50 mW of output power, a spectral resolution of 9–15 cm^{-1} for 15 s, a gamma spectral set up at 400 a, and a 90-3, 500 cm^{-1} 10× objective. The spectrum was collected in triplicate (10 μm of distance between the points) for all bone regions of interest. The spectrum of normal cortical bone, referred to as healthy, was acquired from a region distant from the induced lesion after euthanizing the animals at 15 and 30 days. To compare the Raman spectra of the biomaterials (GelMA and GelMA + *Ximenia americana* L.), with the treated and healthy regions, the raw spectrum in the range of 90–3500 cm^{-1} was processed using the Labspec 5.0 program. Fluorescence was eliminated by applying a fifth-order polynomial fit, and additional preprocessing steps, such as baseline adjustment, were performed.

The obtained spectra were normalized using a normalization vector. This normalization process involved dividing the Raman intensity by the square root of the sum of the calculated square intensities of the entire spectrum. The normalization was performed using Origin 2018 software. After identifying the peaks in the spectra, the integrated areas of the main evaluated peaks were calculated within the range of 957–962 cm^{-1}, which corresponds to the phosphate band and is representative of the mineral content in the bone. This analysis aimed to quantify the bone composition and assess any alterations in the mineral.

To further characterize bone alterations in the mineral, crystallinity was determined by calculating the inverse of the full peak width at half maximum (FWHM) of the υ1 phosphate band peak, which is located around ~960 cm^{-1}. The FWHM represents the width of the peak at its half maximum intensity, and by inverting this value, the crystallinity of the bone can be obtained. This provides insights into the degree of mineralization or structural changes in the bone sample.

2.5.6. Statical Analysis

The analysis of the results was conducted using GraphPad Prism® software (version 8.3.0, Instat Software Inc., La Jolla, CA, USA). Statistical data analyses were performed using ANOVA as a parametric test and the Kruskal–Wallis test as a non-parametric test. A Dunn post-test was applied for further analysis. The significance level was set at $p < 0.005$, indicating statistical significance. The results are presented as means and standard deviations, providing a measure of central tendency and variability, respectively.

3. Results and Discussion

3.1. Production and Characterization of Raw Materials and GelMA and GelMA + Ximenia americana L. Hydrogels

FTIR spectroscopy was performed to characterize the material and evaluate its chemical composition. Figure 1A presents the spectra for the GelMA, *Ximenia americana* L. and GelMA + *Ximenia americana* L. Figure 1A(a) presents the *Ximenia americana* L. spectrum. The following are main bands found and attributed at approximately 3000 to 3800 cm^{-1} band, related to the O-H stretching bond at 1614 and 1517 cm^{-1} bands assigned to the C=C bonds of the aromatic groups; at 1448 and 1388 cm^{-1} bands, related to C-H bonds; at 1300 to 1000 cm^{-1} bands, characteristic of C-O stretching vibration; and at 796 and 667 cm^{-1} bands, corresponding to C-H bonds in aromatics.

The bands were assigned according to the results found [19,24]. Figure 1A(b) presents the GelMA spectrum. The main bands found and assigned were around 3000 and 3600 cm^{-1} bands, referring to the peptide bonds (N-H); at 1650 cm^{-1} bands, corresponding to Amide I, mainly the C=O stretching groups; and at 1490 and 1580 cm^{-1} bands, corresponding to C-N-H folding vibrations. The studies by Santana et al. [19] and Almeida L et al. [24] provided insights into the chemical bonds associated with various functional groups, including ethers, esters and carboxylic acids. These functional groups are commonly found in flavonoids, tannins, anthraquinones and other secondary metabolites present in the extract. The information from these studies helped in identifying and interpreting the specific chemical bonds observed in the spectra. Figure 1A(c) showed that the GelMA + *Ximenia americana* L.

spectrum maintained the same profile of the GelMA spectrum, only observing an increase in the transmittance intensity of the bands. This fact demonstrates that there was an overlapping of the bands of the GelMA and GelMA + *Ximenia americana* L. materials and that this overlap is not indicative of chemical incompatibility.

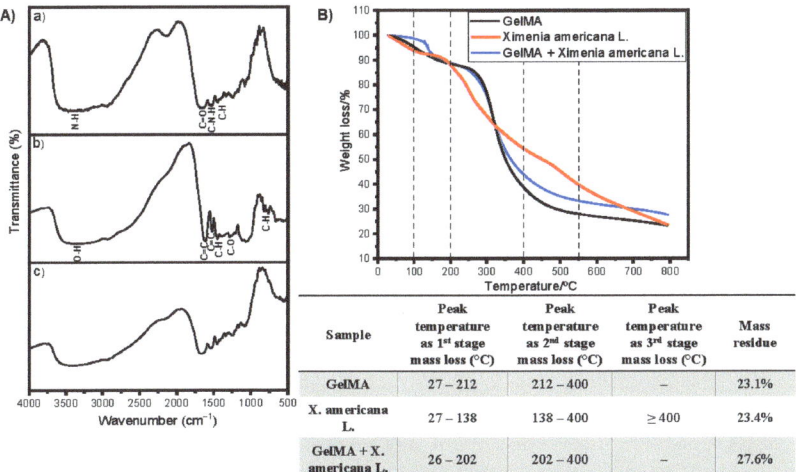

Figure 1. (**A**) FTIR spectra in vibrational regions from 4000 to 500 cm^{-1} for *Ximenia americana* L. (**a**), GelMA, and (**b**) GelMA + *Ximenia americana* L. (**c**). (**B**) Thermal analysis results.

The X-ray diffractograms of the *Ximenia americana* L. samples and the GelMA + *Ximenia americana* L. hydrogel show a high degree of amorphization, and only a very wide band can be seen for both samples in the region between the angles of 10° and 40°, corresponding to pure gelatin [54].

Thermogravimetric results for GelMA, *X. americana* L. and GelMA + *X. americana* L. are shown in Figure 1B. As can be observed, the results for *X. americana* L. showed three decomposition stages, with a mineral residue of ~23.4%. The first event occurs in the temperature range between 27 and 138 °C and can be attributed to the loss of volatile materials, such as the water used in the process. On the other hand, the second and third events occurred at temperatures above 200 °C and 400 °C, respectively, and can be associated with the decomposition of a wide variety of secondary metabolites, mainly the phenolics present in the extract. Equal results were obtained by Santana et al. [19], and by Almeida et al. [24]. The thermal degradation behavior of the GelMA shows two mass loss events: The first occurs in the temperature range between 27 and 212 °C, probably caused by the loss of water molecules, and a second event occurs at temperatures higher than 325 °C, which can be attributed to the degradation of the biopolymer, with a residue of ~23.1% of mass. Similar thermal behavior results were obtained by Aldana et al. [55]. The thermal behavior for the GelMA + *X. americana* L. hydrogel is similar to that obtained for the GelMA. As can be observed, there are two mass loss events for the sample: the first is observed in the temperature range between 26 and 202 °C caused by the loss of water molecules and volatile materials, and the second event occurs at temperatures above 200 °C, which can be attributed to the degradation of the biopolymer and the decomposition of secondary metabolites, and a residue of approximately ~27.6% by mass was observed. Based on the results of the TG/DTG analysis, we can infer that both the GelMA and GelMA + *X. americana* L. have good thermal stability at temperatures up to 200 °C with no significant mass loss (decomposition) in this temperature range. This result enables the application of these materials in this temperature range. More information regarding the thermal behavior of the samples were obtained in the DSC analysis. In the DSC curve of the GelMA, an endothermic band was observed in the range between 30 and 120 °C, and that can be attributed to the glass transition of blocks of amino acids in the peptide chain relative to the amorphous regions of gelatin and to the loss of water and protein breakdown. A similar result was found by Aldana et al. [55] and El-Maghawry et al. [56]. The DSC curve for the GelMA + *X. americana* L. hydrogel shows an endothermic band in the range of 36–110 °C that can be attributed to the glass transition of amino acid blocks in the peptide chain relative to the amorphous regions of gelatin and to the loss of water and degradation of proteins, as seen in the GelMA DSC curve. In the region between 250 and 320 °C, an endothermic band was observed, which can be attributed to the breakage of hydroxyl bonds present in *X. americana* L. A similar phenomenon was observed by De Salvi et al. [57].

3.2. Controlled Release Test of Epicatechin—Main Compound of Ximenia americana L.

The biochemical characterization of *X. americana* L. in most existing studies is concentrated on the investigation of the pulp and seed of the fruit, with rare studies involving the stem, even knowing that this component is widely used in traditional medicine. Figure 2A shows the UV-Vis spectra of the *Ximenia americana* L. stem extract, and a peak centered at 278 nm was observed. According to a study published by Aragão [58], absorption bands centered at 270 nm, 278 nm and 280 nm correspond to the main constituents of the *X. americana* L. stem bark, which are procyanidin B, catechin/epicatechin and procyanidin C, respectively. Among these compounds, epicatechin was found in greater amounts in studies published by Santana et al. [19]. Both studies reported the presence of bands referring to epicatechin between 276 nm and 278 nm. Based on these studies, the band found at 278 nm from the *X. americana* L. extract was attributed to the epicatechin/catechin compound ($C_5H_{14}O_6$).

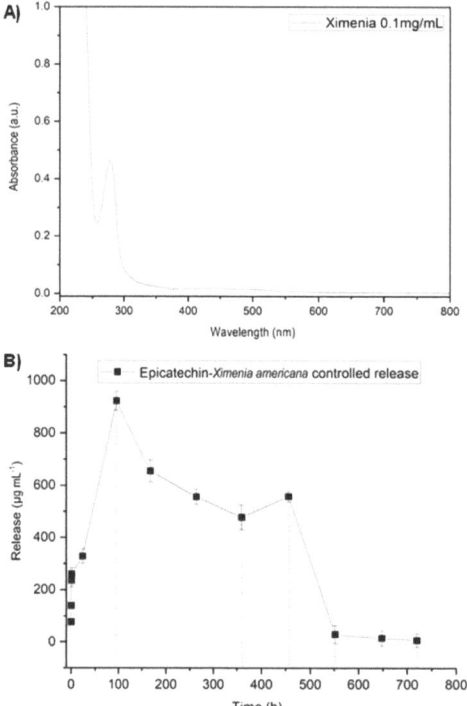

Figure 2. (**A**) UV-Vis spectrum of the *Ximenia americana* L. extract. (**B**) Controlled release of epicatechin as a function of time from the GelMA + *Ximenia americana* L. hydrogel.

Next, to evaluate the epicatechin release time by the GelMA + *X. americana* L., the analytical calibration curve and the controlled release of epicatechin were performed. The obtained analytical curve showed a linear range from 5 to 250 µg/mL, and the interval can be expressed by the equation y = 0.00000296x + 0.001 (R^2 = 0.998). Figure 2B presents the release assay results from the GelMA + *X. americana* L. hydrogel. As can be observed, the release of the extract starts at ~15 min after application and continues upwards until reaching the maximum release peak (922.50 µg/mL^{-1}) after ~4 days. After that, the concentration released starts to decline slowly until ~15 days, and a new release peak occurs at ~19 days (654.9 µg/mL^{-1}), decreasing quickly at ~23 days (0.8296 µg/mL^{-1}). The amount released at the experimental time of 30 days is minimal, constant and close to zero (0.233 µg/mL^{-1}). By not zeroing out and continuing to release even in smaller amounts until the 30th day of the experimental period, it can be concluded that the release of *X. americana* L. is adequate during the period in which the in vivo tests were carried out.

3.3. In Vivo Experiments

Bone healing can indeed be monitored using Raman spectroscopy since it allows for the determination of hydroxyapatite concentration/incorporation, which is an essential component of mineralized bone. Hydroxyapatite is a calcium phosphate mineral that constitutes a major part of the inorganic bone matrix. Through this technique, the hydroxyapatite phosphate band, centered at approximately 960 cm^{-1}, can be monitored [59], and used as a bone repair marker [60–62]. Figure 3 A,B shows the Raman spectra for 15 and 30 days after the surgical procedure, respectively. As can be observed in Figure 3A, the GLEDG (GelMA + LED) and GXG (GelMA + *X. americana* L.) groups showed bands with greater intensity and closer to the healthy one, suggesting an optimized bone regeneration process in these groups, with a high deposition of $\upsilon 1\ PO_4^{3-}$ in a concentration similar to that of healthy bone. On the other hand, the CG showed a lower level of mineralization than the others, indicated by the low relative intensity of the band associated with $\upsilon 1\ PO_4^{3-}$. The greater bone repair observed for the mentioned groups can be explained by the immediate effect of using *X. americana* L. and LED in the GXG and GLEDG groups, respectively. Regarding GXG, we can attribute this optimization of bone repair to the large amount of epicatechin released by the *X. americana* L. in the first days (presented in Figure 2B), where a peak maximum of release was observed at ~4 days. Epicatechin is a flavonoid, which presents antioxidant activity attributed to the phenolic radicals of its structure. These findings corroborate the study by Wan Osman et al. [63], which investigated the use of noni leaves (rich in epicatechin), in bone repair and in combating inflammation of the joint cartilage in rats. The investigation took place through cultures of cartilage explants and preclinical studies. In their results, in a period prior to 30 days, epicatechin suppressed the release of glycosaminoglycan and nitric oxide from the cartilage explant and significantly reduced the amount of mRNA in joint tissues, thus increasing bone formation in addition to improving the structure of joint cartilage and chondrocytes. Regarding the GLEDG (GelMA + LED) group, the improvement can be attributed to the systemic and instantaneous effect resulting from photobiomodulation through LED irradiation to the tissue. Photobiomodulation from LED increases bone metabolism and accelerates fracture healing. Our results corroborate findings in other research studies [38,59,64], which have also found evidence of the optimization of bone repair in fractures in a period prior to 30 days.

From the Raman spectra presented in Figure 3B, it is possible to observe that the relative intensity of the $\upsilon 1\ PO_4^{3-}$ band for the GG, GLEDG and GXG groups has the same intensity to that found for healthy bone. Interestingly, the intensity of the band found for the GXLEDG group exceeded what was shown for healthy bone, suggesting a greater deposition of phosphate (bone) than normal. This result corroborates the large amount of newly formed bone around the fracture shown for these groups, as seen below in the histological analysis.

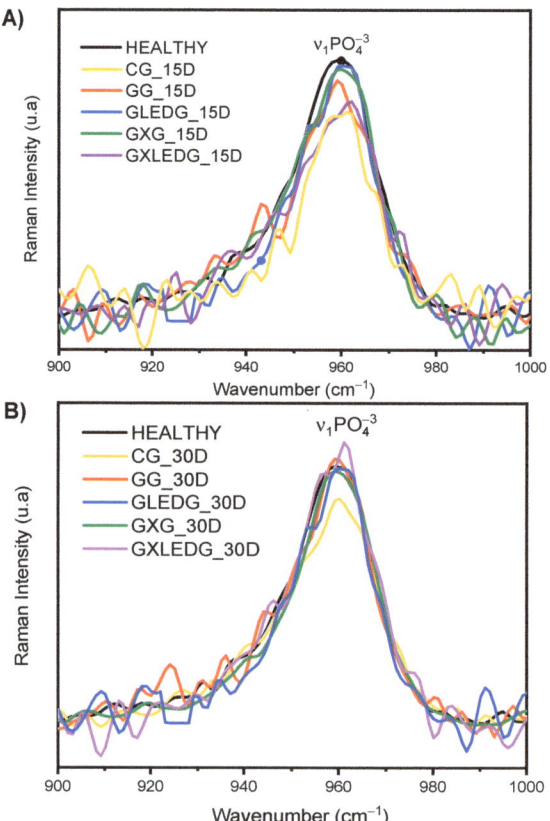

Figure 3. Mean Raman spectra of the bone tissue for the groups at (**A**) 15 days and (**B**) 30 days after the surgical procedure at ~960 cm^{-1}, referring to $\upsilon 1$ PO$_4^{3-}$.

It is known that low intensity laser therapy (LILT) and photobiomodulation have the main purpose of promoting the interaction between biological tissues associated with their optical characteristics, such as reflection, transmission, scattering and absorption [65]. Regarding the effects of photobiomodulation on bone tissue, the therapy aims to stimulate cell proliferation since this resource has the capacity to interact with bone content, favoring the biochemical modulation of bone cells, stimulating mitochondrial respiration, accelerating osteogenic potential through the migration and differentiation of these cells to the irradiation site, stimulating collagen production and the mineralization of the extracellular matrix [66]. On the other hand, the CG presented a lower level of mineralization than the other groups, which was expressed by the low relative intensity of the $\upsilon 1$ PO$_4^{3-}$ band in the same experimental period (30 days).

Figure 4 A,B presents the spectra of the integrated areas of the band centered at 960 cm^{-1} (related to $\upsilon 1$ PO$_4^{3-}$) after 15 and 30 days, respectively, which is related to the carbonated apatite data. On the 15th day of the experiment, a statistical difference was observed when comparing all treated and control groups, suggesting an increase in PO$_4^{3-}$ deposition that is statistically significant ($p < 0.0001$) between the GLEDG (GelMA + LED) and GXG (GelMA + *Ximenia americana* L.) groups, with $p < 0.001$ for the GXLEDG (GelMA + *Ximenia americana* L. + LED) and GG (GelMA), confirming the findings in Figure 3. A difference ($p < 0.05$) was also found between the GG (GelMA) and GXG (GelMA + *Ximenia americana* L.) groups, also noting that the control group had a significantly lower PO$_4^{3-}$ deposition than healthy bone ($p < 0.0001$). After a period of 30 days, a statistical difference comparing all treated and control groups was observed, identifying an increase in PO_4^{3-} deposition, being statistically significant ($p < 0.0001$) between the GXLEDG (GelMA + *Ximenia americana* L. + LED) and control groups, and $p < 0.05$ between the GLEDG (GelMA + LED), GXG (GelMA + *Ximenia americana* L.) and GG (GelMA) groups. A difference ($p < 0.05$), was also found between the GG (GelMA) and GXLEDG (GelMA + *Ximenia americana* L. + LED) groups, also noting that the control group had a lower PO_4^{3-} deposition than healthy bone ($p < 0.001$).

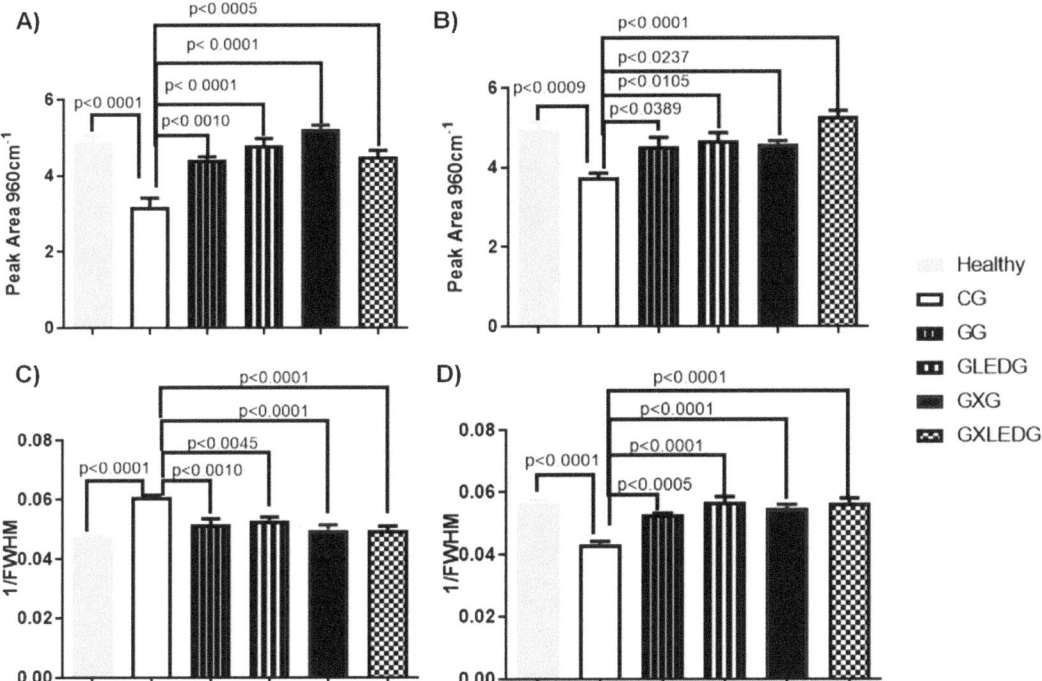

Figure 4. Mean and standard deviation of the integrated areas for bands centered at 960 cm^{-1} (related to υ1 PO_4^{3-}) after 15 (**A**) and 30 days (**B**) of treatment. Mean and standard deviation of crystallinity after 15 (**C**) and 30 days (**D**) of treatment.

Figure 4 C,D presents the spectra for the crystallinity given for the inverse of the width at half height of the peak after 15 and 30 days, respectively. Such data evaluate bone composition by the deposition of new hydroxyapatite crystals in newly formed bone. The crystallinity found in the treated groups ($p < 0.0001$), and of the healthy bone ($p < 0.001$), was significantly higher than that of the control group after 30 days of treatment, with no statistical difference being observed comparing the treated groups. At 15 days of treatment, a statistical difference was observed comparing the healthy group and CG ($p < 0.05$), where the CG had lower crystallinity. The mineral crystallinity results obtained from techniques such as Raman spectroscopy provide valuable information about the size and maturation of mineral crystals in bone tissue, as mentioned in refs. [22,60]. Reduced crystallinity indicates the presence of younger and smaller mineral crystals at the injury site. During the early stages of bone healing, the rapid mineralization process leads to the formation of smaller crystals with lower levels of organization. These crystals may have a higher proportion of non-stoichiometric substitutions and a less defined crystal lattice structure, resulting in reduced crystallinity values. As the bone healing progresses and the tissue matures, the mineral crystals undergo a process of growth and maturation. This is characterized by the replacement of carbonate ions and the incorporation of additional mineral components, leading to larger and more ordered crystals. The increased crystallinity reflects the improved organization and structure of the mineral crystals, indicating a higher degree of maturation [59].

Figure 5 provides a representative histological overview of all the experimental groups at two different time points, specifically 15 days (**A**) and 30 days (**B**) after the bone defect was created. After 15 days, for the CG, GG, GLEDG and GXLEDG groups, the presence of granulation tissue and a slight new bone formation can be observed in the entire defect. However, the GXG group presented a greater presence of new bone tissue sites when compared to the other experimental groups.

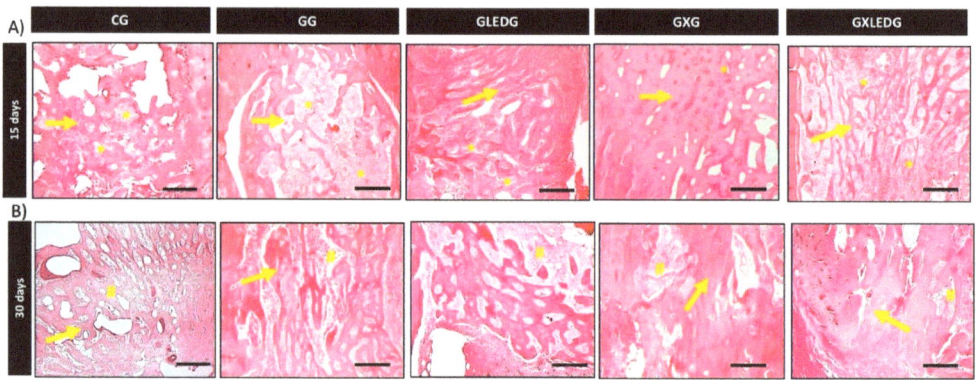

Figure 5. Bone defect photomicrography 15 days (**A**) and 30 days (**B**) after the surgery. Granulation tissue (*); osteoid (#); neoformed bone tissue (→). Bar scale = 500 µm (2.5× image); bar scale = 50 µm (40× image). Used stains: hematoxylin and eosin.

After 30 days, it was possible to observe that for the CG, GG and GLEDG groups, the center of defect was occupied by osteoid tissue and immature newly formed bone cells, exhibiting some interconnected trabeculae. For the GXG and GXLEDG groups, woven formed bone demonstrated a more mature aspect with a well-arranged bundle of bone tissue compared to the other treated groups.

Figure 6 A,B demonstrates the semi-quantitative results of bone repair. In the analysis of the samples at 15 days after surgery, the bone repair score of the GXG group was significantly higher compared to the CG. However, no significant difference comparing the score results for the GG, GLEDG, and GXLEDG groups was observed 15 days after surgery.

Thirty days post-surgery, the GXG and GXLEDG groups had the highest bone repair score when compared to the CG. No other differences were observed in the other experimental groups.

From the findings of the histological analysis, it is possible to suggest that both therapies employed (associated or isolated) provided greater bone trabeculae filling, with the results of bone repair being more expressive in the GXG group at 15 days and in the GXG and GXLEDG groups at 30 days caused by the increased synthesis of osteoblasts and collagen. There are no studies in the literature that have reported the use of *Ximenia americana* L. in bone repair. However, these positive results can be explained by two factors. The first corresponds to the *Ximenia americana* L. itself since several authors [21,22] infer that the stem, as characterized in the present study, has secondary metabolites, such as flavonoids. These metabolites can exert antimicrobial and modulating activities, in addition to anti-inflammatory action, among others [67]. All these properties are inherent to *Ximenia americana* L. when used alone or in association with hydrogels and seem to favor bone repair.

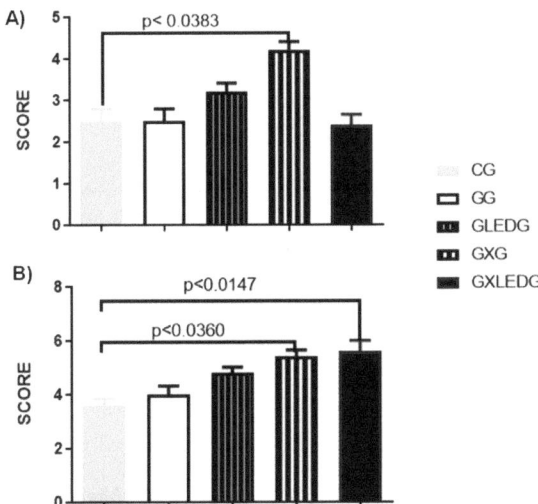

Figure 6. Experimental groups bone repair score 15 (**A**) and 30 days (**B**) after the surgery.

The second factor would be due to the associated treatments, since both the GelMA [68], and photobiomodulation seem to contribute to increased cell metabolism and, consequently, to bone repair. GelMA increases bone tissue due to its inherent bioactivity and physical-chemical adaptability [69], and due to its porous architecture, it promotes migration, proliferation and osteogenic and chondrogenic differentiation [13,70]. In studies reported by Comunian et al. and Ekizer et al. [43,64], who evaluated photobiomodulation in bone repair, it was verified that this modality enabled the improvement of neoformation and the quality of the formed bone tissue. This is because photobiomodulation promotes the increased synthesis of the number of osteocytes, collagen and DNA synthesis, proliferation and the differentiation of osteoblasts, in addition to cell metabolism [43,44]. Therefore, all these factors would also explain the better results obtained by the GXLEDG (GelMA + Ximenia + LED) group at 30 days.

4. Conclusions

The *Ximenia americana* L. stem extract incorporated into the GelMA showed satisfactory results, i.e., it accelerated bone repair in the first 15 days after the fracture. Regarding the association of biomaterial + LED, the group treated with GelMA + *Ximenia americana* L. + LED (GXLEDG) optimized the results by repairing and strengthening the injured bone region in 30 days. Histologically, it was shown that both therapies applied in the study (associated or not), caused greater filling by the bone trabeculae compared to the CG. In 30 days, the GXLEDG and GXG (GelMA + *Ximenia americana* L.) groups presented newly formed bone tissue that is clearly more compact with maturation to bone tissue with a cortical pattern. However, it is possible to observe that the *Ximenia americana* L. extract incorporated into the GelMA, together with the photobiomodulation from the LED, is a potentiator for bone repair in an animal model.

Author Contributions: Conceptualization, methodology, investigation and formal analysis, S.S.L., G.O.d.M.G., V.T.U. and L.S.S.P.; writing—original draft preparation, writing—review and editing, C.R.T. and L.A.; investigation, data curation and formal analysis, A.L.M.M.-F., R.A.d.O. and J.F.-S., writing—review and editing, and supervision, A.O.L., writing—review and editing, and supervision, A.P. All authors have read and agreed to the published version of the manuscript.

Funding: This research was funded by Fundação de Amparo à Pesquisa do Estado de São Paulo (FAPESP) (grant number: 2017/19470-8), Conselho Nacional de Desenvolvimento Científico e Tecnológico (CNPq) e Coordenação de Aperfeiçoamento de Pessoal de Nível Superior- Brasil (CAPES).

Data Availability Statement: The data presented in this study are available from the corresponding author upon request.

Conflicts of Interest: The authors declare no conflict of interest.

References

1. Nicholson, J.A.; Makaram, N.; Simpson, A.H.R.W.; Keating, J.F. Fracture Nonunion in Long Bones: A Literature Review of Risk Factors and Surgical Management. *Injury* **2021**, *52*, S3–S11. [CrossRef]
2. Qiao, K.; Xu, L.; Tang, J.; Wang, Q.; Lim, K.S.; Hooper, G.; Woodfield, T.B.F.; Liu, G.; Tian, K.; Zhang, W.; et al. The Advances in Nanomedicine for Bone and Cartilage Repair. *J. Nanobiotechnol.* **2022**, *20*, 141. [CrossRef]
3. Qi, J.; Yu, T.; Hu, B.; Wu, H.; Ouyang, H. Current Biomaterial-Based Bone Tissue Engineering and Translational Medicine. *Int. J. Mol. Sci.* **2021**, *22*, 10233. [CrossRef]
4. Feng, Y.; Zhu, S.; Mei, D.; Li, J.; Zhang, J.; Yang, S.; Guan, S. Application of 3D Printing Technology in Bone Tissue Engineering: A Review. *Curr. Drug Deliv.* **2020**, *18*, 847–861. [CrossRef]
5. Cui, Z.K.; Kim, S.; Baljon, J.J.; Wu, B.M.; Aghaloo, T.; Lee, M. Microporous Methacrylated Glycol Chitosan-Montmorillonite Nanocomposite Hydrogel for Bone Tissue Engineering. *Nat. Commun.* **2019**, *10*, 3523. [CrossRef]
6. Lin, H.; Sohn, J.; Shen, H.; Langhans, M.T.; Tuan, R.S. Bone Marrow Mesenchymal Stem Cells: Aging and Tissue Engineering Applications to Enhance Bone Healing. *Biomaterials* **2019**, *203*, 96–110. [CrossRef]
7. Dumic-Cule, I.; Peric, M.; Kucko, L.; Grgurevic, L.; Pecina, M.; Vukicevic, S. Bone Morphogenetic Proteins in Fracture Repair. *Int. Orthop.* **2018**, *42*, 2619–2626. [CrossRef]
8. Gao, J.; Liu, X.; Cheng, J.; Deng, J.; Han, Z.; Li, M.; Wang, X.; Liu, J.; Zhang, L. Application of Photocrosslinkable Hydrogels Based on Photolithography 3D Bioprinting Technology in Bone Tissue Engineering. *Regen. Biomater.* **2023**, *10*, rbad037. [CrossRef]
9. Oh, W.T.; Yang, Y.S.; Xie, J.; Ma, H.; Kim, J.M.; Park, K.H.; Oh, D.S.; Park-Min, K.H.; Greenblatt, M.B.; Gao, G.; et al. WNT-Modulating Gene Silencers as a Gene Therapy for Osteoporosis, Bone Fracture, and Critical-Sized Bone Defects. *Mol. Ther.* **2023**, *31*, 435–453. [CrossRef]
10. Ullah, S.; Hussain, Z.; Ullah, I.; Wang, L.; Mehmood, S.; Liu, Y.; Mansoorianfar, M.; Liu, X.; Ma, F.; Pei, R. Mussel Bioinspired, Silver-Coated and Insulin-Loaded Mesoporous Polydopamine Nanoparticles Reinforced Hyaluronate-Based Fibrous Hydrogel for Potential Diabetic Wound Healing. *Int. J. Biol. Macromol.* **2023**, *247*, 125738. [CrossRef]
11. Lantigua, D.; Wu, X.; Suvarnapathaki, S.; Nguyen, M.A.; Camci-Unal, G. Composite Scaffolds from Gelatin and Bone Meal Powder for Tissue Engineering. *Bioengineering* **2021**, *8*, 169. [CrossRef]
12. Goto, R.; Nishida, E.; Kobayashi, S.; Aino, M.; Ohno, T.; Iwamura, Y.; Kikuchi, T.; Hayashi, J.I.; Yamamoto, G.; Asakura, M.; et al. Gelatin Methacryloyl–Riboflavin (Gelma–Rf) Hydrogels for Bone Regeneration. *Int. J. Mol. Sci.* **2021**, *22*, 1635. [CrossRef]
13. Jiang, Q.; Bai, G.; Liu, X.; Chen, Y.; Xu, G.; Yang, C.; Zhang, Z. 3D Gelma Icc Scaffolds Combined with Sw033291 for Bone Regeneration by Modulating Macrophage Polarization. *Pharmaceutics* **2021**, *13*, 1934. [CrossRef]
14. Klotz, B.J.; Gawlitta, D.; Rosenberg, A.J.W.P.; Malda, J.; Melchels, F.P.W. Gelatin-Methacryloyl Hydrogels: Towards Biofabrication-Based Tissue Repair. *Trends Biotechnol.* **2016**, *34*, 394–407. [CrossRef]
15. Miranda, L.L.; Guimarães-Lopes, V.D.P.; Altoé, L.S.; Sarandy, M.M.; Melo, F.C.S.A.; Novaes, R.D.; Gonçalves, R.V. Plant Extracts in the Bone Repair Process: A Systematic Review. *Mediat. Inflamm.* **2019**, *2019*, 1296153. [CrossRef]
16. Park, K.R.; Park, J.E.; Kim, B.; Kwon, I.K.; Hong, J.T.; Yun, H.M. Calycosin-7-o-β-Glucoside Isolated from Astragalus Membranaceus Promotes Osteogenesis and Mineralization in Human Mesenchymal Stem Cells. *Int. J. Mol. Sci.* **2021**, *22*, 11362. [CrossRef]
17. Hanafiah, O.A.; Hanafiah, D.S.; Dohude, G.A.; Satria, D.; Livita, L.; Moudy, N.S.; Rahma, R. Effects of 3% Binahong (Anredera Cordifolia) Leaf Extract Gel on Alveolar Bone Healing in Post-Extraction Tooth Socket Wound in Wistar Rats (Rattus Norvegicus). *F1000Research* **2022**, *10*, 923. [CrossRef]
18. Singh, P.; Gupta, A.; Qayoom, I.; Singh, S.; Kumar, A. Orthobiologics with Phytobioactive Cues: A Paradigm in Bone Regeneration. *Biomed. Pharmacother.* **2020**, *130*, 110754. [CrossRef]
19. Santana, C.P.; Medeiros, F.D.; Correia, L.P.; Diniz, P.H.G.D.; Véras, G.; Medeiros, A.C.D. Dissolution and Uniformity of Content of Tablets Developed with Extract of *Ximenia americana* L. *PLoS ONE* **2018**, *13*, e0197323. [CrossRef]
20. Leal, S.S.; Uchôa, V.T.; Figuerêdo-Silva, J.; Soares, R.B.; Mota, D.M.; De Alencar, R.C.; Filho, A.L.M.M.; Sant'Ana, A.E.G.; Beltrame Junior, M. Eficácia Da Fonoforese Com *Ximenia americana* L. Na Inflamação de Tendão de Ratos. *Rev. Bras. Med. Esporte* **2016**, *22*, 355–360. [CrossRef]
21. da Silva, K.M.A.; Chaves, T.P.; Santos, R.L.; Brandão, D.O.; Fernandes, F.H.A.; de Ramos Júnior, F.J.L.; dos Santos, V.L.; de Felismino, D.C.; Medeiros, A.C.D. Modulation of the Erythromycin Resistance in Staphylococcus Aureus by Ethanolic Extracts of *Ximenia americana* L. and Schinopsis Brasiliensis Engl. *Boletín Latinoam. Caribe Plantas Med. Aromáticas* **2015**, *14*, 92–98.

22. Silva, M.S.P.; Brando, D.O.; Chaves, T.P.; Formiga Filho, A.L.N.; Costa, E.M.M.D.B.; Santos, V.L.; Medeiros, A.C.D. Study Bioprospecting of Medicinal Plant Extracts of the Semiarid Northeast: Contribution to the Control of Oral Microorganisms. Evidence-based Complement. *Altern. Med.* **2012**, *2012*, 681207. [CrossRef]
23. Da Palma, A.F.M.; Marques, L.K.M.; Carneiro, R.D.S.; Carvalho, G.F.S.; Ferreira, D.C.L.; Sant'Ana, A.E.G.; Maia Filho, A.L.M.; Marques, R.B.; Alves, W.D.S.; Uchôa, V.T. Evaluation of Hydroalcoholic Extracts of Stem and Leaves of *Ximenia americana* L. In the Healing of Excisional Acute Wounds in Mice. *Rev. Virtual Quim.* **2020**, *12*, 37–50. [CrossRef]
24. Almeida, L.; Júnior, J.A.O.; Silva, M.; Nóbrega, F.; Andrade, J.; Santos, W.; Ribeiro, A.; Conceição, M.; Veras, G.; Medeiros, A.C. Tablet of *Ximenia americana* L. Developed from Mucoadhesive Polymers for Future Use in Oral Treatment of Fungal Infections. *Polymers* **2019**, *11*, 379. [CrossRef]
25. Dias, T.L.M.F.; Melo, G.M.A.; Da Silva, Y.K.C.; Queiroz, A.C.; Goulart, H.F.; Alexandre-Moreira, M.S.; Santana, A.E.G.; Uchôa, V.T. Antinociceptive and Anti-Inflammatory Activities of the Ethanolic Extract, of Fractions and of Epicatechin Isolated from the Stem Bark of *Ximenia americana* L. (Oleacaceae). *Rev. Virtual Quim.* **2018**, *10*, 86–101. [CrossRef]
26. Jin, Y.; Koh, R.H.; Kim, S.H.; Kim, K.M.; Park, G.K.; Hwang, N.S. Injectable Anti-Inflammatory Hyaluronic Acid Hydrogel for Osteoarthritic Cartilage Repair. *Mater. Sci. Eng. C* **2020**, *115*, 111096. [CrossRef]
27. Gao, Z.R.; Feng, Y.Z.; Zhao, Y.Q.; Zhao, J.; Zhou, Y.H.; Ye, Q.; Chen, Y.; Tan, L.; Zhang, S.H.; Feng, Y.; et al. Traditional Chinese Medicine Promotes Bone Regeneration in Bone Tissue Engineering. *Chin. Med.* **2022**, *17*, 86. [CrossRef]
28. Ortiz, A.d.C.; Fideles, S.O.M.; Reis, C.H.B.; Bellini, M.Z.; Pereira, E.d.S.B.M.; Pilon, J.P.G.; de Marchi, M.Â.; Detregiachi, C.R.P.; Flato, U.A.P.; Trazzi, B.F.d.M.; et al. Therapeutic Effects of Citrus Flavonoids Neohesperidin, Hesperidin and Its Aglycone, Hesperetin on Bone Health. *Biomolecules* **2022**, *12*, 626. [CrossRef]
29. Sun, W.; Li, M.; Zhang, Y.; Huang, Y.; Zhan, Q.; Ren, Y.; Dong, H.; Chen, J.; Li, Z.; Fan, C.; et al. Total Flavonoids of Rhizoma Drynariae Ameliorates Bone Formation and Mineralization in BMP-Smad Signaling Pathway Induced Large Tibial Defect Rats. *Biomed. Pharmacother.* **2021**, *138*, 111480. [CrossRef]
30. Carlos Rodríguez-Merchán, E. The Molecular Mechanisms of Bone Healing. *Int. J. Mol. Sci* **2021**, *22*, 767. [CrossRef]
31. Zuo, Y.; Li, Q.; Xiong, Q.; Li, J.; Tang, C.; Zhang, Y.; Wang, D. Naringin Release from a Nano-Hydroxyapatite / Collagen Tissue Reconstruction. *Polymers* **2022**, *14*, 3260. [CrossRef] [PubMed]
32. Uchôa, V.T.; Sousa, C.M.M.; Carvalho, A.A.; Sant'Ana, A.E.G.; Chaves, M.H. Free Radical Scavenging Ability of *Ximenia americana* L. Stem Bark and Leaf Extracts. *J. Appl. Pharm. Sci.* **2016**, *6*, 091–096. [CrossRef]
33. Carvalho, G.F.S.; Marques, L.K.; Sousa, H.G.; Silva, L.R.; Leão Ferreira, D.C.; Pires de Moura do Amaral, F.; Martins Maia Filho, A.L.; Figueredo-Silva, J.; Alves, W.d.S.; Oliveira, M.d.D.A.d.; et al. Phytochemical Study, Molecular Docking, Genotoxicity and Therapeutic Efficacy of the Aqueous Extract of the Stem Bark of *Ximenia americana* L. in the Treatment of Experimental COPD in Rats. *J. Ethnopharmacol.* **2020**, *247*, 112259. [CrossRef] [PubMed]
34. Carneiro, R.d.S.; Canuto, M.R.; Ribeiro, L.K.; Ferreira, D.C.L.; Assunção, A.F.C.; Costa, C.A.C.B.; de Freitas, J.D.; Rai, M.; Cavalcante, L.S.; Alves, W. dos S.; et al. Novel Antibacterial Efficacy of ZnO Nanocrystals/Ag Nanoparticles Loaded with Extract of Ximenia americana L. (Stem Bark) for Wound Healing. *S. Afr. J. Bot.* **2022**, *151*, 18–32. [CrossRef]
35. Deniz, E.; Arslan, A.; Diker, N.; Olgac, V.; Kilic, E. Evaluation of Light-Emitting Diode Photobiomodulation on Bone Healing of Rat Calvarial Defects. *Biotechnol. Biotechnol. Equip.* **2015**, *29*, 758–765. [CrossRef]
36. dos Santos, S.A.; dos Santos Vieira, M.A.; Simões, M.C.B.; Serra, A.J.; Leal-Junior, E.C.; de Carvalho, P.d.T.C. Photobiomodulation Therapy Associated with Treadmill Training in the Oxidative Stress in a Collagen-Induced Arthritis Model. *Lasers Med. Sci.* **2017**, *32*, 1071–1079. [CrossRef]
37. Mostafavinia, A.; Razavi, S.; Abdollahifar, M.; Amini, A.; Ghorishi, S.K.; Rezaei, F.; Pouriran, R.; Bayat, M. Evaluation of the Effects of Photobiomodulation on Bone Healing in Healthy and Streptozotocin-Induced Diabetes in Rats. *Photomed. Laser Surg.* **2017**, *35*, 537–545. [CrossRef]
38. Pinheiro, A.L.B.; Soares, L.G.P.; da Silva, A.C.P.; Santos, N.R.S.; da Silva, A.P.L.T.; Neves, B.L.R.C.; Soares, A.P.; Gerbi, M.E.M.M.; dos Santos, J.N. The Use of Photobiomodulation Therapy or LED and Mineral Trioxide Aggregate Improves the Repair of Complete Tibial Fractures Treated with Wire Osteosynthesis in Rodents. *Lasers Med. Sci.* **2021**, *36*, 735–742. [CrossRef]
39. Chen, A.C.H.; Huang, Y.Y.; Sharma, S.K.; Hamblin, M.R. Effects of 810-Nm Laser on Murine Bone-Marrow-Derived Dendritic Cells. *Photomed. Laser Surg.* **2011**, *29*, 383–389. [CrossRef]
40. Barbosa, D.; Villaverde, A.G.J.B.; LoschiavoArisawa, E.Â.; de Souza, R.A. Laser Therapy in Bone Repair in Rats: Analysis of Bone Optical Density. *Acta Ortop. Bras.* **2014**, *22*, 71–74. [CrossRef]
41. Sella, V.R.G.; do Bomfim, F.R.C.; Machado, P.C.D.; da Silva Morsoleto, M.J.M.; Chohfi, M.; Plapler, H. Effect of Low-Level Laser Therapy on Bone Repair: A Randomized Controlled Experimental Study. *Lasers Med. Sci.* **2015**, *30*, 1061–1068. [CrossRef]
42. Mayer, L.; Freddo, A.L.; Blaya, D.S. Effects of Low-Level Laser Therapy on Distraction Osteogenesis: A Histological Analysis. *RFO UPF* **2012**, *17*, 326–331.
43. Ekizer, A.; Uysal, T.; Güray, E.; Akkuş, D. Effect of LED-Mediated-Photobiomodulation Therapy on Orthodontic Tooth Movement and Root Resorption in Rats. *Lasers Med. Sci.* **2015**, *30*, 779–785. [CrossRef]
44. Kloukos, D. The Effect of Light-Emitting Diode Phototherapy on Rate of Orthodontic Tooth Movement: A Split Mouth, Controlled Clinical Trial. *J. Orthod.* **2015**, *42*, 271. [CrossRef]

45. Lv, L.; Cheng, W.; Wang, S.; Lin, S.; Dang, J.; Ran, Z.; Zhu, H.; Xu, W.; Huang, Z.; Xu, P.; et al. Poly(β-Amino Ester) Dual-Drug-Loaded Hydrogels with Antibacterial and Osteogenic Properties for Bone Repair. *ACS Biomater. Sci. Eng.* **2023**, *9*, 1976–1990. [CrossRef]
46. Nichol, J.W.; Koshy, S.; Bae, H.; Hwang, C.M.; Khademhosseini, A. 2010 Biomaterials Ali. Cell-Laden Microengineered Gelatin Methacrylate Hydrogels. *Biomaterials* **2011**, *31*, 5536–5544. [CrossRef]
47. Lee, J.Y.; Son, S.J.; Son, J.S.; Kang, S.S.; Choi, S.H. Bone-Healing Capacity of PCL/PLGA/Duck Beak Scaffold in Critical Bone Defects in a Rabbit Model. *BioMed Res. Int.* **2016**, *2016*, 2136215. [CrossRef]
48. Schlickewei, C.; Klatte, T.O.; Wildermuth, Y.; Laaff, G.; Rueger, J.M.; Ruesing, J.; Chernousova, S.; Lehmann, W.; Epple, M. A Bioactive Nano-Calcium Phosphate Paste for In-Situ Transfection of BMP-7 and VEGF-A in a Rabbit Critical-Size Bone Defect: Results of an In Vivo Study. *J. Mater. Sci.* **2019**, *30*, 15. [CrossRef]
49. Kido, H.W.; Brassolatti, P.; Tim, C.R.; Gabbai-Armelin, P.R.; Magri, A.M.P.; Fernandes, K.R.; Bossini, P.S.; Parizotto, N.A.; Crovace, M.C.; Malavazi, I.; et al. Porous Poly (D,L-Lactide-Co-Glycolide) Acid/Biosilicate® Composite Scaffolds for Bone Tissue Engineering. *J. Biomed. Mater. Res.-Part B Appl. Biomater.* **2017**, *105*, 63–71. [CrossRef]
50. Alves, A.M.M.; de Miranda Fortaleza, L.M.; Filho, A.L.M.M.; Ferreira, D.C.L.; da Costa, C.L.S.; Viana, V.G.F.; Santos, J.Z.L.V.; de Oliveira, R.A.; de Meira Gusmão, G.O.; Soares, L.E.S. Evaluation of Bone Repair after Application of a Norbixin Membrane Scaffold with and without Laser Photobiomodulation (λ 780 Nm). *Lasers Med. Sci.* **2018**, *33*, 1493–1504. [CrossRef]
51. Nascimento, L.D.E.S.; Nicolau, R.A.; Filho, A.L.M.M.; Santos, J.Z.L.V.; Fonseca, K.M.; Ferreira, D.C.L.; de Sousa, R.C.; Viana, V.G.F.; Carvalho, L.F.M.; Figueredo-Silva, J. Effect of Norbixin-Based Poly(Hydroxybutyrate) Membranes on the Tendon Repair Process after Tenotomy in Rats. *Acta Cir. Bras.* **2019**, *34*, e201901101. [CrossRef]
52. Cardoso, Á.B. *Estudo Histomofométrico Comparativo Da Reparação Óssea Em Ratos Após o Uso de Biomateriais de Origem Bovina e Sintética*; Universidade Federal do Pernambuco: Recife, Brazil, 2008.
53. Kido, H.W.; Bossini, P.S.; Tim, C.R.; Parizotto, N.A.; da Cunha, A.F.; Malavazi, I.; Renno, A.C.M. Evaluation of the Bone Healing Process in an Experimental Tibial Bone Defect Model in Ovariectomized Rats. *Aging Clin. Exp. Res.* **2014**, *26*, 473–481. [CrossRef]
54. Radev, L.; Fernandes, M.H.V.; Salvado, I.M.; Kovacheva, D. Organic/Inorganic Bioactive Materials Part III: In Vitro Bioactivity of Gelatin/Silicocarnotite Hybrids. *Cent. Eur. J. Chem.* **2009**, *7*, 721–730. [CrossRef]
55. Aldana, A.A.; Malatto, L.; Ur Rehman, M.A.; Boccaccini, A.R.; Abraham, G.A. Fabrication of Gelatin Methacrylate (GelMA) Scaffolds with Nano-and Micro-Topographical and Morphological Features. *Nanomaterials* **2019**, *9*, 120. [CrossRef] [PubMed]
56. El-Maghawry, E.; Tadros, M.I.; Elkheshen, S.A.; Abd-Elbary, A. Eudragit®-S100 Coated Plga Nanoparticles for Colon Targeting of Etoricoxib: Optimization and Pharmacokinetic Assessments in Healthy Human Volunteers. *Int. J. Nanomed.* **2020**, *15*, 3965–3980. [CrossRef] [PubMed]
57. De Salvi, D.T.B.; da Barud, H.S.; Treu-Filho, O.; Pawlicka, A.; Mattos, R.I.; Raphael, E.; Ribeiro, S.J.L. Preparation, Thermal Characterization, and DFT Study of the Bacterial Cellulose: Triethanolamine System. *J. Therm. Anal. Calorim.* **2014**, *118*, 205–215. [CrossRef]
58. Aragão, Ticiana Parente. ATIVIDADE GASTROPROTETORA DA CASCA DO CAULE DE *Ximenia americana* L. (Ameixa de Espinho) (OLACACEAE) EM RATOS, 2019. Available online: https://repositorio.ufpe.br/handle/123456789/33692 (accessed on 5 July 2023).
59. Aciole, J.; Barbosa, P. Avaliação Da Fotobiomodulação Laser/LED Em Defeito Ósseo No Fêmur de Ratas Osteoporóticas: Estudo Histológico, Histomorfométrico e Por Espectroscopia Raman Em Modelo Animal, 2016. Available online: https://repositorio.ufba.br/handle/ri/20782 (accessed on 5 July 2023).
60. Akkus, O.; Adar, F.; Schaffler, M.B. Age-Related Changes in Physicochemical Properties of Mineral Crystals Are Related to Impaired Mechanical Function of Cortical Bone. *Bone* **2004**, *34*, 443–453. [CrossRef] [PubMed]
61. Awonusi, A.; Morris, M.D.; Tecklenburg, M.M.J. Carbonate Assignment and Calibration in the Raman Spectrum of Apatite. *Calcif. Tissue Int.* **2007**, *81*, 46–52. [CrossRef] [PubMed]
62. Morris, M.D.; Mandair, G.S. Raman Assessment of Bone Quality. *Clin. Orthop. Relat. Res.* **2011**, *469*, 2160–2169. [CrossRef] [PubMed]
63. Wan Osman, W.N.F.; Che Ahmad Tantowi, N.A.; Lau, S.F.; Mohamed, S. Epicatechin and Scopoletin Rich Morinda Citrifolia (Noni) Leaf Extract Supplementation, Mitigated Osteoarthritis via Anti-Inflammatory, Anti-Oxidative, and Anti-Protease Pathways. *J. Food Biochem.* **2019**, *43*, e12755. [CrossRef]
64. Comunian, C.R.; Custódio, A.L.N.; de Oliveira, L.J.; Dutra, C.E.A.; D'almeida Ferreira Neto, M.; Rezende, C.M.F. Photobiomodulation with LED and Laser in Repair of Mandibular Socket Rabbit: Clinical Evaluation, Histological, and Histomorphometric. *Oral Maxillofac. Surg.* **2017**, *21*, 201–206. [CrossRef] [PubMed]
65. de Freitas, L.F.; Hamblin, M.R. Proposed Mechanisms of Photobiomodulation or Low-Level Light Therapy. *IEEE J. Sel. Top. Quantum Electron.* **2016**, *22*, 348–364. [CrossRef] [PubMed]
66. Patrocínio-Silva, T.L.; de Souza, A.M.F.; Goulart, R.L.; Pegorari, C.F.; Oliveira, J.R.; Fernandes, K.R.; Magri, A.M.P.; Pereira, R.M.R.; Ribeiro, D.A.; Nagaoka, M.R.; et al. Low-Level Laser Therapy Associated to a Resistance Training Protocol on Bone Tissue in Diabetic Rats. *Arch. Endocrinol. Metab.* **2016**, *60*, 457–464. [CrossRef] [PubMed]
67. Chaves, T.P.; Santana, C.P.; Véras, G.; Brandão, D.O.; Felismino, D.C.; Cláudia, A.; Medeiros, D.; De, D.M.; Trovão, B.M. Seasonal Variation in the Production of Secondary Metabolites and Antimicrobial Activity of Two Plant Species Used in Brazilian Traditional Medicine. *Afr. J. Biotechnol.* **2013**, *12*, 847–853. [CrossRef]

68. Nogueira Albino Calland, F.; de Castro Brito, G.; Fernandes de Sousa, G.; de Carvalho Oliveira, F.; Roberta Marciano, F.; Oliveira Lobo, A. Evaluation of Wound Healing Activity of GelMA/PCLMA Fibrous Composites in Diabetic Model Rats. *Mater. Lett.* **2023**, *336*, 133893. [CrossRef]
69. Yue, K.; Trujillo-de Santiago, G.; Alvarez, M.M.; Tamayol, A.; Annabi, N.; Khademhosseini, A. Synthesis, Properties, and Biomedical Applications of Gelatin Methacryloyl (GelMA) Hydrogels. *Biomaterials* **2015**, *73*, 254–271. [CrossRef]
70. Jiang, G.; Li, S.; Yu, K.; He, B.; Hong, J.; Xu, T.; Meng, J.; Ye, C.; Chen, Y.; Shi, Z.; et al. A 3D-Printed PRP-GelMA Hydrogel Promotes Osteochondral Regeneration through M2 Macrophage Polarization in a Rabbit Model. *Acta Biomater.* **2021**, *128*, 150–162. [CrossRef]

Disclaimer/Publisher's Note: The statements, opinions and data contained in all publications are solely those of the individual author(s) and contributor(s) and not of MDPI and/or the editor(s). MDPI and/or the editor(s) disclaim responsibility for any injury to people or property resulting from any ideas, methods, instructions or products referred to in the content.

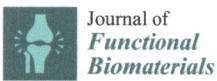 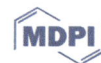

Article

Exploring CVD Method for Synthesizing Carbon–Carbon Composites as Materials to Contact with Nerve Tissue

Aneta Fraczek-Szczypta [1,*], Natalia Kondracka [2], Marcel Zambrzycki [1], Maciej Gubernat [1], Pawel Czaja [3], Miroslawa Pawlyta [4], Piotr Jelen [1], Ryszard Wielowski [1] and Danuta Jantas [5]

1. Faculty of Materials Science and Ceramics, AGH University of Science and Technology in Krakow, Mickiewicza 30 Av., 30-059 Krakow, Poland; zambrzycki@agh.edu.pl (M.Z.); maciej.gubernat@agh.edu.pl (M.G.); pjelen@agh.edu.pl (P.J.); rwielows@agh.edu.pl (R.W.)
2. Faculty of Electrical Engineering, Automatics, Computer Science and Biomedical Engineering, AGH University of Science and Technology in Krakow, Mickiewicza 30 Av., 30-059 Krakow, Poland; n.kondracka98@gmail.com
3. Institute of Metallurgy and Materials Science, Polish Academy of Science, Reymonta 25 St., 30-059 Krakow, Poland; czaja.p@imim.pl
4. Materials Research Laboratory, Faculty of Mechanical Engineering, Silesian University of Technology, Akademicka 2A Str., 44-100 Gliwice, Poland; mpawlyta@polsl.pl
5. Department of Experimental Neuroendocrinology, Maj Institute of Pharmacology, Polish Academy of Sciences, Smetna 12 Str., 31-343 Krakow, Poland; jantas@if-pan.krakow.pl
* Correspondence: afraczek@agh.edu.pl; Tel.: +48-126174738

Abstract: The main purpose of these studies was to obtain carbon–carbon composites with a core built of carbon fibers and a matrix in the form of pyrolytic carbon (PyC), obtained by using the chemical vapor deposition (CVD) method with direct electrical heating of a bundle of carbon fibers as a potential electrode material for nerve tissue stimulation. The methods used for the synthesis of PyC proposed in this paper allow us, with the appropriate selection of parameters, to obtain reproducible composites in the form of rods with diameters of about 300 μm in 120 s (CF_PyC_120). To evaluate the materials, various methods such as scanning electron microscopy (SEM), scanning transmission electron microscope (STEM), high-resolution transmission electron microscopy (HRTEM), selected area electron diffraction (SAED), Raman spectroscopy, X-ray photoelectron spectroscopy (XPS), and tensiometer techniques were used to study their microstructural, structural, chemical composition, surface morphology, and surface wettability. Assessing their applicability for contact with nervous tissue cells, the evaluation of cytotoxicity and biocompatibility using the SH-SY5Y human neuroblastoma cell line was performed. Viability and cytotoxicity tests (WST-1 and LDH release) along with cell morphology examination demonstrated that the CF_PyC_120 composites showed high biocompatibility compared to the reference sample (Pt wire), and the best adhesion of cells to the surface among all tested materials.

Keywords: carbon fibers; pyrolytic carbon; C/C composites; materials for nerve stimulation; CVD method

1. Introduction

The nervous system acts as a complex management center for the human body, relying on multiple factors like genetics, external influences, and aging for proper functioning. Neurodegenerative diseases, including Alzheimer's, ALS, Huntington's, and Parkinson's, are examples of nervous system malfunctions [1–3]. These conditions lead to a gradual loss of nerve cells in different brain regions, causing nervous system dysfunction [3].

Treating neurodegenerative diseases involves pharmacological methods as well as deep brain stimulation (DBS) [4–6]. DBS utilizes implanted electrodes in specific brain areas, customized to the disease type, along with a neurostimulator. This system works to inhibit abnormal neuron activity [5,7]. DBS has been employed for many years to treat severe movement disorders like Parkinson's, tremors, dystonias, and chorea, as well as central pain syndromes, epilepsy, and certain mental disorders [5,7]. The most commonly used materials for DBS electrodes are various metals and metal alloys, like platinum or platinum–iridium (Pt-Ir) [8]. These materials are preferred for their ability to stimulate neurons effectively and their biocompatibility.

Current neuromodulation techniques for DBS have several major drawbacks. These include the large size of the implanted devices, with electrode diameters exceeding 1 mm. There is also a lack of feedback monitoring of brain electrical activity, high demand for electrical current, and the risk of brain hemorrhage due to the numerous microelectrodes passing through the brain [9,10]. Another significant issue with DBS electrodes is the formation of glial scar tissue around them. This leads to an increase in electrical resistance between the electrodes and nerve tissue, requiring a higher voltage and current for nerve stimulation [11–14]. As a result, the battery drains faster, shortening the electrodes' lifespan. Additionally, glial scar tissue can cause brain trauma due to long-term inflammation [15]. Furthermore, the stiffness of the electrodes, typically greater than the surrounding tissue, can result in tissue detachment [16].

Challenges in electrode use and design include the size of the electrodes, their diameter-to-length ratio, and achieving miniaturization [9,17]. Optimal electrode size influences the quality and effectiveness of brain stimulation, while the diameter-to-length ratio impacts the area affected by the stimulation. Carbon materials, due to the variety of forms, allotropes, and the resulting very different properties, are often considered potential materials for electrodes or substrates for stimulation and regeneration of nervous tissue. Among these materials, we can mention carbon nanomaterials such as nanotubes (CNT), graphene and its derivatives, carbon nanofibers (CNF), and finally, carbon fibers (CF) and their composites [18–26]. Especially, carbon fibers (CF) with diameters of single micrometers are potential materials for electrodes and microelectrodes for brain stimulation.

Carbon fibers with diameters ranging from 4 to 10 μm allow precise control when combined into cylindrical electrodes [27]. Their various thicknesses, stiffnesses, and surface profiles make customization for specific tissues possible [28]. The superior properties of polyacrylonitrile-based carbon fibers (PAN-based carbon fibers), including tensile strength, thermal and chemical resistance, and electrical conductivity, surpass other options. The carbon surface can be easily modified for desired outcomes, impacting biocompatibility and reducing scar tissue formation [29]. Carbon fiber electrodes, smaller than conventional metal wire electrodes, show better capabilities for chronic neural recording and cause less tissue damage [30]. They also offer promise for magnetic resonance (MR) compatibility, ensuring safety during MR acquisitions [31,32]. Adverse implant interactions, such as heating, forces, induction, and MR artifacts, are important considerations [26]. Precise electrode positioning is vital for therapy effectiveness, using imaging methods like magnetic resonance imaging (MRI) during surgery [10]. Post-procedure, the electrode location is closely monitored [8]. Hence, MR compatibility is crucial to avoid artifacts and heating during imaging.

Carbon fiber shows promise as an electrode material with a wide range of research and application possibilities [25,26]. It can be used for neurotransmitter detection, monitoring, and recording signals from the nervous system [26,30,33,34]. Microelectrodes based on carbon fibers outperform conventional electrodes, ensuring stable neural recording without signal deterioration over time [30]. Graphitized fibers (GF) have also been tested for neuronal stimulation, exhibiting low impedance, a wide electrochemical window, and stability for 24 days [35]. In rats with Parkinson's disease, GF showed the ability to stimulate cells and alleviate symptoms.

While carbon fibers offer numerous advantages for nervous tissue applications, they are highly mechanically fragile [36]. Their limited insertion depth in cortex regions, less than 2 mm, is due to the individual fibers' insufficient stiffness to penetrate deeper brain regions despite their high mechanical properties [30,36]. Improving the durability and stiffness of individual fibers is crucial. One method reported in the literature is the application of DLC-based carbon coatings or diamond, obtained through the CVD method [25,29,36]. Pyrolytic carbon (PyC), another option similar to DLC, can also enhance carbon fibers' stiffness and usability. Low-temperature pyrolytic carbon is a well-known and highly biocompatible material used in medicine [37].

Pyrolytic carbon is usually obtained in the form of layers of varying thicknesses on various substrates [38]. Depending on their designation, they can perform various functions, e.g., they may improve the biocompatibility of modified materials in contact with blood or improve the wear resistance of friction elements in joint endoprostheses [39–41]. Among the materials available for mechanical heart valve prostheses, pyrolytic carbon has the best combination of blood compatibility, physical and mechanical properties, and durability [37,39]. Pyrolytic carbons can be obtained by, among other methods, CVD, where hydrocarbons, e.g., methane or propane are used as carbon-containing compounds [38,42]. What is interesting is that pyrolytic carbon can have a variety of structures, such as smooth and dark laminar or isotropic [43]. The structure of the pyrolytic carbon is controlled by the gas flow rate, hydrocarbon species, temperature, and bed surface area. Pyrolytic carbon can also be obtained as a matrix in carbon-carbon (C/C) composites using the chemical vapor infiltration (CVI) method belonging to the family of CVD methods [44,45]. In contrast to CVD, in CVI the deposition takes place within porous preforms usually made of fibers. Thus, the gaseous precursor penetrates through the preform pores and undergoes a chemical reaction thereby depositing in the pores [46]. In this way, the matrix material grows into a fibrous porous structure (preform) in a continuous layer-by-layer way, thus forming the composite matrix [37].

One significant drawback of obtaining pyrolytic carbon through CVD methods is the long synthesis time, which can extend to several thousand hours, depending on the sample's size. To address this, the researchers in this work used the CVD method with direct heating of the sample to prepare C/C composites. This method is very poorly covered in the literature and so far only one article has described this technique [47]. They created a dedicated system for synthesizing rod-shaped composites, using a fiber bundle as the core and pyrolytic carbon as the matrix. This method allows for the rapid synthesis of pyrolytic carbon (several minutes) to obtain a composite with a controlled diameter and length.

While pyrolytic carbon is known in cardiac surgery and orthopedics, it represents a novelty in the field of neurosurgery. Also, to the best of our knowledge, the concept of C/C composites in the area of stimulation of nerve tissue cells has never been previously studied and is yet to appear in the literature. In addition, the CVD method with direct electrical heating of a bundle of carbon fibers proposed in this work is also a very interesting and innovative tool for the synthesis of C/C composites.

The main goal of this pioneering study on carbon electrodes in the form of rods for stimulating nerve tissue cells was to optimize the electrode production process, assess the microstructural and structural properties of the materials obtained, and evaluate their initial biocompatibility in vitro with SH-SY5Y human neuroblastoma cells. The optimization focused on the quantity of fibers in the composite, affecting the electrode diameter, and the synthesis time for pyrolytic carbon (PyC). Scanning microscopy examinations characterized the microstructure, fiber bundle filling with pyrocarbon, and porosity. The functional properties of the composites were influenced by the structure of pyrolytic carbon, and evaluated using high-resolution transmission microscopy (HRTEM), selected area electron diffraction (SAED), and Raman spectroscopy. Surface chemistry and wettability were measured using the XPS technique and a tensiometer, respectively. To utilize these C/C composite-based electrodes in the future, cytotoxicity and cell viability assessments were essential. The SH-SY5Y cell line was chosen for this purpose, as it is commonly used in neurodegenerative disorder models and neurological research experiments [48–51]. This study marks the first step towards further research on carbon electrodes based on carbon fibers and PyC for stimulating nerve tissue cells.

2. Materials and Methods

2.1. Materials

2.1.1. Carbon Fibers

In order to obtain carbon–carbon (C/C) composites, high-modulus carbon fibers (CF) obtained from a polyacrylonitrile (PAN) precursor by Celanese Co., USA were used. The basic parameters of the CF from the datasheet are: the number of filaments in a bundle of 250, tensile strength of 1.8 GPa, and Young's modulus of 500 GPa. The carbon fibers used for the study have a dog-bone-like shape (Figure 1). The longer diameter of the fiber is about 12.42 ± 0.79 µm, and the shorter diameter is about 4.38 ± 0.41 µm (Figure 1, arrows). The main factor determining the selection of this type of fiber was the initial small number of carbon fibers in the bundle and the low specific resistance of these materials. Additionally, it was advisable to use CF based on the polyacrylonitrile precursor, and not based on pitch, although the latter have higher electrical conductivity. The low number of fibers in the bundles facilitates their formation and separation in order to obtain C/C composites with a small diameter.

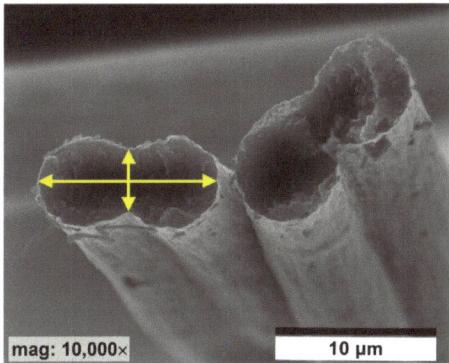

Figure 1. SEM image of dog-bone-shaped CFs cross-sectional.

2.1.2. CVD Method with Direct Electrical Heating of Carbon Fibers

Carbon–carbon (C/C) composites were obtained as a result of pyrolysis of a gaseous precursor (methane) in order to obtain pyrolytic carbon (PyC). The synthesis method is an upgraded version of the chemical vapor deposition (CVD) method using direct electric heating of a bundle of carbon fibers. This method allows for very quick heating (single seconds) of a bundle of fibers to a predetermined temperature thanks to the use of a DC generator in the reactor into which the carbonaceous gas is introduced directly. Direct heating of fibers causes the gas pyrolysis process to take place in the hottest zone, in this case directly on the surface of the fibers or a short distance from their surface, which makes the pyrolytic yield much higher than in the case of the classic CVD method or the CVI method. The latter is very effective in the process of obtaining C/C composites, but it requires many densification cycles, which makes it long-lasting and expensive. In addition, the method proposed in this work allows one to obtain a large amount of pyrocarbon in a short time, i.e., up to 0.5–3 minutes, depending on the amount of carbonaceous gas introduced. The device was manufactured specifically for the project and the production of C/C composites in the form of thin rods and is called CFCPP-1100, carbon fiber pyrolytic carbon coating by Fine Instruments, Poland. The circuit diagram is shown in the image below (Figure 2). The system consists of a quartz glass reactor, a system for assembling fiber samples (two pairs of graphite elements between which a bundle of carbon fibers was introduced and through which the current was passed), a vacuum pump, a DC generator, a system for gas supply and extraction, a flow counter, gas cylinders and a pyrometer to control the temperature of the fiber bundle.

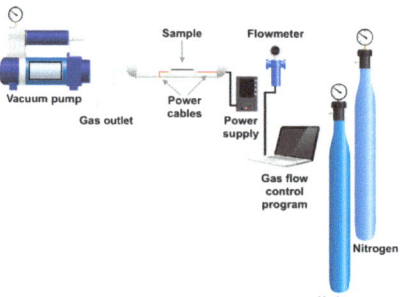

Figure 2. Scheme of the system for the synthesis of pyrolytic carbon using the CVD method with direct electrical heating of the sample.

For the purpose of synthesis, a bundle of carbon fibers with the appropriate number of fibers in the bundle was placed between graphite elements and heated to the set temperature in the range of 1100–1200 °C. The image below shows a bundle of fibers before and during heating (Figure 3A,B). Prior to the CVD synthesis process, a vacuum is created to better remove air from the reactor as well as from the spaces between the individual fibers in the bundle. Then, an inert gas (N_2) is introduced into the reactor and the vacuum is removed. The reactor is flushed with N_2 for 60 seconds. After this time, a carbonaceous gas (CH_4) is introduced into the reactor while the flow of N_2 is maintained. The amount of CH_4 introduced into the reactor is 2 L/h, while the amount of N_2 is 10 L/h. The gas injection time varies, i.e., from 30 s to 180 s. In the next stage, the sample is kept at the synthesis temperature for 30 s in an inert atmosphere, without the flow of carbonaceous gas. Finally, the system is cooled to room temperature (RT) by reducing the voltage on the DC power supply to zero. The total time needed to carry out the entire synthesis from the introduction of the sample into the reactor to its removal after synthesis is a maximum of 6–7 min.

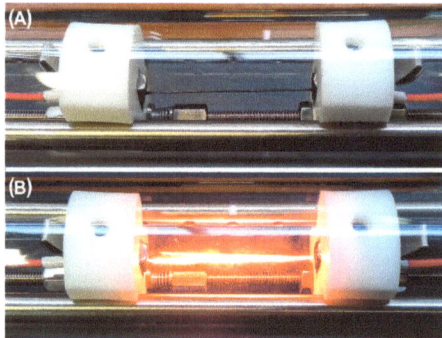

Figure 3. Bundle of fibers before (**A**) and during (**B**) synthesis.

Using this method, the following 4 types of C/C composites were produced:
- CF_PyC30—rod-shaped C/C composite based on carbon fiber and PyC obtained after 30 s of synthesis.
- CF_PyC60—rod-shaped C/C composite based on carbon fiber and PyC obtained after 60 s of synthesis.
- CF_PyC120—rod-shaped C/C composite based on carbon fiber and PyC obtained after 120 s of synthesis.
- CF_PyC180—rod-shaped C/C composite based on carbon fiber and PyC obtained after 180 s of synthesis.

- CF—bundle of carbon fibers.

Each bundle of fibers synthesized by CVD had between 200 to 220 individual fibers per bundle. The number of fibers was dictated by the need to obtain a rod-shaped C/C composite with a diameter of less than 1 mm and good handiness.

2.2. Methods

2.2.1. SEM and Digital Microscope

The evaluation of the microstructure and morphology of carbon fibers and C/C composites was performed using Nova NanoSEM 200 (FEI Europe Company, Eindhoven, The Netherlands) scanning electron microscope and Thermo Fisher Scientific (Waltham, MA, USA) SCIOS II Dual Beam scanning electron microscopes (SEM). The acceleration voltage was 10 kV. The SEM images were also used to evaluate the diameter of carbon fibers and C/C composites and also to evaluate diameters of ball-like protuberances characteristic for pyrocarbon after using ImageJ v1.53e software, developed at the National Institutes of Health and the Laboratory for Optical and Computational Instrumentation (LOCI, University of Wisconsin), USA, public domain. In total, 70 protuberance measurements were made on the surface of PyC. Moreover, the porosity of all C/C composites was established based on SEM microphotographs using ImageJ software. For porosity thresholding of SEM images was performed. Thresholding is a type of image segmentation where the pixels of an image are changed to make the image easier to analyze. In thresholding, the images are converted from color or grayscale into a binary image, i.e., one that is simply black and white. A digital microscope (VHX-900F, Keyence Co., Mechelen, Belgium) was also used to analyze the surface morphology of the samples. Equipped with two lenses, a standard lens, and a Z500T lens, it allows images at $20\times$–$200\times$ and $500\times$–$5000\times$ magnification. The working distance is 4.4 mm.

2.2.2. TEM and HRTEM

Detailed characterization of microstructure and structure was performed with a Thermo Fisher Scientific (Waltham, MA, USA) Titan Themis Cs corrected 200 kV XFEG transmission electron microscope (TEM). Thin foils for TEM inspection were cut out with a focused ion beam (FIB) technique employing Thermo Fisher Scientific SCIOS II Dual Beam scanning electron microscopes. Thin lamellas for TEM inspection were cut out from cross-sections of carbon rods, from the boundary separating the matrix and the inner rod. The voltage applied was 30 kV, while the current was initially set to 30 nA during regular cross-section milling, and subsequently it was reduced down to 3 nA. Once the lamellae were cut out it was transferred onto a copper grid with a lift-out omniprobe system. The lamella was welded to the grid with Pt and further thinned with the beam current gradually decreasing from 3 nA to 50 pA. Then it was transferred onto a TEM holder and examined.

2.2.3. Selected Area Electron Diffraction (SAED)

The obtained SAED images were used to quantify the degree of preferred orientation, the so-called orientation angle, OA. The procedure included the following steps:

- Determining the position of the center of the diffraction pattern and the radius of the diffraction ring with indices (002);
- Determining (using a self-developed script in Python) the profile of intensity changes along the perimeter of a circle with a predetermined center and radius (values read in 0.2 degree steps);
- Fitting two Gaussian curves to the obtained profile, the maximum values of which occur at points of the circle (located on opposite sides) with the highest intensity, and determining the half-width FWHM of these curves [52,53];
- Determination of their average value, equal to orientation angle OA.

2.2.4. Raman Spectroscopy

Raman spectroscopy measurements were performed using a WITec Alpha 300 M + apparatus with a 600 g/mm grating, a 488 nm diode laser, and a 50× lens. A total of 10 accumulations with 20 s integration times were recorded for each point in the line measurement. Fityk 0.8.0 software was used for the spectra analysis. Spectral deconvolution was performed using the Voigt function [54]. It allowed us to distinguish characteristic bands corresponding to vibrations of carbon structures in samples. The I_D/I_G ratio was determined from the total intensities of the D and G bands as a coefficient describing the degree of crystallinity of the carbons. Additionally, the size of the L_a crystallite was also determined using the Cançado equation [55]:

$$L_a = \left(2.4 \times 10^{-10}\right) \times \lambda^4 \times \left(\frac{I_D}{I_G}\right)^{-1} \quad (1)$$

where L_a is a crystallite size (nm), λ is the radiation wavelength (nm) and I_D/I_G are the intensity of Raman D and G bands.

2.2.5. XPS

The surface chemistry of the samples was determined using the X-ray photoelectron spectroscopy (XPS) spectroscope PHI VersaProbe II Scanning XPS system working with a monochromatic Al source—line Kα (1486.6 eV). Energy pass was set to 117.50 eV for the survey scan and 46.95 eV for core-level spectra. The charge compensation was ensured with a dual beam of 7 eV Ar$^+$ ions and 1 eV electrons. The operating pressure in the analytical chamber was $< 3 \times 10^{-9}$ mbar, and the area of focus of X-rays was 100 µm. Estimated depth of analytical information was about 5 nm. The shift of energy due to the charging effects was calibrated assuming binding energy of C1s line = 285 eV. Fitting of core-level spectra and background subtraction using the Shirley method were performed using PHI MultiPak software (v.9.9.2).

2.2.6. Contact Angle Measurement

The contact angle 20 µm, measuring range: 0–180° and resolution 0.01°. The proposed method of assessing wettability is a dynamic method in which the so-called advancing angle (θ_{Adv}) between a liquid (water) and a solid is determined [56]. The system also allows the measurement of the contact angle of the fiber bundle, which has already been described in the publications of other authors [57,58]. During the measurements, the sample (in the form of fiber/rod) is stationary, and the vessel holder moves up (advancing cycle) and down (receding cycle). Each sample was repeatedly dipped in and withdrawn from the liquid vessel three times to measure a series of dynamic advancing contact angles. The dynamic contact angles at constant advancing velocities can be calculated from the Wilhelmy equation [59]:

$$F = L \times \gamma \times \cos\theta_{Adv} \quad (2)$$

where F is the force detected by the microbalance, L is the wetted length of the sample, θ_{Adv} is the dynamic contact angle.

2.2.7. In Vitro Study

Cell Culture and Experimental Groups

Human neuroblastoma SH-SY5Y cells (ATCC CRL-2266, Manassas, VA, USA) were cultured in high glucose DMEM (Life Technologies Ltd., Paisley, UK) supplemented with a 10% fetal bovine serum (FBS, Life Technologies Ltd., Paisley, UK) and 1% penicillin + streptomycin solution (Life Technologies Ltd., Paisley, UK). Cells were propagated in sterile cell culture flasks (75 cm^2) and kept at 37 °C in a saturated humidity atmosphere containing 5% CO_2. After reaching 80% confluency the cells were trypsinized (0.05% trypsin/EDTA, Life Technologies Ltd.)), counted (Bürker chamber) and seeded at a density of 8×10^4 into 48-well plates containing the investigated materials (CF_FF, Pt wire, CF, and CF_PyC120) which were immobilized in the wells by quartz rings. Pt wire was used as a reference due to being the material from which conventional DBS electrodes are currently made whereas CF_FF, made of a core in the form of CF and a matrix in the form of phenol formaldehyde resin, was used as a positive control sample in the form of a rod of a size comparable to the investigated samples. Before cell seeding, the plates with materials and rings were sterilized with UV for 30 min. The control experimental group involved seeding wells containing only quartz rings. There were 3 replicates for each experimental group.

Cytotoxicity Assay

Twenty-four and forty-eight hours after cell seeding, 50 µL from each cell culture well was collected in a 96-well plate format to assess the potential cytotoxic effect of the studied materials in comparison to the control group. This parameter was measured by the Cytotoxicity Detection Kit (RocheDiagnostic, Mancheim, Germany) described previously [60]. The absorbance of each sample was measured after 15 min from reagent addition (25 µL/well) with a multi-well plate reader (Infinite® M200 PRO, Tecan, Mannedorf, Switzerland) at 490 nm. After the subtraction of blank value (absorbance of cell culture medium) the data were normalized to the control group and are presented as the mean ± S.E.M. from three replicates.

Live Cell Imaging

Twenty-four and forty-eight hours after cell seeding the plates were imaged using the differential interference contrast (DIC) light microscopy method. For this purpose, an inverted microscope AxioObserver (Carl Zeiss, Jena, Germany) was used, which was equipped with a white–black camera (Axio-CamMRm, Carl Zeiss, Jena, Germany). One microphotograph was taken for each well.

Cell Viability Assay

Forty-eight hours after cell seeding, the WST-1 reagent was added to all experimental groups (in 2 replicates) as described previously [61]. After 60 min of incubation with the substrate, 100 µL of probe from each experimental group (in 2 replicates) was transferred to a 96-well plate. The absorbance of samples was measured with a multi-well plate reader (Infinite® M200 PRO, Tecan) at 440 nm (measurement wavelength) and 630 nm (reference wavelength). Data (calculated difference between measurement and reference measurement) after subtraction for blank value (total damage, 1% Triton X-100 for 15 min) were normalized to the control group and are expressed as a percentage of the control ± S.E.M.

Scanning Electron Microscopy

At 48 h after cell seeding, the SH-SY5Y cells were fixed in 4% paraformaldehyde and then the samples were washed with PBS, treated with a 25% glutaraldehyde and 8% formaldehyde solution in a cacodylate buffer overnight, and then washed in cacodylate buffer. Next, the samples were dehydrated in increasing concentrations of ethanol (from 5% to 100%). All the dehydration steps were carried out at RT. The samples were finally dried using a CO_2 critical point dryer, attached to the holders, and coated with a thin layer of carbon. Neuronal cells were analyzed using scanning electron microscopy (SEM) (NovaNanoSEM 200, FEI).

Statistical Analysis

Data were analyzed using Statistica software [62]. The analysis of variance (one- or two-way ANOVA) and post hoc Duncan test for multiple comparisons were used to show statistical significance with assumed $p < 0.05$.

3. Results and Discussion

3.1. Morphology and Microstructure of Rod-Shaped C/C Composite

The morphology and microstructure of the obtained C/C composites were shown both in digital and SEM images (Figures 4 and 5). The surface morphology of the C/C composites is rough, containing numerous ball-like protuberances characteristic of pyrocarbon [63]. The size of the spherical structures increases with the length of the synthesis time. The smallest of them are present in the case of PyC synthesis for 30 s (Figure 4B,E), and the largest at 180 s (Figure 4H,J). Also, with the increase in synthesis time, an increase in the PyC thickness on the surface is observed, which translates into an increase in the diameter of the C/C composites (Figure 4K). In addition, in the case of composites obtained in the time from 30 to 120 s, the morphology is preserved to some extent reflecting the fibrous form of the substrate itself. An increase in the synthesis time to 180 s causes the disappearance of this tendency, which is most likely related to a large increase in the thickness of the PyC. All composites were characterized by significant stiffness when compared to the bundle of carbon fibers (Figure 4A,D). This was observed especially at synthesis times of 60 s and more (Figure 4C,F–J).

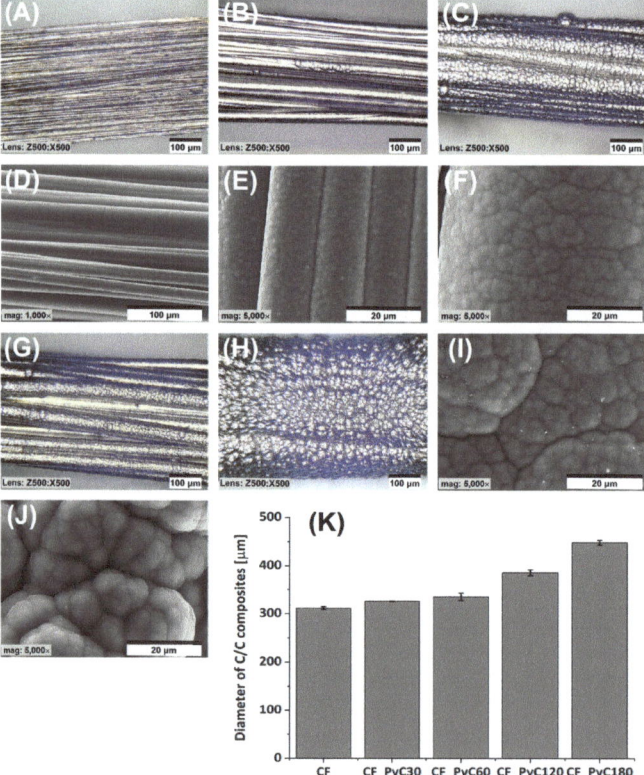

Figure 4. Morphology of a bundle of carbon fibers (**A,D**) and C/C composites after different durations of PyC synthesis (**B,E**) 30 s, (**C,F**) 60 s, (**G,I**) 120 s and (**H,J**) 180 s, diameter of C/C composites (**K**).

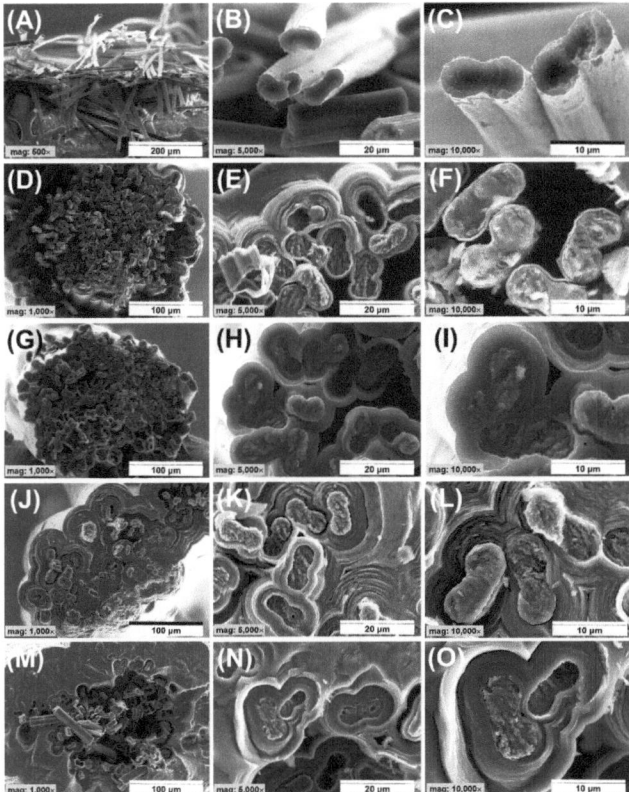

Figure 5. SEM analysis of cross-sections of the obtained C/C composites depending on the time of PyC synthesis, (**A–C**) bundle of CF, (**D–F**) CF_PyC30, (**G–I**) CF_PyC60, (**J–L**) CF_PyC120, (**M–O**) CF_PyC 180.

The main factor that determined the choice of pyrocarbon synthesis conditions was to obtain C/C composites in which PyC would fill the spaces between individual fibers in the bundle, allowing on the one hand an increase in stiffness, while at the same time minimizing any increase in diameter of the material obtained in the form of rods. An important study allowing the observation of the degree of composite densification was the preparation of fractures and their examination using SEM (Figure 5). The analysis of the cross-sections of the obtained composites shows a significant difference between the samples, strongly correlated with the PyC synthesis time. Synthesis of PyC using the CVD method as a result of direct heating of a bundle of carbon fibers allowed us to observe that in the range of synthesis time from 30 s to 60 s a significant degree of porosity can be observed in the volume of a bundle of carbon fibers (Figure 5D–I).

The pore size for these samples varies and is strongly dependent on the synthesis time. The highest porosity was observed for the shortest synthesis time, i.e., for 30 s, where the total porosity was about 20%. In turn, the lowest porosity was characteristic of the sample obtained at 120 s and was below 1% (Figure 6A). The decrease in porosity is closely related to the filling of the space between the individual fibers, which is also confirmed by the increase in the thickness of the PyC layers between the individual fibers in the volume of the bundle (Figure 6A). A short synthesis time means that the amount of synthesized PyC around the fibers is the smallest. It increases proportionally to the synthesis time and after 120 s, the spaces between the fibers are filled (Figure 5J–L), and the amount of pyrocarbon on the surface of the composites begins to increase (Figure 6B).

An unquestionably unfavorable effect is observed after 180 s when the amount of PyC deposit significantly increases (Figures 5M and 6B). Such an effect is undesirable due to a significant increase in the diameter of the composite, and the appearance of cracks in the layer (Figure 7 arrows), which may adversely affect the mechanical properties of the composite. In addition, such a large layer of pyrocarbon no longer fulfills the assumed requirements, i.e., creating a matrix in which carbon fibers are embedded. The pyrolytic carbon in these samples has a distinct laminar structure which promotes crack propagation extending along the laminar structure, parallel to the fiber surface. Crack propagation is even more likely as the thickness of the pyrocarbon layers increases. Crack propagation in laminar PyC has also been mentioned in other literature [46,64,65].

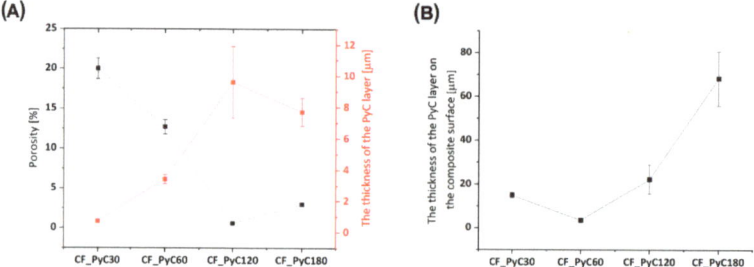

Figure 6. Porosity and thickness of the PyC around the fibers inside the bundle in a C/C composite (**A**); the thickness of the PyC layer on the composite surface (**B**).

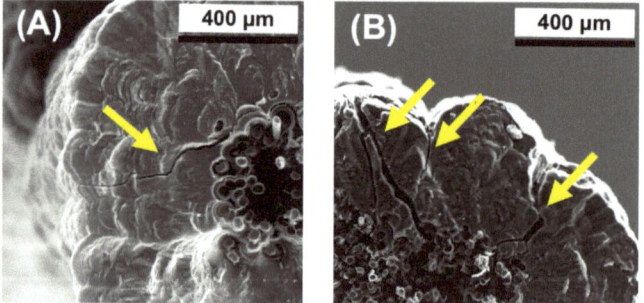

Figure 7. Crack propagation in the PyC layer in different places (**A**,**B**).

Analyzing the results of the assessment of the morphology and microstructure of the obtained C/C composites, the most favorable in terms of homogeneity of PyC distribution, is characterized by the CF_PyC120 sample. This composite was also characterized by the best handiness among the obtained samples in the form of a rod. It is this composite that will be subjected to further tests.

3.2. Structure of Rod-Shaped C/C Composite

The structure and properties of the interface determine the adhesion between the fiber and the matrix. The mechanical properties of C/C composites are highly dependent on the load transfer at the fiber/matrix interface. A weak interface may impair the integrity of composites, whereas a strong bond may induce brittle fracture behavior [44,66]. For analyzing the microstructures close to the CF and PyC interface, SEM, TEM, and high-resolution TEM (HRTEM) were used. The analysis of the interface between the carbon fiber and the deposited PyC layer indicates good adhesion at the interface. The SEM microphotography indicates that the carbon fibers are surrounded by concentric pyrocarbon layers, and the boundary between these two phases is continuous (Figure 8A,B). It demonstrates that there is relatively good adhesion between the CF and the PyC. This is more visible from the scanning TEM HAADF-STEM micrographs shown in Figure 8C,D. As can be seen in the images the interface is continuous and free from any structural distortions. This is very evident from the area selected for illustration of the electron diffraction pattern (SAED) in the inset in Figure 9D. The corresponding orientation angles (OA), determined by the SAED pattern, indicate the existence of two different textures namely smooth laminar (SL) also called medium textured, OA = 76 ± 2° and dark laminar (DL) also called low textured, OA = 93 ± 2°. SL pyrocarbon is composed of wavy graphene layers, with strong distortions and curvatures. DL pyrolytic carbon is classified as isotropic carbon, although the preferred orientation of the pyrolytic carbon domains (texture) in this type of PyC is between typical isotropic (ISO) and that of typical low-textured ones, i.e., smooth laminar (SL) [43]. In the SEM images, we do not observe a clear difference in pyrocarbon morphology that would allow for a clear distinction between the SL and the DL pyrocarbons. SEM images indicate to a greater extent the presence of pyrocarbon SL (Figure 8A,B), which is characterized by a higher degree of texture parallel to the surface of the fiber [46,65].

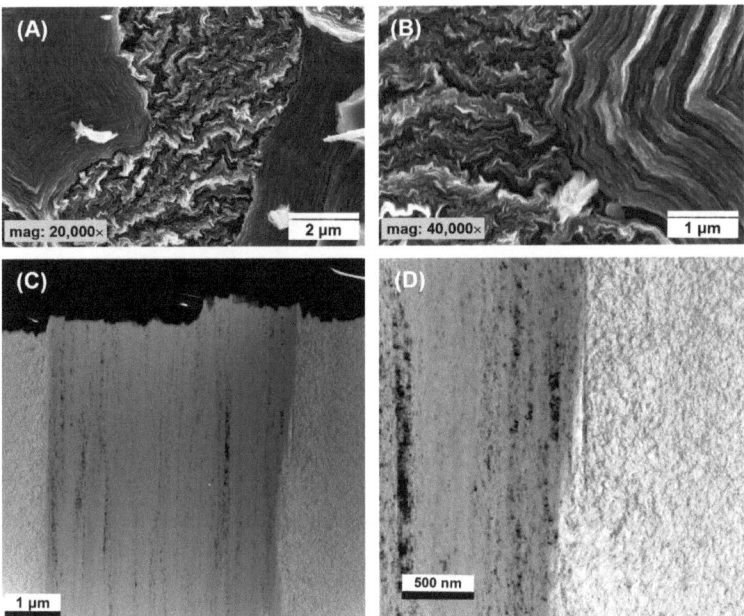

Figure 8. SEM (**A**,**B**) and STEM (**C**,**D**) morphologies of fracture surface of C/C composites.

Only the analysis of HRTEM images of the interface between the CF and PyC, as well as of the PyC itself, shows some differences in its structure and allows us to distinguish regions characteristic of SL and DL matrices (Figure 9). The analysis of HRTEM images of the PyC matrix clearly indicates the areas of occurrence of two types of pyrocarbon, i.e., with low and medium texturing (Figure 9B). In the HRTEM images, we can observe the interface between the fiber and the pyrocarbon. As in the case of TEM and SEM images, the interface between the phases is homogeneous, but there is a significant difference between the structure of the CF itself and the PyC (Figure 9A). The PyC matrix contains both low- and medium-textured domains, while the carbon fiber is characterized by high anisotropy and the clear arrangement of graphene layers parallel to the axis of the fiber (Figure 9C). The crystallographic structure of CF and PyC was assessed using the SAED technique (Figure 9) without the corresponding BF images; instead, the SAEDs are shown together with sample HRTEM micrographs to illustrate the structural features. The recorded diffraction patterns were characterized by the presence of three diffraction rings with scattering vectors of 3.0 nm^{-1}, 4.8 nm^{-1}, and 8.1 nm^{-1}, assigned to the carbon planes (002), (100), and (110), respectively [67]. The diffraction rings in the case of CF showed a certain directional intensity distribution related to the (002) planes, indicating the anisotropic orientation of the crystal domains. In contrast, PyC showed a generally uniform intensity distribution with some slight direction indicating the isotropic orientation of the crystalline domains. The d_{002} value estimated from the diffraction patterns for CF was 3.39 Å, while for PyC it was 3.42 Å. The smaller value of the interplanar distances indicates a better ordering of the carbon structure in CF than in PyC, which is probably also related to the synthesis temperature of both types of carbon [68,69]. The carbon fibers were obtained at a temperature of 2000 °C, while the PyC synthesis temperature is between 1100–1200 °C.

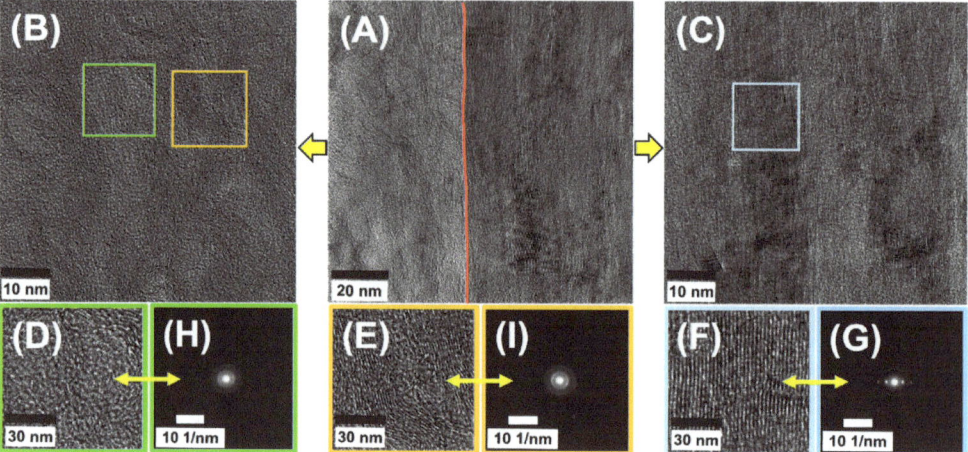

Figure 9. HRTEM images CF_PyC120 at the border between CF and PyC (**A**) composite, PyC in the CF_PyC120 composite (**B,D,E**), and CF in the CF_PyC120 composite (**C,F**) and SAEDs taken independently of HRTEM from two regions of PyC (**H,I**) and CF (**G**).

The high-resolution TEM HRTEM images, given for illustration in Figure 9, were taken with no objective aperture. In Figure 9A–C they are shown in a large field of view for a better illustration of the interface between the CF and PyC. The small squares marked in the images (Figure 9B) and (Figure 9C) indicate areas from which fast Fourier transforms (FFTs) were taken (Figure 9G,H). The FFTs are well in accordance with selected area electron diffraction patterns (SADPs), not shown, which were taken for statistics from different areas of the thin foil, from the respective regions corresponding to CF and PyC. Both the SADPs and FFTs indicate considerable changes in the structure between both phases. The results indicated more texture features and structural organization in the CF relative to PyC. The latter appeared more disarrayed and randomly organized. Regardless of the structural differences between both phases, however, the interface between the CF and PyC appeared largely coherent. It can be observed that some layers of graphene in the CF and smooth laminar pyrocarbon undulated together in the bonding area. This can improve the bond strength of the fiber with the pyrocarbon matrix acting like a hook. Therefore, the strength of the interfacial bonding of the fiber–PyC matrix can be strong [44].

When analyzing the possible mechanism of pyrocarbon growth in contact with a heated substrate, in this case, carbon fiber, the literature most often pays attention to such control parameters of the PyC deposition process as hydrocarbon concentration, residence time, surface area to volume of pore ratio (A/V) and temperature [70,71]. Initially, most of the work focused on the maturation of gases and the evolution of hydrocarbon pyrolysis decomposition products into small linear particles, which subsequently coalesced and combined into the synthesis of polycyclic aromatic hydrocarbons (PAHs) [70]. Over time, however, attention was paid to the role of the A/V ratio, and the concept of a nucleation and growth mechanism based on gas maturation and the concentration ratio between small linear molecules and polycyclic aromatic hydrocarbons (PAHs) was suggested [46,70–72]. The growth mechanism, usually obtained with short residence times and high A/V ratios, is based on the chemisorption of molecules (C_2 or PAHs) in active sites at the edge of the graphene layer [73,74]. The second mechanism, i.e., nucleation, occurs most often in processes carried out with long residence times, high temperatures, and high concentrations of precursors and is associated with the physisorption of large PAH molecules on the surface of the substrate [72,74,75].

The PyC synthesis process takes place in the temperature range of 1100–1200 °C, however, it may be accompanied by various effects. In general, this temperature is relatively low, which is not sufficient to allow the maturation of the intermediate forms to produce large amounts of PAHs. Hence, the concentration of small linear/aromatic molecules increases, possibly reducing the formation of soot particles, and may also prevent the formation of five-member rings. This change in concentration will result in the deposition of PyC with a higher level of texture [70]. On the other hand, as was also described in one of the publications [70], if the PyC synthesis temperature is even lower, e.g., in the range of 1000–1100 °C, the amount of energy and intermediate compounds will not be enough to produce large aromatic molecules. This lack of large aromatic molecules will lead to the formation of five-member rings [72], thus producing PyC with lower levels of texture. At this stage, PyC formation will be completely controlled by the chemisorption of intermediate species at the graphene edges. Thus, in our particular case, we cannot clearly state which of the mechanisms is dominant, because, firstly, PyC deposition takes place in a temperature range that allows both nucleation and growth mechanisms to appear, and besides, temperature is not the only factor affecting this process. In addition to the aforementioned factors, the type of mechanism and microstructure may also depend on the construction of the reactor, and the distance between the nozzle and the substrate on which the deposition takes place, which has already been confirmed in the publications of other authors [70,71]. Therefore, in our case, the synthesis of PyC takes place through both mechanisms, as evidenced by the different microstructure of the obtained PyC.

Raman spectroscopy was performed in order to evaluate the structure of the C/C composites and compare their properties to CF which is issued as the core of the composite. The Raman spectra of C/C composites (CF_PyC120) and carbon fibers are shown in Figure 10.

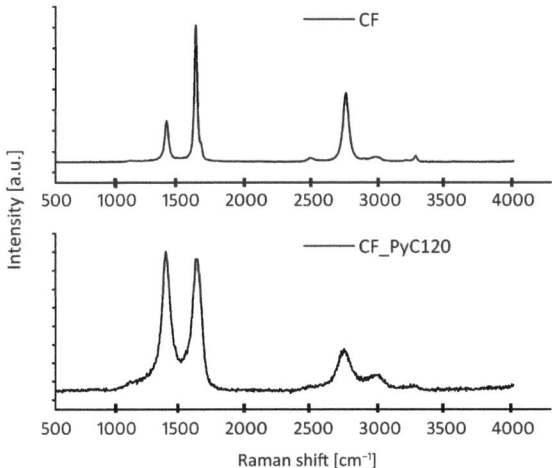

Figure 10. Raman spectra of carbon fibers (CF) and CF_PyC120 composite.

Based on the Raman spectra, two characteristic D and G bands were observed for all samples. In the Raman spectra of carbon materials, two ranges of bands are observed, the first in the range of 1000–2000 cm^{-1} and the second in the range of 2000–3500 cm^{-1}. In the former, there are two characteristic bands D and G. The D band occurs at the Raman shift of about 1350 cm^{-1} and is associated with the presence of defects that break the translational symmetry of the graphene sheet. The G band at about 1590 cm^{-1} is induced by the in-plane stretching vibrations of C=C bonds, which are attributed to longitudinal optical phonon mode at the center of the Brillouin zone of graphite. Near the G band, at Raman shift around 1620 cm^{-1}, also the weak shoulder peak occurs, known as D' band. This line originates from the double resonance intravalley scattering Raman processes activating phonons around Γ of the Brillouin zone of graphite, and it is one of the spectral feature characteristics of defective carbon materials. The separated D' band is clearly visible only in the case of the CF sample, but it is present also in CF_PyC120, covered by the broadened G peak due to the lattice disorder. The exact contribution of this component was obtained using the Sadetzky five-band model described elsewhere [76]. In the second range of Raman spectra, there is a characteristic band at about 2650 cm^{-1}, often also denoted as 2D, due to two phonons with opposite momentum in the highest optical branch near the K point of the Brillouin zone [77–81]. It is related to the stacking order of graphene sheets, sensitive to the electronic structure of carbon, and its intensity increases with the number of graphene layers [78,82]. In the second order region, weak overtone bands are also present for both samples—D+D' ($\sim$2900 cm^{-1}), D+D'' ($\sim$2450 cm^{-1}), and 2D' ($\sim$3200 cm^{-1}). Table 1 summarizes the structural parameters extracted from the Raman spectra of CF and CF_PyC120 samples.

Table 1. Structural parameters obtained from Raman spectra of CF and CF_PyC120.

Sample	I_D	I_G	I_{2D}	I_D/I_G	I_{2D}/I_G	L_a [nm]
CF	6148	17,107	15,937	0.36	0.93	37.88
CF_PyC120	7102	6844	3739	1.04	0.55	13.12

The values of L_a were obtained from Cancado Equation (1).

The results of Raman carbon fiber studies confirm the results obtained from high-resolution transmission microscopy (HRTEM) (Figure 9). Sharp and narrow characteristic bands testify to the highly crystalline character of the carbon fiber sample. The CF selected as a core of the C/C composite component is high-modulus, highly crystalline with high structural order. Such a structure of CF is evidenced by the greater intensity of the G band than the D band and the ratio of the integral intensities of the D and G bands (I_D/I_G) which is 0.36. This parameter is generally considered to be the basic indicator of the structural order of sp^2 carbons, closely related to their electronic structure and crystallinity [80]. An additional parameter, often analyzed to determine the structure of the tested material, is the ratio of the integral intensities of the 2D and G bands (I_{2D}/I_G). A high value for this parameter indicates a three-dimensional long-range order and changes in the electronic structure associated with an increase in the concentration of charge carriers, as well as a large number of graphene layers in the tested material [81,82]. Structurally, C/C composites differ significantly from carbon fibers which are the core of these composites. PyC obtained by the CVD method at a temperature of 1100–1200 °C is characterized by a much lower structural order than carbon fibers, as evidenced by the I_D/I_G and I_{2D}/I_G parameters. The difference in the structure of the composite and carbon fibers is also evidenced by the size of the crystallite, namely the average lateral elongation of the graphene planes, which is more than four times greater in carbon fibers than in the C/C composite (Table 1).

In order to answer the question of whether the conditions prevailing during the CVD synthesis affect the changes in the pyrolytic carbon structure, an analysis of the PyC at a depth was carried out. Optical focus depth profiling with a Raman confocal microscope was used to analyze the PyC from the outer surface to a depth of 24 µm (Figure 11B). The analyzed thickness in the case of PyC was dictated by its thickness on the surface of the fibers in the composite, which ranged between 20–30 μm. The same profiling was also carried out on carbon fiber, but to a depth of 8 μm, due to the diameter (longer diagonal) of the fiber (Figure 11A). For pyrolytic carbon, there is a slight decrease in signal intensity with increasing depth of focal, resulting mainly from the absorption of radiation depending on the absorption coefficient of the material, the depth of the optical focus, and the in-depth probe response parameter [77,83]. In order to quantify the structural changes at the depth of the PyC layer, the I_D/I_G parameters were determined. Determination of these parameters did not cause problems, because no significant changes in peak broadening caused by noise were observed at the tested depth, therefore band areas were used to determine them (Figure 11B,C). There was a similar situation in the case of carbon fibers (Figure 11A,C).

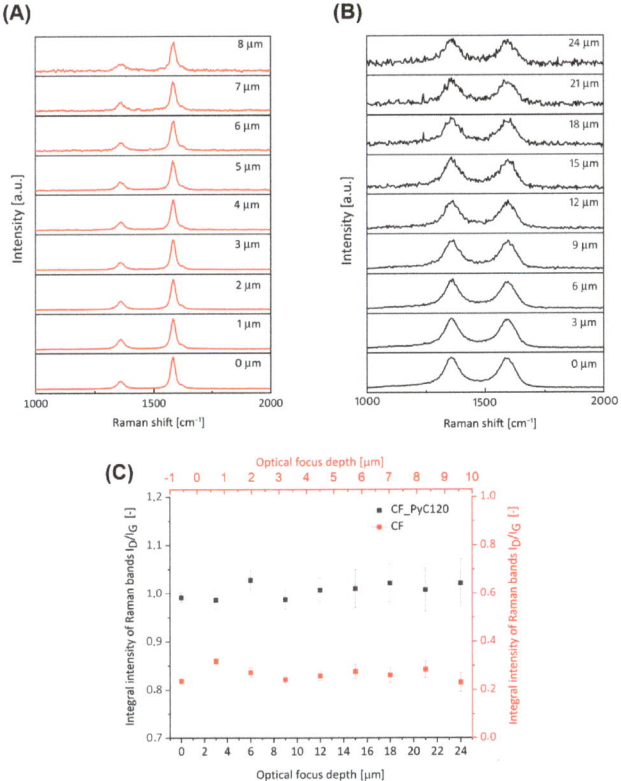

Figure 11. First-order Raman spectra of CF (**A**) and CF_PyC120 (**B**) composites collected at the various optical focus depths. (**C**) Depth profiles of the I_D/I_G (areas) of CF and CF_PyC120 composite.

The values of the I_D/I_G parameters are at a similar level along with the depth of profiling of the tested samples. The obtained results confirm the structural homogeneity of the fibers themselves, which means that it is a commercial product. Whereas the results for the composite may confirm that the structural layer of PyC synthesized on the surface of carbon fibers is uniform in thickness throughout (Figure 11C). The obtained results are also confirmed by tests performed with the use of transmission electron microscopy (Figure 9).

3.3. Surface Chemistry of Rod-Shaped C/C Composite

The surface chemical composition of the carbon fibers (CF) and C/C composites (CF_PyC120) determined by the XPS is shown in Table 2. The main elements detected on the surfaces of these samples are carbon (C1s line) and oxygen (O1s line). The C1s core-level spectra for all samples were fitted with six components corresponding to C=C (sp^2) type bonds (284.5 eV), C-C (sp^3) bonds (285.3 eV), C-OH/C-O-C bonds (286.1 eV), C=O/O-C-O bonds (287.0 eV), O-C=O groups (288.5 eV) and $\pi \rightarrow \pi^*$ satellite (291.0 eV) [12,31]. The latter is correlated with the graphitic character of the samples. The peak fitting of the C1s core level for CF and CF_PyC120 is presented in Figure 12.

Table 2. Surface chemistry of CF and CF_PyC120 obtained from XPS analysis.

Sample	Elemental Composition (%)		(-)	Deconvolution of the C1s Spectra (%)					
	C	O	O/C	284.5 eV C=C (sp^2)	285.3 eV C-C (sp^3)	286.1 eV C-O, C-OH	287.0 eV C=O, O-C-O	288.5 eV O-C=O	291.0 eV $\pi \rightarrow \pi^*$
CF	87.60	12.40	0.14	65.90	14.20	3.10	2.00	0.90	1.50
CF_PyC120	90.30	9.70	0.11	56.10	23.10	2.80	3.40	1.60	3.30

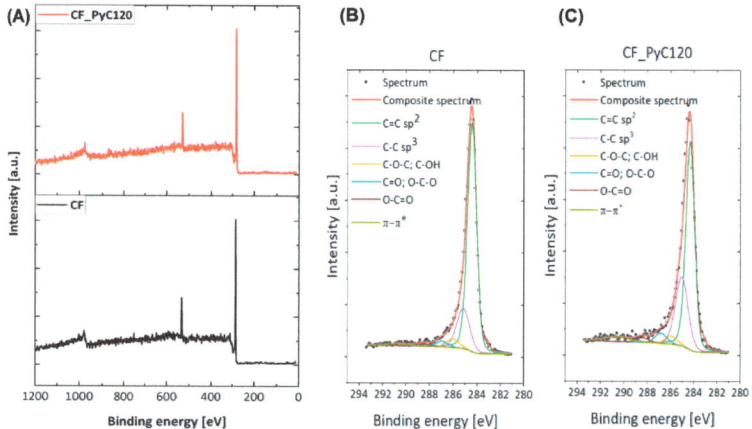

Figure 12. (**A**) XPS survey spectra of CF and CF_PyC120. Deconvoluted C1s peaks at (**B**) CF, (**C**) CF_PyC120.

The total carbon content in both analyzed samples is at a similar level. Nonetheless, analysis of the C1s peak indicates a higher content of carbon in hybridization sp^2 in the CF as compared with CF_PyC120. The percentage of sp^2 bonds is strictly related to the degree of graphitization of carbon and correlates well with the results obtained from HRTEM and Raman spectroscopy (Figures 9 and 10). At the same time, for graphitized CF, the percentage of sp^3 (C–C) bonds associated with the presence of defects in the carbon structure is lower than for the CF_PyC120 composite sample. Interestingly, in the case of carbon fibers, we observe a relatively high oxygen content, mainly in the form of C-O, C=O, and O-C-O bonds, higher than for the composite with a pyrolytic carbon matrix. On the one hand, this may indicate the presence of sizing in this type of fiber, but it may also be related to the presence of structural defects on the surface of the fiber, for example in the form of dangling bonds capable of reacting with atmospheric oxygen. The presence of defects on the fibers' surface may also be evidenced by the presence of a rather large amount of bonds with sp^3 hybridization (14.20%) for graphitized fibers.

In order to assess the wettability of the surface of the tested materials, the Wilhelmy method was used, applying a tensiometer with a holder for testing single fibers with a diameter above 20 µm. This method is dedicated primarily to the analysis of solid samples, but it can also be used for bundles of fibers, as in the case of CF tow [57,58]. Wettability was evaluated for three types of samples, namely C/C composites, carbon fibers as the main reinforcing and directivity component of the composite, and a platinum (Pt) wire. The Pt wire was chosen because in the next study (in vitro study) it will be used as a reference due to the fact that it is currently the material from which electrodes for deep brain stimulation are most often made. The figures for individual values of the dynamic contact angle relative to the position during immersion of the samples in water and the results of the average values of the advancing angle θ_{Adv} are presented below (Figure 13).

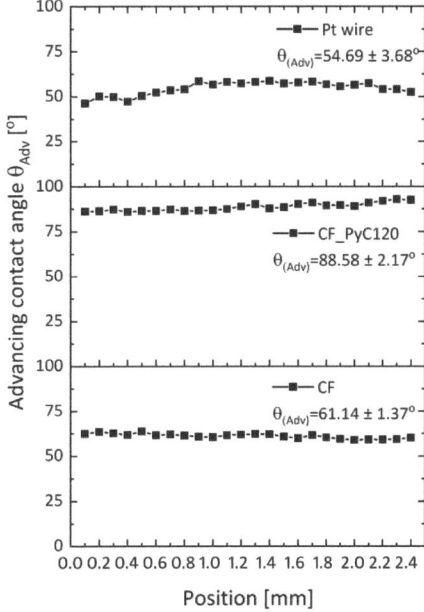

Figure 13. Typical measured θ_{Adv} versus position (mm) curves for CF tow, CF_PyC120, and Pt wire samples in water.

The highest value of the contact angle is observed for the composite sample, which is $88.58 \pm 2.17°$. The values of the water contact angle for pyrolytic carbon, used primarily in medicine as a coating on the surface of bileaflet mechanical heart valve prostheses, are in the range of 86–110°. The exact value mainly depends on the synthesis temperature, types of precursor, and the presence of other elements, such as Si, used to improve mechanical parameters, mainly hardness and abrasion resistance [69,84,85]. In medicine, in particular for covering mechanical heart valves, low-temperature pyrolytic carbons are obtained at a temperature below 1500 °C [41]. Low-temperature isotropic carbon differs from isotropic carbon obtained at temperatures above 2000 °C not only in the degree of ordering of the carbon structure but also in the presence of heteroatoms which may affect, among other things, the degree of wettability of pyrolytic carbon. LTI carbon is characterized by a contact angle of about 90°; therefore, the value of the contact angle for PyC in CF_PyC120 composite confirms that we are dealing with low-temperature PyC. The wettability of the fiber bundle is higher than that of the composite sample, which is most likely due to the presence of sizing on the surface of carbon fibers. The presence of sizing on the surface of the fibers is also confirmed by the XPS test results. The value of the water contact angle for the tested fibers is about $61.14 \pm 1.37°$, which is consistent with the values presented in the literature for water contact angles of carbon fibers with sizing. The most frequently presented values of these angles in the literature are 62.5°, 65.8°, and about 71° depending on the research method used [57,58,86,87]. The first two values refer to the dynamic method, as in this paper. The lower contact angle of CF compared to the C/C composite may also be evidenced by the presence of oxygen groups associated with sizing as well as in combination with structural defects on the fiber surface, which is confirmed by the XPS test results (Table 2, Figure 12). A higher oxygen content in the CF sample is evidenced by, for example, a higher O/C ratio (Table 2).

The wettability of the Pt wire is 54.69 ± 3.68° and confirms data in the literature indicating the hydrophilic character of this material [88].

3.4. Biocompatibility of Rod-Shaped C/C Composite

The in vitro biological tests were aimed at the preliminary assessment of cytotoxicity and cell viability in contact with the manufactured materials. The SH-SY5Y cell line is derived from human neuroblastoma cells and is a widely accepted model of human neuronal-like cells [89,90]. This cell line, being of catecholaminergic phenotype, is often used as an in vitro model for neurotoxicity and neurodegenerative disorders. This line was selected for in vitro biological studies due to the intention to use the manufactured composites in the brain. The SH-SY5Y cell line is an excellent model for screening for the first assessment of the biocompatibility of the obtained C/C composites. To date, there have not been any studies in the literature regarding the preparation of such composites in the form of rods intended for the stimulation of nervous tissue cells, and equally so biological studies assessing their potential cytotoxicity. That is why these tests are so important, and the choice of the SH-SY5Y line in this case is certainly justified.

The in vitro tests were carried out for three types of samples, i.e., CF, CF_PyC120 composite, and Pt wire, which served as a reference sample. In addition, a positive control sample (CF_F-F composite) and a negative control sample (PS) were used. Both qualitative tests, i.e., mainly imaging in light (Figure 14) and scanning electron microscope (SEM) (Figure 15), were performed for the tested samples, as well as quantitative tests, i.e., viability using the WST-1 test and cytotoxicity using the lactate dehydrogenase (LDH) release test (Figure 16).

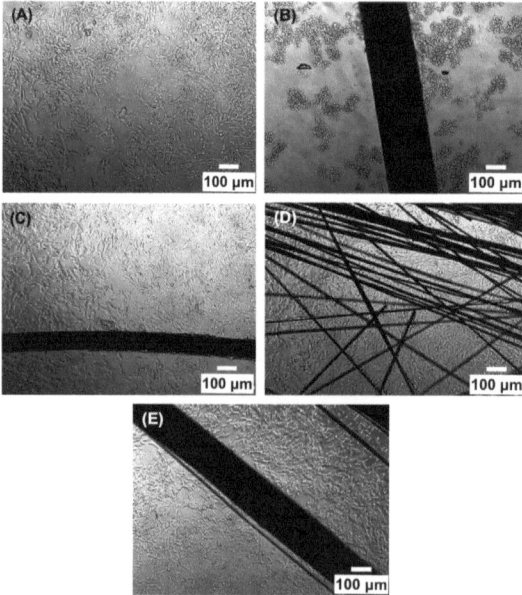

Figure 14. Differential interference contrast (DIC) images of SH-SY5Y cells in contact with (**A**) PS—negative control, (**B**) CF_FF—positive control, (**C**) Pt wire, (**D**) CF and (**E**) CF_PyC120 samples acquired 48 h after cell seeding.

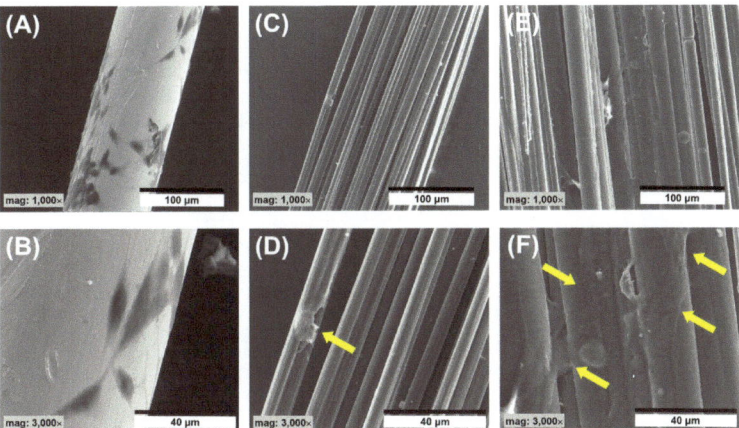

Figure 15. SEM micrographs of sample surfaces in contact with SH-SY5Y cells, (**A,B**) Pt wire, (**C,D**) CF, and (**E,F**) CF_PyC120.

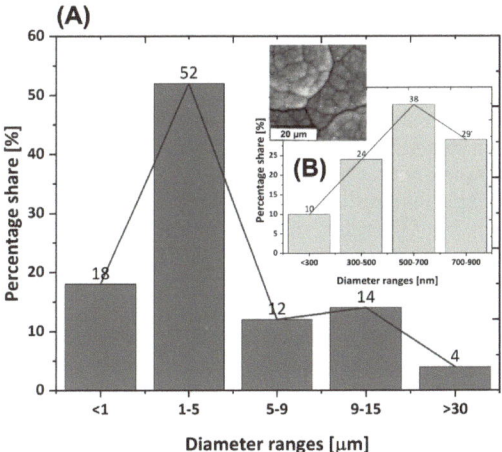

Figure 16. Size distribution of ball-like protuberances on the surface of CF-PyC120 composites; (**A**) size distribution of ball-like protuberances above 1 μm, (**B**) size distribution of ball-like protuberances above and below 1 μm. The numbers above the bars mean percentage share of ball-like protuberances on the surface of CF-PyC120 composites.

Based on the microscopic images shown in Figure 14, the morphology of SH-SY5Y cells in contact with samples can be assessed. Most of the cells in contact with a negative control sample (PS) have a polygonal, star shape; these cells are flattened, form clusters, and strongly adhere to the PS surface (Figure 14A). Cells in contact with the tested materials CF and CF_PyC120 after 48 h of culture also have a flattened, star shape, very similar in morphology to the cells on the PS control samples. Similar results can be observed for cells in contact with Pt wire. No morphological changes were observed in close or distant proximity to the sample compared to the negative control sample. In order to exclude the influence of the size and amount of the sample on the cellular response, a positive control sample (CF_FF) in the form of a rod of a size comparable to the analyzed samples was also prepared. Three repetitions were made for each test sample; in all three the amount of a given sample in the form of rods in each culture well was the same and amounted to three pieces. Significant differences in cell morphology and structure were observed for the positive control sample (CF_FF) compared to the negative control sample as well as to other samples. In this sample, the cells are showing signs of severe damage, evidenced by a smaller size, rounded shape, loose attachment to the surface, and agglomeration (Figure 14B). The negative impact of the positive sample is also evidenced by the results of cytotoxicity studies carried out using the LDH assay and cell viability in contact with samples (Figure 17).

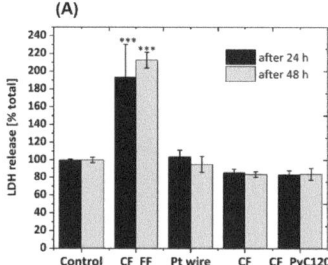
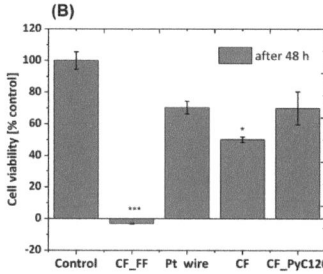

Figure 17. Quantitative biosafety assessment of the tested materials using cytotoxicity (**A**) and cell viability (**B**) biochemical assays. Cytotoxicity was assessed by LDH release assay and cell viability by WST-1 assay (detail in Material and Methods section). The data were normalized to the control group and are presented as a mean S.E.M. Two-way (**A**) and one-way (**B**) ANOVA. with post hoc Duncan test was used with * $p < 0.05$ and *** $p < 0.001$ vs. control group.

In addition, the analysis of SEM images allowed the observation of the behavior of cells in contact with the surface of the tested samples (Figure 15). Three types of samples were used for the tests, namely, a Pt wire as a reference, CFs, and a C/C composite. On the surface of the Pt wire, the presence of single flattened cells can be observed (Figure 15A,B). Due to the difference in the electron density of the tested materials, the SEM images of the cells on the surface of the Pt wire are by far the most visible. In the case of a sample of CFs, the number of cells adhering to the surface of the sample is much smaller compared to the Pt wire (Figure 15C,D). In this case, a single cell is seen, relatively flattened on the surface of the fiber bundle (Figure 15D, arrow). In the case of composite samples, it can be observed that the cells on the surface of the sample cover quite a large area and are well spread out (Figure 15E,F). The SEM images show the presence of single pseudopodia (Figure 15F arrows) of cells occupying more distant areas of the sample, which may indicate good SH-SY5Y cell adhesion to the sample surface. It can even be observed that the surface area occupied by the cells in contact with the CF_PyC120 sample is larger when compared to the reference sample (Pt wire).

One probable reason for the better adhesion of cells to the surface of the composite sample is the larger diameter of this sample compared to carbon fibers, in which the diameter of a single fiber is between 4 μm and 12 μm (depending on the direction) (Figure 1). On such a surface, the cell has more opportunities for proper anchoring and better adhesion than on the surface of a sample with a small diameter and which is also elongated. When analyzing the influence of the surface properties of the tested samples on the adhesion of cells, the first parameter that appears is wettability. The highest wettability can be observed for carbon fibers, although the remaining samples also have a hydrophilic surface (Figure 13). The surface of the C/C composite sample is the least wettable but having analyzed the behavior of cells on this surface, it can be concluded that this is not the most important parameter determining the cellular response. The surface of the CF_PyC120 sample also contains some ball-like protuberances, cauliflower-like structures of different sizes (Figure 16), which may contribute to better adhesion by creating additional sites for cell attachment to the sample surface. In the tested C/C composite sample, we can talk about hierarchical roughness containing both precipitates with dimensions of several to several dozen micrometers (form 1 μm to >30 μm, Figure 16A), as well as roughness in the nanometric scale (in the range from <300 nm to 900 nm, Figure 16B). Analyzing the data from the literature, the presence of roughness in the micro- and nanoscale seems to be the most desirable property with regard to cellular response and the effect on cell adhesion [91–93].

The cytotoxicity of the tested materials was determined on the basis of the LDH release test. Two-way ANOVA statistical analysis of LDH test results demonstrated the effects of the types of materials investigated, but not the time of incubation with the tested materials. We demonstrated a significant cytotoxic effect of the (CF_FF) sample at both of the studied time points (24 and 48 h), whereas the other materials were non-cytotoxic to SH-SY5Y cells when compared to the control group (Figure 17A).

The one-way ANOVA statistical analysis of cell viability data confirmed the severe cell-damaging effect of CF_FF found in the LDH test and light microscopy. Moreover, a significant reduction (about 50%) was observed for the CF samples and some tendency towards the reduction of cell viability (by about 30%) was also noted for the Pt wire and CF_PyC120 samples (Figure 17B). This was probably induced by the presence of material in the wells which blocked cell proliferation when compared to the control group. On this basis, it can be concluded that the PyC obtained by the CVD method in the resistance heating system improves cell viability compared to high-modulus CF without any modification. In turn, the high level of cytotoxicity for the CF_FF control sample also results in a significant decrease in cell viability, which confirms the negative effect of this sample on cellular response. Analyzing the effect of the individual components of the C/C composite on the cellular response, it can be concluded that none of them, i.e., neither carbon fiber nor pyrolytic carbon, have a negative impact on the cellular response of SH-SY5Y cells. Carbon fibers have been of interest in various areas of medicine for many years; these are primarily applications in the area of bone, cartilage, ligament, and tendon reconstructions [83]. In this area, the use of fibrous forms alone met with great enthusiasm at first, but over time it turned out that the biocompatibility of these materials is limited, this results primarily from the types of fiber used. Therefore, further applications of carbon fibers focused on their use as reinforcements in polymer composites. Lower cell viability in contact with CF compared to Pt and C/C composites may be, as mentioned earlier, the result of poorer cell adhesion to their surface, which was observed by analyzing the SEM results. Another factor that may also affect cell viability is the structure of the tested CFs. In the literature on the biocompatibility of CFs, attention is paid to the type of carbon fiber, whether they are high-modulus fibers, i.e., high-crystalline, or low-modulus, i.e., low-crystalline. Generally, the more crystalline the samples of carbon fibers and the more ordered their structure, the worse the biological response [94]. The authors of these papers indicated that carbon fibers with higher crystallinity and a better-organized graphite structure were assimilated by the body with more difficulty, and small particles coming from these materials were found in the regional lymph nodes. The carbon fibers used in this work are high-modulus fibers with a high degree of crystallinity, which was confirmed by HRTEM tests and Raman spectroscopy (Figures 9 and 10). These fibers are also dominated by carbon with sp^2 hybridization, which proves the ordered structure of this material. Pyrolytic carbon constituting the matrix of the C/C composite, in turn, is characterized by a more amorphous structure and a higher content of carbon with sp^3 hybridization than in the case of carbon fibers (Table 2). This amorphous structure is associated with the presence of structural defects, capable of interacting with the surrounding environment, including protein in the culture medium or on cellular membranes [95–97]. Therefore, these factors may also affect cell viability and demonstrate higher biocompatibility of C/C composites with PyC matrix. While carbon fibers in applications for the stimulation of nervous tissue as microelectrodes have been the subject of research [25,26], so far pyrolytic carbon has not been tested in relation to nervous tissue cells, so these results can be considered pioneering.

4. Conclusions

This study is focused on creating carbon–carbon composites using carbon fibers and pyrolytic carbon in the form of rods. These composites are being investigated as potential materials for use with nerve tissue cells. Since these materials have not been previously considered for treating neurodegenerative diseases, each step of their preparation is crucial. The first objective was to develop a method for obtaining rod-shaped C/C composites with dimensions below 1 mm. To achieve this, a non-standard approach using direct electrical heating of a bundle of carbon fibers in the CVD method was employed. The study examined the influence of different synthesis times (30 s, 60 s, 120 s, and 180 s) on the quality of the resulting composites. The surface of the cross-sections of the samples was analyzed through SEM to assess sample compaction, porosity, PyC layer thickness, and composite rod diameters. Based on these analyses, the most suitable conditions for the synthesis of C/C composites were identified, specifically a sample designated as CF_PyC_120, synthesized for 120 s using methane as the carbonaceous gas.

Another essential aspect of the research was the evaluation of the structure of the obtained composite rods, particularly the PyC matrix. High-resolution transmission electron microscopy (HRTEM), selected area electron diffraction (SAED), and Raman spectroscopy were employed to determine the degree of crystallinity in the pyrocarbon structure, measure interplanar distance (d_{002}), and establish the size of crystallites in both the PyC phase and fibers. The orientation angle (OA), which indicates the texture of PyC, was also analyzed, revealing the presence of two distinct textures: smooth laminar and dark laminar. The interface structure influences the adhesion between the fibers and matrix, which can significantly impact the mechanical properties of C/C composites and load transfer at the fiber/matrix interface. Understanding the structural parameters also affects the electrical properties of the composites, which will be studied in subsequent research stages.

In addition to structural parameters, the study investigated the morphology and microstructure of the surface of the C/C composites in the form of rods, as well as their surface chemistry, which affects factors like sample wettability and cellular response in vitro. The X-ray photoelectron spectroscopy (XPS) method and tensiometer were used to determine these parameters. Furthermore, since these materials had not been tested before for their response to nerve tissue cells, it was crucial to assess their toxicity and viability against neural cells. The SH-SY5Y cell line, commonly used in neurological experiments, was used as a model for this purpose. Cytotoxicity was examined using the LDH release test, while viability studies were conducted using the WST-1 test. The results showed that both carbon fibers and pyrolytic carbon in the C/C composites did not negatively impact the cellular response of SH-SY5Y cells. Cell viability on the surface of the composite was at a similar level to that of the reference sample, which was a Pt wire. In turn, assessing the morphology of cells in contact with the tested CF_PyC_120 composite using SEM and DIC light microscopy methods, it can be concluded that after culture they have a flattened and star-like shape, morphologically very similar to the cells on the PS control samples. Also, no morphological changes were observed in close or distant proximity to the sample when compared to the negative control sample. Interestingly, in the case of the C/C composite samples, it can also be observed that the cells are well distributed on their surface, with visible single pseudopodia of cells occupying more distant areas of the sample, which may indicate good adhesion of SH-SY5Y cells to the sample surface. It can even be observed that the surface occupied by cells in contact with the CF_PyC120 sample is larger than on the reference sample (Pt wire). Good adhesion of cells to the surface of the CF_PyC_120 composite may be determined by the hierarchical roughness of the composite surface as well as its amorphous character, manifested by the presence of structural defects, such as dangling bonds capable of interacting with the surrounding biological environment.

Author Contributions: Writing—original draft, A.F.-S., M.Z. and D.J.; conceptualization, A.F.-S.; investigation, A.F.-S., N.K., M.Z., M.G., P.C., P.J. and D.J.; methodology, A.F.-S., N.K., M.Z., M.G. and D.J.; data curation, A.F.-S.; funding acquisition, A.F.-S.; editing, A.F.-S.; supervision, A.F.-S.; formal analysis, P.C., P.J., M.P. and D.J.; software, M.P.; editing, R.W.; visualization, A.F.-S. and R.W.; writing—review and editing, A.F.-S., M.Z., M.P., P.J. and R.W. All authors have read and agreed to the published version of the manuscript.

Funding: This research was funded in whole by the National Science Centre, Poland, grant number: UMO-2020/39/B/ST5/02126. Hybrid carbon composites for stimulation of cells of the central nervous system. For the purpose of Open Access, the author has applied a CC-BY public copyright license to any Author Accepted Manuscript (AAM) version arising from this submission.

Data Availability Statement: The data presented in this study are available from the corresponding author upon request.

Conflicts of Interest: The authors have no conflict of interest to declare that are relevant to the content of this article.

References

1. Brown, R.C.; Lockwood, A.H.; Sonawane, B.R. Neurodegenerative Diseases: An Overview of Environmental Risk Factors. *Environ. Health Perspect.* **2005**, *113*, 1250–1256. [CrossRef] [PubMed]
2. Checkoway, H.; Lundin, J.I.; Kelada, S.N. Neurodegenerative diseases. *IARC Sci. Publ.* **2011**, *163*, 407–419.
3. Chi, H.; Chang, H.-Y.; Sang, T.-K. Neuronal Cell Death Mechanisms in Major Neurodegenerative Diseases. *Int. J. Mol. Sci.* **2018**, *19*, 3082. [CrossRef] [PubMed]
4. Poddar, K.M.; Chakraborty, A.; Banerjee, S. Neurodegeneration: Diagnosis, Prevention, and Therapy. In *Oxidoreductase*; IntechOpen: London, UK, 2021.
5. Hariz, M.; Blomstedt, P. Deep brain stimulation for Parkinson's disease. *J. Intern. Med.* **2022**, *292*, 764–778. [CrossRef] [PubMed]
6. Kim, E.; Kim, S.; Kwon, Y.W.; Seo, H.; Kim, M.; Chung, W.G.; Park, W.; Song, H.; Lee, D.H.; Lee, J.; et al. Electrical stimulation for therapeutic approach. *Interdiscip. Med.* **2023**, *1*, e20230003. [CrossRef]
7. Malek, N. Deep Brain Stimulation in Parkinson's Disease. *Neurol. India* **2019**, *67*, 968. [CrossRef] [PubMed]
8. Kolaya, E.; Firestein, B.L. Deep brain stimulation: Challenges at the tissue-electrode interface and current solutions. *Biotechnol. Prog.* **2021**, *37*, e3179. [CrossRef] [PubMed]
9. Arcot Desai, S.; Gutekunst, C.-A.; Potter, S.M.; Gross, R.E. Deep brain stimulation macroelectrodes compared to multiple microelectrodes in rat hippocampus. *Front. Neuroeng.* **2014**, *7*, 16. [CrossRef]
10. Hickey, P.; Stacy, M. Deep Brain Stimulation: A Paradigm Shifting Approach to Treat Parkinson's Disease. *Front. Neurosci.* **2016**, *10*, 173. [CrossRef]
11. Polikov, V.S.; Block, M.L.; Fellous, J.-M.; Hong, J.-S.; Reichert, W.M. In vitro model of glial scarring around neuroelectrodes chronically implanted in the CNS. *Biomaterials* **2006**, *27*, 5368–5376. [CrossRef]
12. McConnell, G.C.; Rees, H.D.; Levey, A.I.; Gutekunst, C.-A.; Gross, R.E.; Bellamkonda, R.V. Implanted neural electrodes cause chronic, local inflammation that is correlated with local neurodegeneration. *J. Neural Eng.* **2009**, *6*, 056003. [CrossRef] [PubMed]
13. Wellman, S.M.; Li, L.; Yaxiaer, Y.; McNamara, I.; Kozai, T.D.Y. Revealing Spatial and Temporal Patterns of Cell Death, Glial Proliferation, and Blood-Brain Barrier Dysfunction Around Implanted Intracortical Neural Interfaces. *Front. Neurosci.* **2019**, *13*, 493. [CrossRef] [PubMed]
14. Usoro, J.O.; Sturgill, B.S.; Musselman, K.C.; Capadona, J.R.; Pancrazio, J.J. Intracortical Microelectrode Array Unit Yield under Chronic Conditions: A Comparative Evaluation. *Micromachines* **2021**, *12*, 972. [CrossRef]
15. Cherry, J.D.; Olschowka, J.A.; O'Banion, M.K. Neuroinflammation and M2 microglia: The good, the bad, and the inflamed. *J. Neuroinflamm.* **2014**, *11*, 98. [CrossRef] [PubMed]
16. Karumbaiah, L.; Saxena, T.; Carlson, D.; Patil, K.; Patkar, R.; Gaupp, E.A.; Betancur, M.; Stanley, G.B.; Carin, L.; Bellamkonda, R.V. Relationship between intracortical electrode design and chronic recording function. *Biomaterials* **2013**, *34*, 8061–8074. [CrossRef] [PubMed]
17. Mohammed, M.; Ivica, N.; Bjartmarz, H.; Thorbergsson, P.T.; Pettersson, L.M.E.; Thelin, J.; Schouenborg, J. Microelectrode clusters enable therapeutic deep brain stimulation without noticeable side-effects in a rodent model of Parkinson's disease. *J. Neurosci. Methods* **2022**, *365*, 109399. [CrossRef]
18. Tian, G.; Yang, D.; Chen, C.; Duan, X.; Kim, D.-H.; Chen, H. Simultaneous Presentation of Dexamethasone and Nerve Growth Factor via Layered Carbon Nanotubes and Polypyrrole to Interface Neural Cells. *ACS Biomater. Sci. Eng.* **2023**, *9*, 5015–5027. [CrossRef]
19. Rodrigues, A.F.; Tavares, A.P.M.; Simões, S.; Silva, R.P.F.F.; Sobrino, T.; Figueiredo, B.R.; Sales, G.; Ferreira, L. Engineering graphene-based electrodes for optical neural stimulation. *Nanoscale* **2023**, *15*, 687–706. [CrossRef]
20. Lim, J.; Lee, S.; Kim, J.; Hong, J.; Lim, S.; Kim, K.; Kim, J.; Yang, S.; Yang, S.; Ahn, J.-H. Hybrid graphene electrode for the diagnosis and treatment of epilepsy in free-moving animal models. *NPG Asia Mater.* **2023**, *15*, 7. [CrossRef]

21. Nekounam, H.; Samadian, H.; Golmohammadi, H.; Asghari, F.; Shokrgozar, M.A.; Ahadian, S.; Majidi, R.F. Carbon nanofibers fabrication, surface modifications, and application as the innovative substrate for electrical stimulation of neural cell differentiation. *Surf. Interfaces* **2023**, *40*, 102926. [CrossRef]
22. Hejazi, M.A.; Tong, W.; Stacey, A.; Soto-Breceda, A.; Ibbotson, M.R.; Yunzab, M.; Maturana, M.I.; Almasi, A.; Jung, Y.J.; Sun, S.; et al. Hybrid diamond/carbon fiber microelectrodes enable multimodal electrical/chemical neural interfacing. *Biomaterials* **2020**, *230*, 119648. [CrossRef]
23. Dresvyanina, E.N.; Tagandurdyyeva, N.A.; Kodolova-Chukhontseva, V.V.; Dobrovol'skaya, I.P.; Kamalov, A.M.; Nashchekina, Y.A.; Nashchekin, A.V.; Ivanov, A.G.; Yukina, G.Y.; Yudin, V.E. Structure and Properties of Composite Fibers Based on Chitosan and Single-Walled Carbon Nanotubes for Peripheral Nerve Regeneration. *Polymers* **2023**, *15*, 2860. [CrossRef]
24. Pi, W.; Zhang, Y.; Li, L.; Li, C.; Zhang, M.; Zhang, W.; Cai, Q.; Zhang, P. Polydopamine-coated polycaprolactone/carbon nanotube fibrous scaffolds loaded with brain-derived neurotrophic factor for peripheral nerve regeneration. *Biofabrication* **2022**, *14*, 035006. [CrossRef]
25. Hejazi, M.; Tong, W.; Ibbotson, M.R.; Prawer, S.; Garrett, D.J. Advances in Carbon-Based Microfiber Electrodes for Neural Interfacing. *Front. Neurosci.* **2021**, *15*, 658703. [CrossRef] [PubMed]
26. Devi, M.; Vomero, M.; Fuhrer, E.; Castagnola, E.; Gueli, C.; Nimbalkar, S.; Hirabayashi, M.; Kassegne, S.; Stieglitz, T.; Sharma, S. Carbon-based neural electrodes: Promises and challenges. *J. Neural Eng.* **2021**, *18*, 041007. [CrossRef] [PubMed]
27. Bhatt, P.; Goe, A. Carbon Fibres: Production, Properties and Potential Use. *Mater. Sci. Res. India* **2017**, *14*, 52–57. [CrossRef]
28. Gillis, W.F.; Lissandrello, C.A.; Shen, J.; Pearre, B.W.; Mertiri, A.; Deku, F.; Cogan, S.; Holinski, B.J.; Chew, D.J.; White, A.E.; et al. Carbon fiber on polyimide ultra-microelectrodes. *J. Neural Eng.* **2018**, *15*, 016010. [CrossRef] [PubMed]
29. Manciu, F.S.; Oh, Y.; Barath, A.; Rusheen, A.E.; Kouzani, A.Z.; Hodges, D.; Guerrero, J.; Tomshine, J.; Lee, K.H.; Bennet, K.E. Analysis of Carbon-Based Microelectrodes for Neurochemical Sensing. *Materials* **2019**, *12*, 3186. [CrossRef]
30. Lee, Y.; Kong, C.; Chang, J.W.; Jun, S.B. Carbon-Fiber Based Microelectrode Array Embedded with a Biodegradable Silk Support for In Vivo Neural Recording. *J. Korean Med. Sci.* **2019**, *34*, e24. [CrossRef]
31. Dunn, J.F.; Tuor, U.I.; Kmech, J.; Young, N.A.; Henderson, A.K.; Jackson, J.C.; Valentine, P.A.; Teskey, G.C. Functional brain mapping at 9.4T using a new MRI-compatible electrode chronically implanted in rats. *Magn. Reson. Med.* **2009**, *61*, 222–228. [CrossRef]
32. Cruttenden, C.E.; Taylor, J.M.; Hu, S.; Zhang, Y.; Zhu, X.-H.; Chen, W.; Rajamani, R. Carbon nano-structured neural probes show promise for magnetic resonance imaging applications. *Biomed. Phys. Eng. Express* **2017**, *4*, 015001. [CrossRef] [PubMed]
33. Huffman, M.L.; Venton, B.J. Carbon-fiber microelectrodes for in vivo applications. *Analyst* **2009**, *134*, 18–24. [CrossRef]
34. Letner, J.G.; Patel, P.R.; Hsieh, J.-C.; Smith Flores, I.M.; della Valle, E.; Walker, L.A.; Weiland, J.D.; Chestek, C.A.; Cai, D. Post-explant profiling of subcellular-scale carbon fiber intracortical electrodes and surrounding neurons enables modeling of recorded electrophysiology. *J. Neural Eng.* **2023**, *20*, 026019. [CrossRef]
35. Zhao, S.; Li, G.; Tong, C.; Chen, W.; Wang, P.; Dai, J.; Fu, X.; Xu, Z.; Liu, X.; Lu, L.; et al. Full activation pattern mapping by simultaneous deep brain stimulation and fMRI with graphene fiber electrodes. *Nat. Commun.* **2020**, *11*, 1788. [CrossRef]
36. Bennet, K.E.; Tomshine, J.R.; Min, H.-K.; Manciu, F.S.; Marsh, M.P.; Paek, S.B.; Settell, M.L.; Nicolai, E.N.; Blaha, C.D.; Kouzani, A.Z.; et al. A Diamond-Based Electrode for Detection of Neurochemicals in the Human Brain. *Front. Hum. Neurosci.* **2016**, *10*, 102. [CrossRef] [PubMed]
37. More, R.B.; Haubold, A.D.; Bokros, J.C. Pyrolytic Carbon for Long-Term Medical Implants. In *Biomaterials Science*; Elsevier: Amsterdam, The Netherlands, 2013; pp. 209–222.
38. Li, A.; Norinaga, K.; Zhang, W.; Deutschmann, O. Modeling and simulation of materials synthesis: Chemical vapor deposition and infiltration of pyrolytic carbon. *Compos. Sci. Technol.* **2008**, *68*, 1097–1104. [CrossRef]
39. Forti, S.; Lunelli, L.; Della Volpe, C.; Siboni, S.; Pasquardini, L.; Lui, A.; Canteri, R.; Vanzetti, L.; Potrich, C.; Vinante, M.; et al. Hemocompatibility of pyrolytic carbon in comparison with other biomaterials. *Diam. Relat. Mater.* **2011**, *20*, 762–769. [CrossRef]
40. Daecke, W.; Veyel, K.; Wieloch, P.; Jung, M.; Lorenz, H.; Martini, A.-K. Osseointegration and Mechanical Stability of Pyrocarbon and Titanium Hand Implants in a Load-Bearing In Vivo Model for Small Joint Arthroplasty. *J. Hand Surg. Am.* **2006**, *31*, 90–97. [CrossRef]
41. Stanley, J.; Klawitter, J.; More, R. Replacing joints with pyrolytic carbon. In *Joint Replacement Technology*; Elsevier: Amsterdam, The Netherlands, 2008; pp. 631–656.
42. Norinaga, K.; Deutschmann, O.; Saegusa, N.; Hayashi, J. Analysis of pyrolysis products from light hydrocarbons and kinetic modeling for growth of polycyclic aromatic hydrocarbons with detailed chemistry. *J. Anal. Appl. Pyrolysis* **2009**, *86*, 148–160. [CrossRef]
43. Drescher, M.; Hüttinger, K.J.; Dormann, E. Pyrolytic carbon layers—An electron spin resonance analysis. *Carbon* **2003**, *41*, 773–783. [CrossRef]
44. He, Y.-G.; Li, K.-Z.; Li, H.-J.; Wei, J.-F.; Fu, Q.-G.; Zhang, D.-S. Effect of interface structures on the fracture behavior of two-dimensional carbon/carbon composites by isothermal chemical vapor infiltration. *J. Mater. Sci.* **2010**, *45*, 1432–1437. [CrossRef]
45. Oku, T. Carbon/Carbon Composites and Their Properties. In *Carbon Alloys*; Elsevier: Amsterdam, The Netherlands, 2003; pp. 523–544.
46. Reznik, B.; Gerthsen, D.; Hüttinger, K.J. Micro- and nanostructure of the carbon matrix of infiltrated carbon fiber felts. *Carbon* **2001**, *39*, 215–229. [CrossRef]

47. Xu, X.; Ouyang, T.; Zeng, L.; Chai, L. Study on the Pyrolytic Carbon Generated by the Electric Heating CVD Method. *J. Wuhan Univ. Technol. Sci. Ed.* **2018**, *33*, 409–413. [CrossRef]
48. Kovalevich, J.; Langford, D. Considerations for the Use of SH-SY5Y Neuroblastoma Cells in Neurobiology. *Methods Mol. Biol.* **2013**, *1078*, 9–21. [PubMed]
49. Jantas, D.; Chwastek, J.; Malarz, J.; Stojakowska, A.; Lasoń, W. Neuroprotective Effects of Methyl Caffeate against Hydrogen Peroxide-Induced Cell Damage: Involvement of Caspase 3 and Cathepsin D Inhibition. *Biomolecules* **2020**, *10*, 1530. [CrossRef]
50. Ruffels, J.; Griffin, M.; Dickenson, J.M. Activation of ERK1/2, JNK and PKB by hydrogen peroxide in human SH-SY5Y neuroblastoma cells: Role of ERK1/2 in H_2O_2-induced cell death. *Eur. J. Pharmacol.* **2004**, *483*, 163–173. [CrossRef] [PubMed]
51. Jantas, D.; Piotrowski, M.; Lason, W. An Involvement of PI3-K/Akt Activation and Inhibition of AIF Translocation in Neuroprotective Effects of Undecylenic Acid (UDA) Against Pro-Apoptotic Factors-Induced Cell Death in Human Neuroblastoma SH-SY5Y Cells. *J. Cell. Biochem.* **2015**, *116*, 2882–2895. [CrossRef] [PubMed]
52. Reznik, B.; Hüttinger, K. On the terminology for pyrolytic carbon. *Carbon* **2002**, *40*, 621–624. [CrossRef]
53. Meadows, P.J.; López-Honorato, E.; Xiao, P. Fluidized bed chemical vapor deposition of pyrolytic carbon—II. Effect of deposition conditions on anisotropy. *Carbon* **2009**, *47*, 251–262. [CrossRef]
54. Meier, R.J. On art and science in curve-fitting vibrational spectra. *Vib. Spectrosc.* **2005**, *39*, 266–269. [CrossRef]
55. Cançado, L.G.; Takai, K.; Enoki, T.; Endo, M.; Kim, Y.A.; Mizusaki, H.; Jorio, A.; Coelho, L.N.; Magalhães-Paniago, R.; Pimenta, M.A. General equation for the determination of the crystallite size La of nanographite by Raman spectroscopy. *Appl. Phys. Lett.* **2006**, *88*, 163106. [CrossRef]
56. Tiab, D.; Donaldson, E.C. Wettability. In *Petrophysics*; Elsevier: Amsterdam, The Netherlands, 2012; pp. 371–418.
57. Qiu, S.; Fuentes, C.A.; Zhang, D.; Van Vuure, A.W.; Seveno, D. Wettability of a Single Carbon Fiber. *Langmuir* **2016**, *32*, 9697–9705. [CrossRef] [PubMed]
58. Wang, J.; Fuentes, C.A.; Zhang, D.; Wang, X.; Van Vuure, A.W.; Seveno, D. Wettability of carbon fibres at micro- and mesoscales. *Carbon* **2017**, *120*, 438–446. [CrossRef]
59. Yuan, Y.; Lee, T.R. Contact Angle and Wetting Properties. In *Surface Science Techniques*; Springer: Berlin/Heidelberg, Germany, 2013; pp. 3–34.
60. Fraczek-Szczypta, A.; Jantas, D.; Ciepiela, F.; Grzonka, J. Graphene oxide-conductive polymer nanocomposite coatings obtained by the EPD method as substrates for neurite outgrowth. *Diam. Relat. Mater.* **2020**, *102*, 107663. [CrossRef]
61. Jantas, D.; Malarz, J.; Le, T.N.; Stojakowska, A. Neuroprotective Properties of Kempferol Derivatives from Maesa membranacea against Oxidative Stress-Induced Cell Damage: An Association with Cathepsin D Inhibition and PI3K/Akt Activation. *Int. J. Mol. Sci.* **2021**, *22*, 10363. [CrossRef]
62. StatSoft. *Statistica*, Version 13.3; Tibco Software Inc.: Palo Alto, CA, USA, 2017.
63. Reznik, B.; Norinaga, K.; Gerthsen, D.; Deutschmann, O. The effect of cooling rate on hydrogen release from a pyrolytic carbon coating and its resulting morphology. *Carbon* **2006**, *44*, 1330–1334. [CrossRef]
64. Ren, J.; Li, K.; Zhang, S.; Yao, X.; Tian, S. Preparation of carbon/carbon composite by pyrolysis of ethanol and methane. *Mater. Des.* **2015**, *65*, 174–178. [CrossRef]
65. López-Honorato, E.; Meadows, P.J.; Xiao, P.; Marsh, G.; Abram, T.J. Structure and mechanical properties of pyrolytic carbon produced by fluidized bed chemical vapor deposition. *Nucl. Eng. Des.* **2008**, *238*, 3121–3128. [CrossRef]
66. Tezcan, J.; Ozcan, S.; Gurung, B.; Filip, P. Measurement and analytical validation of interfacial bond strength of PAN-fiber-reinforced carbon matrix composites. *J. Mater. Sci.* **2008**, *43*, 1612–1618. [CrossRef]
67. Schierholz, R.; Kröger, D.; Weinrich, H.; Gehring, M.; Tempel, H.; Kungl, H.; Mayer, J.; Eichel, R.-A. The carbonization of polyacrylonitrile-derived electrospun carbon nanofibers studied by in situ transmission electron microscopy. *RSC Adv.* **2019**, *9*, 6267–6277. [CrossRef]
68. Zambrzycki, M.; Piech, R.; Raga, S.R.; Lira-Cantu, M.; Fraczek-Szczypta, A. Hierarchical carbon nanofibers/carbon nanotubes/NiCo nanocomposites as novel highly effective counter electrode for dye-sensitized solar cells: A structure-electrocatalytic activity relationship study. *Carbon* **2023**, *203*, 97–110. [CrossRef]
69. Boehm, R.D.; Jin, C.; Narayan, R.J. Carbon and Diamond. In *Comprehensive Biomaterials II*; Elsevier: Amsterdam, The Netherlands, 2017; pp. 145–164.
70. López-Honorato, E.; Meadows, P.J.; Xiao, P. Fluidized bed chemical vapor deposition of pyrolytic carbon—I. Effect of deposition conditions on microstructure. *Carbon* **2009**, *47*, 396–410. [CrossRef]
71. Hu, Z.J.; Zhang, W.G.; Hüttinger, K.J.; Reznik, B.; Gerthsen, D. Influence of pressure, temperature and surface area/volume ratio on the texture of pyrolytic carbon deposited from methane. *Carbon* **2003**, *41*, 749–758. [CrossRef]
72. Dong, G.L.; Hüttinger, K.J. Consideration of reaction mechanisms leading to pyrolytic carbon of different textures. *Carbon* **2002**, *40*, 2515–2528. [CrossRef]
73. De Pauw, V.; Collin, A.; Send, W.; Hawecker, J.; Gerthsen, D.; Pfrang, A.; Schimmel, T. Deposition rates during the early stages of pyrolytic carbon deposition in a hot-wall reactor and the development of texture. *Carbon* **2006**, *44*, 3091–3101. [CrossRef]
74. Hu, Z.J.; Hüttinger, K.J. Mechanisms of carbon deposition—A kinetic approach. *Carbon* **2002**, *40*, 624–628. [CrossRef]
75. Vignoles, G.L.; Langlais, F.; Descamps, C.; Mouchon, A.; Le Poche, H.; Reuge, N.; Bertrand, N. CVD and CVI of pyrocarbon from various precursors. *Surf. Coatings Technol.* **2004**, *188–189*, 241–249. [CrossRef]

76. Sadezky, A.; Muckenhuber, H.; Grothe, H.; Niessner, R.; Pöschl, U. Raman microspectroscopy of soot and related carbonaceous materials: Spectral analysis and structural information. *Carbon* **2005**, *43*, 1731–1742. [CrossRef]
77. Zambrzycki, M.; Łoś, S.; Fraczek-Szczypta, A. Structure and electrical transport properties of carbon nanofibres/carbon nanotubes 3D hierarchical nanocomposites: Impact of the concentration of acetylacetonate catalyst. *Ceram. Int.* **2021**, *47*, 4020–4033. [CrossRef]
78. Zambrzycki, M.; Jeleń, P.; Fraczek-Szczypta, A. Structure and electrical transport properties of electrospun carbon nanofibers/carbon nanotubes 3D hierarchical nanocomposites: Effect of the CCVD synthesis conditions. *J. Mater. Sci* **2022**, *57*, 9334–9356. [CrossRef]
79. Ferrari, A.C.; Basko, D.M. Raman spectroscopy as a versatile tool for studying the properties of graphene. *Nat. Nanotechnol.* **2013**, *8*, 235–246. [CrossRef] [PubMed]
80. Schuepfer, D.B.; Badaczewski, F.; Guerra-Castro, J.M.; Hofmann, D.M.; Heiliger, C.; Smarsly, B.; Klar, P.J. Assessing the structural properties of graphitic and non-graphitic carbons by Raman spectroscopy. *Carbon* **2020**, *161*, 359–372. [CrossRef]
81. Ma, B.; Rodriguez, R.D.; Ruban, A.; Pavlov, S.; Sheremet, E. The correlation between electrical conductivity and second-order Raman modes of laser-reduced graphene oxide. *Phys. Chem. Chem. Phys.* **2019**, *21*, 10125–10134. [CrossRef]
82. Ferrari, A.C. Raman spectroscopy of graphene and graphite: Disorder, electron–phonon coupling, doping and nonadiabatic effects. *Solid State Commun.* **2007**, *143*, 47–57. [CrossRef]
83. Zhou, J.; Sun, G.; Zhan, Z.; An, J.; Zheng, L.; Xie, E. Probing structure and strain transfer in dry-spun carbon nanotube fibers by depth-profiled Raman spectroscopy. *Appl. Phys. Lett.* **2013**, *103*, 031912. [CrossRef]
84. Torrisi, L.; Scolaro, C. Blood Wettability of Haemocompatible Carbon-based Materials. *J. Adv. Chem. Eng.* **2017**, *7*. [CrossRef]
85. Vigano, G.; Ten Brink, G.; Pollack, D.K.M.; Mariani, M.A.; Kooi, B.J. Wettability Properties of Standard Pyrolytic Carbon Bileaflet Mechanical Heart Valve Prostheses. *Struct. Hear.* **2020**, *4*, 41. [CrossRef]
86. Xie, J.; Xin, D.; Cao, H.; Wang, C.; Zhao, Y.; Yao, L.; Ji, F.; Qiu, Y. Improving carbon fiber adhesion to polyimide with atmospheric pressure plasma treatment. *Surf. Coatings Technol.* **2011**, *206*, 191–201. [CrossRef]
87. An, F.; Lu, C.; Guo, J.; He, S.; Lu, H.; Yang, Y. Preparation of vertically aligned carbon nanotube arrays grown onto carbon fiber fabric and evaluating its wettability on effect of composite. *Appl. Surf. Sci.* **2011**, *258*, 1069–1076. [CrossRef]
88. Contact Angle of Water on Smooth Surfaces and Wettability. Available online: http://www.uskino.com/articleshow_113.html (accessed on 9 August 2023).
89. Lopez-Suarez, L.; Al Awabdh, S.; Coumoul, X.; Chauvet, C. The SH-SY5Y human neuroblastoma cell line, a relevant in vitro cell model for investigating neurotoxicology in human: Focus on organic pollutants. *Neurotoxicology* **2022**, *92*, 131–155. [CrossRef]
90. Xie, H.; Hu, L.; Li, G. SH-SY5Y human neuroblastoma cell line: In vitro cell model of dopaminergic neurons in Parkinson's disease. *Chin. Med. J.* **2010**, *123*, 1086–1092.
91. Majhy, B.; Priyadarshini, P.; Sen, A.K. Effect of surface energy and roughness on cell adhesion and growth—Facile surface modification for enhanced cell culture. *RSC Adv.* **2021**, *11*, 15467–15476. [CrossRef]
92. Zhu, L.; Luo, D.; Liu, Y. Effect of the nano/microscale structure of biomaterial scaffolds on bone regeneration. *Int. J. Oral Sci.* **2020**, *12*, 6. [CrossRef] [PubMed]
93. Giljean, S.; Bigerelle, M.; Anselme, K. Roughness statistical influence on cell adhesion using profilometry and multiscale analysis. *Scanning* **2014**, *36*, 2–10. [CrossRef]
94. Robinson, D.; Efrat, M.; Mendes, D.G.; Halperin, N.; Nevo, Z. Implants composed of carbon fiber mesh and bone-marrow-derived chondrocyte-enriched cultures for joint surface reconstruction. *Bull. Hosp. Jt. Dis.* **1993**, *53*, 75–82.
95. Sengupta, B.; Gregory, W.E.; Zhu, J.; Dasetty, S.; Karakaya, M.; Brown, J.M.; Rao, A.M.; Barrows, J.K.; Sarupria, S.; Podila, R. Influence of carbon nanomaterial defects on the formation of protein corona. *RSC Adv.* **2015**, *5*, 82395–82402. [CrossRef] [PubMed]
96. Atilhan, M.; Costa, L.T.; Aparicio, S. On the interaction between carbon nanomaterials and lipid biomembranes. *J. Mol. Liq.* **2019**, *295*, 111714. [CrossRef]
97. Baoukina, S.; Monticelli, L.; Tieleman, D.P. Interaction of Pristine and Functionalized Carbon Nanotubes with Lipid Membranes. *J. Phys. Chem. B* **2013**, *117*, 12113–12123. [CrossRef] [PubMed]

Disclaimer/Publisher's Note: The statements, opinions and data contained in all publications are solely those of the individual author(s) and contributor(s) and not of MDPI and/or the editor(s). MDPI and/or the editor(s) disclaim responsibility for any injury to people or property resulting from any ideas, methods, instructions or products referred to in the content.

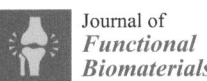

Journal of
Functional
Biomaterials

Review

The Effects of Platelet-Rich Fibrin in the Behavior of Mineralizing Cells Related to Bone Tissue Regeneration—A Scoping Review of In Vitro Evidence

Renata de Lima Barbosa [1,2], Emanuelle Stellet Lourenço [1], Julya Vittoria de Azevedo dos Santos [1,2], Neilane Rodrigues Santiago Rocha [1,2], Carlos Fernando Mourão [3,*] and Gutemberg Gomes Alves [1,2]

[1] Clinical Research Unit, Antonio Pedro Hospital, Fluminense Federal University, Niteroi 24033-900, Brazil
[2] Graduate Program in Science and Biotechnology, Fluminense Federal University, Niteroi 24210-201, Brazil
[3] Department of Periodontology, Tufts University School of Dental Medicine, Boston, MA 02111, USA
* Correspondence: carlos.mourao@tufts.edu; Tel.: +1-(617)-636-0958

Abstract: Platelet-rich fibrin (PRF) is a second-generation blood concentrate that serves as an autologous approach for both soft and hard tissue regeneration. It provides a scaffold for cell interaction and promotes the local release of growth factors. PRF has been investigated as an alternative to bone tissue therapy, with the potential to expedite wound healing and bone regeneration, though the mechanisms involved are not yet fully understood. This review aims to explore the in vitro evidence of PRF's effects on the behavior of mineralizing cells related to bone tissue regeneration. A systematic electronic search was conducted up to August 2023, utilizing three databases: PubMed, Web of Science, and Scopus. A total of 76 studies were selected, which presented in vitro evidence of PRF's usefulness, either alone or in conjunction with other biomaterials, for bone tissue treatment. PRF membranes' influence on the proliferation, differentiation, and mineralization of bone cells is linked to the constant release of growth factors, resulting in changes in crucial markers of bone cell metabolism and behavior. This further reinforces their therapeutic potential in wound healing and bone regeneration. While there are some notable differences among the studies, the overall results suggest a positive effect of PRF on cell proliferation, differentiation, mineralization, and a reduction in inflammation. This points to its therapeutic potential in the field of regenerative medicine. Collectively, these findings may help enhance our understanding of how PRF impacts basic physiological processes in bone and mineralized tissue.

Keywords: review; osteoblast; cell therapy; PRF; platelet concentrates

1. Introduction

In recent years, there has been significant advancement in bone tissue engineering, where damaged or diseased bones are repaired using materials that closely replicate the properties of natural bones while being safe for the body. A wide range of both synthetic and natural biomaterials have been extensively studied, each with its unique strengths and limitations. Being aware of the differences between these materials is vital for harnessing their respective benefits and pushing the boundaries of this field [1–3].

Various artificially crafted (alloplastic) materials can be customized to meet specific medical requirements nowadays. These synthetic biomaterials made from metals, ceramics, and polymers can be manufactured reproducibly on a large scale, with tunable physical and chemical properties. Nevertheless, these materials usually lack the intricate structure and biological components found in natural materials of biological origin, such as xenografts, allografts, and autografts [1,3]. As a result, these materials of natural origin often have some advantages over synthetic biomaterials, such as increased biocompatibility, biodegradability, and biological activity.

In this context, the development of autologous blood-derived aggregates, such as platelet-rich fibrin (PRF) or leukocyte- and platelet-rich fibrin (L-PRF), has garnered significant interest in the medical and dental fields for its importance in tissue regeneration [2]. PRF stands out as a promising choice for natural biomaterial due to its remarkable compatibility with the human body. As a second-generation blood concentrate, PRF has undergone significant advancements since its inception. It has built on the foundations of platelet-rich plasma (PRP) from the late 1990s and boasts enhanced attributes that make it valuable in numerous surgical procedures [4–7]. Its concentration of essential cytokines and growth factors facilitates cell growth, migration, proliferation, and differentiation, allowing for smooth integration with native tissues [1–3].

Produced through the straightforward centrifugation of a patient's blood without the need for anticoagulants or activating agents, PRF manifests as a dense fibrin matrix rich in leukocytes, platelets, and a myriad of proteins pivotal for wound healing. This autologous biomaterial has been hailed for fostering angiogenesis, promoting cell specialization and differentiation, and serving as a supportive scaffold for bone cells, thereby expediting the bone healing and formation process [3]. Furthermore, the polymerization of PRF results in a membrane with a favorable physiological structure, offering a robust framework for osteoprogenitor cells to adhere to and facilitating the continuous release of vital growth factors such as fibroblast growth factors (FGFs), vascular endothelial growth factors (VEGFs), transforming growth factors (TGFs), and platelet-derived growth factors (PDGFs) [8–10] (Figure 1). These are important cytokines that regulate various aspects of bone regeneration. While the VEGF stimulates angiogenesis and osteogenesis, the PDGF promotes chemotaxis and the proliferation of mesenchymal stem cells and osteoblasts, the FGF enhances osteoblast differentiation and bone matrix formation, and the TGF modulates inflammation and immune response. These cytokines act synergistically to enhance bone healing and repair, and their delivery to bone defects can improve the outcome of bone regeneration therapies [11–14].

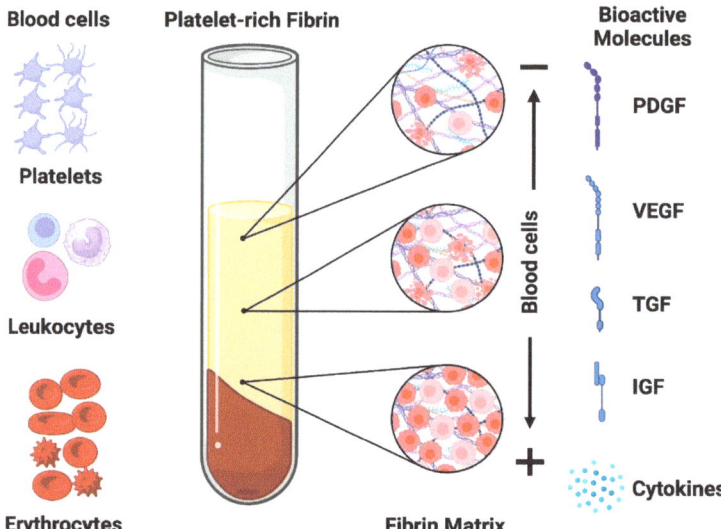

Figure 1. The platelet-rich fibrin membranes consist of cells, structural proteins, and regulatory mediators, such as cytokines and growth factors.

Despite the promising attributes of PRF, the scientific community continues to explore and debate its clinical efficacy compared to other biomaterials or conventional techniques. Particularly, inquiries concerning its direct positive influence on mineralizing cells, such as osteoblasts, have spurred numerous in vitro studies aimed at unraveling the biological mechanisms and impacts of PRF on mineralized tissues [8,10]. This scoping review aimed to elucidate the understanding of the biological basis of the applicability of different PRF derivations with potential use in bone therapy, compiling and comparing their effects on events such as proliferation, differentiation, and mineralization capacity of bone cells from evidence provided by controlled in vitro studies.

2. Materials and Methods

2.1. Protocol and Registry

This scoping review was conducted based on the Preferred Reporting Items for Systematic Reviews and Meta-Analysis (PRISMA) Statement and its extension for Scoping Reviews (PRISMA-ScR) [15]. The present research protocol is registered in the Open Science Framework database.

2.2. Information Sources and Search Strategy

The search strategy was developed based on a PICOS framework, where the following aspects were considered. Population: cell lines involved in bone regeneration; intervention: exposure to second-generation autologous platelet aggregates (PRFs); comparison: cells not exposed to PRFs; outcome: positive effect on parameters related to regeneration (proliferation, differentiation, mineralization); and setting: in vitro assessments.

The search was conducted up to August 2023 in three different electronic databases: PubMed, Web of Science, and Scopus. The search key employed for each database is described in Table 1. Adaptations were performed to fit the same terms into the different search engines and in combination with specific database filters when available. The entries were sent to Mendeley Desktop (Elsevier) software (version 2.98.0) to eliminate replicas and thus consolidate the list of references for subsequent analysis.

Table 1. The search key employed in the three consulted databases.

DATABASE	Search Key
PubMed (https://pubmed.ncbi.nlm.nih.gov/, accessed on 14 August 2023)	(PRF OR "platelet rich fibrin" OR L-PRF OR i-PRF OR "Sticky bone" OR "concentrated growth factors" OR CGF) AND (Bone OR osteoblast* OR MSC OR "mesenchymal stem cell" OR "bone marrow" OR "Bone and bones" [mh] OR "bone cell" OR preosteoblast* OR Skeleton) AND ("in vitro" OR In Vitro Techniques" [mh] OR "Cell Lineage" [mh] OR "Cells, Cultured" [mh]).
Web of Science (https://www.webofscience.com/, accessed on 14 August 2023)	((PRF OR "platelet rich fibrin" OR L-PRF OR i-PRF OR "Sticky bone" OR "concentrated growth factors" OR CGF) AND (Bone OR osteoblast OR MSC OR "mesenchymal stem cell" OR "bone marrow" OR "Bone and bones" OR "bone cell" OR preosteoblast OR PDL OR "periodontal ligament OR mineralization) AND ("in vitro" OR "In Vitro Techniques" OR "Cell Lineage" OR "Cells, Cultured")) Refined by DOCTYPE: (ARTICLE).
Scopus (https://www.scopus.com/search/form.uri?display=basic, accessed on 14 August 2023)	TITLE-ABS-KEY (prf OR "platelet rich fibrin" OR l-prf OR i-prf OR "Sticky bone" OR "concentrated growth factors" OR cgf) AND TITLE-ABS-KEY (bone OR osteoblast OR MSC OR "mesenchymal stem cell" OR "bone marrow" OR "Bone and bones" OR "bone cell" OR preosteoblast OR pdl OR "periodontal ligament OR mineralization) AND TITLE-ABS-KEY (("in vitro" OR "In Vitro Techniques" OR "Cell Lineage" OR "Cell Culture") AND (LIMIT TO (DOCTYPE, "ar"))).

2.3. Study Selection

The eligibility criteria for the studies included the use of cell lines for bone regeneration, second-generation autologous platelet aggregate (PRF) exposure to cells, and a positive effect on parameters related to regeneration in vitro. Exclusion criteria comprised study designs and publication types that used other autologous materials that did not involve cell exposure or were case reports, exposure limited to non-mineralizing cells, such as fibroblasts and osteoclasts, articles that did not represent complete primary sources of evidence (abstracts, reviews, editorial letters, opinion letters, commentary articles), and in vivo or clinical studies. Subjects related to other research topics, such as meniscus, cartilage, cancer treatments, drug studies, and in vitro delivery, were considered "off-topic". There was no restriction on the publication date or language of publication.

Two reviewers (R.L.B. and E.S.L.) read all the titles and abstracts of the articles retrieved from the search after performing piloting and calibrating on data collection with a Cohen kappa of 0.97 concordances. They analyzed and selected articles according to the eligibility criteria described above, eliminating duplicates. Any disagreement on study eligibility was resolved through discussion and consensus or a third reviewer (G.G.A.) to make the final decision.

2.4. Critical Appraisal

The selected studies were evaluated by 3 reviewers (R.L.B., N.R.S.R., and G.G.A.) using the ToxRTool (Toxicological Data Reliability Assessment Tool) to assess the quality and reliability of in vitro data at the methodological level [16]. This tool includes 18 criteria that describe important aspects for developing reliable articles regarding the methodology applied and how the study was conducted. The checklist includes a description of the methodological aspects of each study, such as substance identification, test system, study design, and documentation of results. Each criterion corresponds to one point, where the article receives one point if it meets the criterion and zero points if it does not. Finally, the scores are summed, generating a final score. Articles with scores less than 11 are considered unreliable, studies with scores between 11 and 14 are considered reliable with possible restrictions, and studies with scores between 15 and 18 are considered reliable without restrictions.

2.5. Data Extraction

For data extraction, scientific and technical information were tabulated and analyzed using Microsoft Office Excel 2013. The data extracted included the authors and year of publication, cell type, growth factors detected, the presence of association/modification/addition with PRF membranes, conditions of exposure of cells to PRF (time, volume), biological parameters evaluated, and main findings for the outcomes. These data were used for a qualitative evaluation and synthesis of evidence.

3. Results

From the search key developed according to each database, 1157 articles were retrieved, and 429 duplicate records were excluded. Thus, 728 articles were evaluated for eligibility, applying the inclusion and exclusion criteria. Of these, 652 articles were excluded from the review because they did not meet the eligibility criteria (Figure 2). Therefore, 76 articles were evaluated in detail and used in the qualitative analysis of this review.

The ToxRTool was employed to assess the inherent quality of the selected studies of toxicological data reported in a publication or a test report, with a reliability categorization performed as shown in Table 2. Among the 76 selected articles, around half (52%) achieved the maximum score (18 points), while a further 48% (36 studies) presented only a few reporting limitations, with scores ranging from 15 to 17, rending a total of 100% of the studies classified as reliable without restrictions (Table 2).

Of these, many articles did not specify the amount of medium used for membrane cultivation/extraction of PRF membranes, the number of replicates, or the passage of cells used in the experiments. These factors can influence the interpretation of the biological response, as the time of cultivation and sequential passages can affect the behavior of cells, changing their morphological, functional, and molecular characteristics, which may compromise the quality and reliability of the results obtained with in vitro cultured cells.

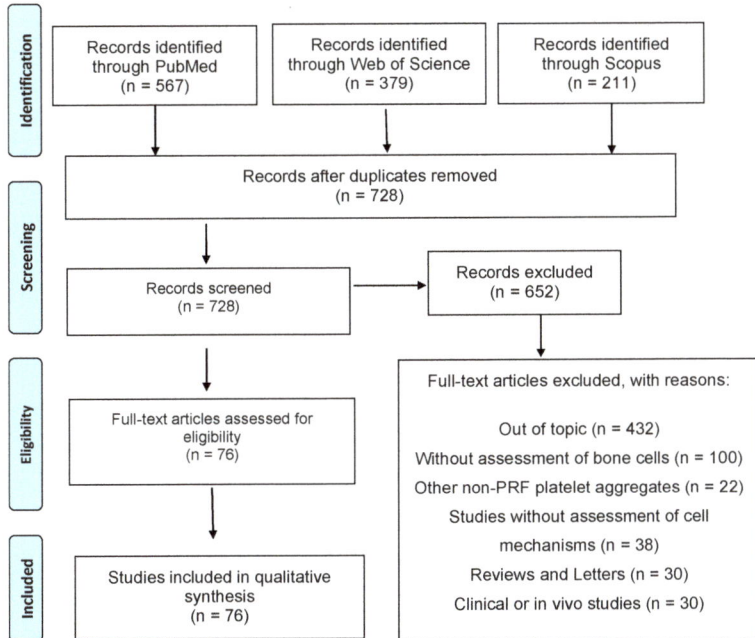

Figure 2. The screening process, selection, and systematic steps according to the PRISMA Statement.

Table 2. Critical appraisal of the selected studies, performed according to the ToxRTool [16].

Publication	Group I: Test Substance	Group I: Test Substance	Group II: Test System Characterization (3)	Group III: Study Design Description (6)	Group IV: Study Results Documentation (3)	Group V: Plausibility of Study Design and Data (2)	Total (18)
Al-Maawi et al., 2021 [17]	4	3	6	3	2	18
Al-Maawi et al., 2022 [18]	4	3	6	3	2	18
Bagio et al., 2021 [19]	3	3	6	3	2	17
Banyatworakul et al., 2021 [20]	4	3	6	3	2	18
Bi et al., 2020 [21]	4	3	6	3	2	18
Blatt et al., 2021 [22]	4	3	5	3	2	17
Chang, Tsai, and Chang, 2010 [23]	4	2	5	3	2	16
Chen et al., 2015 [24]	4	3	6	3	2	18
Cheng et al., 2022 [25]	4	3	5	3	2	17
Chi et al., 2019 [26]	4	3	5	3	2	17
Clipet et al., 2012 [27]	4	3	6	3	2	18
Dohan Ehrenfest et al., 2010 [28]	4	1	5	3	2	15
Dohle et al., 2018 [29]	4	3	6	3	2	18
Douglas et al., 2012 [30]	4	1	5	3	2	15
Duan et al., 2018 [31]	4	1	5	3	2	15
Ehrenfest et al., 2009 [32]	4	1	5	3	2	15
Esmaeilnejad et al., 2022 [33]	4	3	6	3	2	18
Fernandez-Medina et al., 2019 [34]	4	3	6	3	2	18

Table 2. *Cont.*

Publication	Group I: Test Substance	Group I: Test Substance	Group II: Test System Characterization (3)	Group III: Study Design Description (6)	Group IV: Study Results Documentation (3)	Group V: Plausibility of Study Design and Data (2)	Total (18)
Gassling et al., 2009 [35]	4	1	5	3	2		15
Gassling et al., 2010 [36]	4	3	5	3	2		17
Gassling et al., 2013 [37]	4	3	6	3	2		18
Gassling et al., 2013 [38]	4	3	5	3	2		17
Girija and Kavitha, 2020 [39]	2	3	5	2	1		13
He et al., 2009 [40]	4	3	5	3	2		17
Hong, Chen, and Jiang, 2018 [41]	4	3	6	3	2		18
Huang et al., 2010 [42]	4	3	6	3	2		18
Irastorza et al., 2019 [43]	4	3	6	3	2		18
Isobe et al., 2017 [44]	4	1	6	3	2		16
Ji et al., 2015 [45]	4	3	6	3	2		18
Kang et al., 2011 [46]	4	3	6	3	2		18
Kardos et al., 2018 [47]	4	2	5	3	2		16
Kim et al., 2017 [48]	4	2	5	3	2		16
Kim et al., 2017 [49]	4	3	5	3	2		17
Kosmidis et al., 2023 [50]	4	3	6	3	2		18
Koyanagi et al., 2022 [51]	4	3	5	3	2		17
Kyyak et al., 2020 [52]	4	3	6	3	2		18
Kyyak et al., 2021 [53]	4	3	6	3	2		18
Li et al., 2013 [54]	4	2	6	3	2		17
Li et al., 2014 [55]	4	3	6	3	2		18
Li et al., 2018 [56]	4	3	6	3	2		18
Li et al., 2018 [57]	4	3	6	3	2		18
Liang et al., 2021 [58]	3	3	6	3	2		17
Liu et al., 2019 [59]	4	3	6	3	2		18
Liu et al., 2022 [60]	4	3	6	3	2		18
Lo Monaco et al. 2020 [61]	4	3	6	3	2		18
Marchetti, 2020 [62]	4	3	6	3	2		18
Moradian et al., 2017 [63]	4	2	5	3	2		16
Nguyen et al., 2022 [64]	4	3	6	3	2		18
Nie et al., 2020 [65]	4	3	6	3	2		18
Nugraha et al., 2018 [66]	4	2	5	3	2		16
Nugraha et al., 2018 [67]	4	2	5	3	2		16
Nugraha et al., 2018 [68]	4	2	5	3	2		16
Nugraha et al., 2019 [69]	4	2	5	3	2		16
Rastegar et al., 2021 [70]	4	3	6	3	2		18
Shah et al., 2021 [71]	4	2	4	3	2		15
Song et al., 2018 [72]	4	3	6	3	2		18
Steller et al., 2019 [73]	4	3	6	3	2		18
Steller et al., 2019 [74]	4	3	6	3	2		18
Sui et al., 2023 [75]	4	3	6	3	2		18
Thanasrisuebwong et al., 2020 [76]	4	2	6	3	2		16
Verboket et al., 2019 [77]	4	2	6	3	2		17
Wang et al., 2015 [78]	4	3	6	3	2		18
Wang et al., 2018 [79]	4	3	6	3	2		18
Wang et al., 2022 [80]	4	3	5	3	2		17
Wang et al., 2023 [81]	4	3	5	3	2		17
Wong et al., 2021 [7]	4	3	6	3	2		18

Table 2. Cont.

Publication	Group I: Test Substance	Group I: Test Substance	Group II: Test System Characterization (3)	Group III: Study Design Description (6)	Group IV: Study Results Documentation (3)	Group V: Plausibility of Study Design and Data (2)	Total (18)
Wong et al., 2021 [82]	4		3	6	3	2	18
Woo et al., 2016 [83]	4		1	5	3	2	15
Wu et al., 2012 [84]	4		3	5	3	2	16
Yu et al., 2016 [85] Yu et al., 2023 [86]	4		3	6	3	2	18
Zhang et al., 2019 [87]	4		3	6	3	2	18
Zhang et al., 2023 [88]	4		3	5	3	2	17
Zhao et al., 2013 [89]	4		2	5	3	2	16
Zheng et al., 2015 [90]	4		1	5	3	2	15
Zheng et al., 2020 [91]	4		3	6	3	2	18

Table 3 shows the main data extracted from the selected studies regarding the effects of different protocols of PRF production on bone-related cells. Various studies propose ways to obtain and use PRF to optimize its handling characteristics and storage and develop new application possibilities. These include the tube type, time and speed of centrifugation, mode of application, and even association with other materials.

More than half (56%) of the studies investigated the classical L-PRF protocol proposed by Choukx, which forms a thick clotted yellow, Jell-O-like moldable scaffold. Advanced PRF (A-PRF) is another type of platelet concentrate produced by centrifuging blood at a low speed and for a longer time, which results in a fibrin clot with a rich content of platelets, growth factors, and other bioactive molecules, which was studied in nine (12%) of the selected studies. Further, nine studies investigated the effects of exposure to injectable PRF (i-PRF), which is usually prepared by centrifuging blood samples at 1060 rpm for 14 min, forming a thinner unclotted liquid that can be injected into various sites where bone grafts have been placed or where infections have occurred. Two other studies assessed the biological properties of H-PRF, which is produced by horizontal centrifugation. Finally, nine studies (12%) investigated the impact of freezing or lyophilizing L-PRF membranes on the effects of these materials on mineralizing cells. A few of the selected studies (six) compared the biological properties of two or more of these protocols, as will be discussed in the next section of this review.

One of the challenges in studying the effects of PRF on cell behavior is to choose the appropriate method of exposure. About half (51%) of the selected studies employed indirect exposure of cells to eluates, while the other 42% (32 studies) cultivated cells in co-culture or directly seeded into PRF matrices. The difference between direct and indirect in vitro exposure of cells to PRF eluates or co-cultures is that the former simulates the initial contact of cells with PRF, while the latter mimics the long-term interaction of cells with PRF. The direct exposure of cells to PRF eluates can assess the cytotoxicity, inflammation, and differentiation potential of PRF, while the co-culture of cells with PRF can evaluate the proliferation, migration, and mineralization ability of cells in the presence of PRF.

Table 3. The main biological information of the selected studies.

Publication	PRF Protocol	Mineralizing Cell Type	Exposure Time	Exposure Method	Biological Parameters	Results
Al-Maawi et al., 2021 [17]	A-PRF	Primary human osteoblasts	After 3 and 7 days	Eluate	VEGF; TGF-β1; PDGF, OPG, IL-8; OPN; ALP activity.	PRF produced according to the low-speed centrifugation concept, associated with a polymeric scaffold, had a significant effect on osteogenic markers of osteoblasts.
Al-Maawi et al., 2022 [18]	L-PRF and H-PRF	Primary human osteoblasts (pOBs)	24 h	Eluate	Cell adhesion.	Osteoblasts exposed to PRF produced with fixed-angle rotors presented higher adhesion than those exposed to PRF produced with variable angles.
Bagio et al., 2021 [19]	A-PRF	Human dental pulp stem cells	5, 12 and 24 h	Eluate	VEGF-A.	5% A-PRF extracts increased VEGF-A expression by hDPSCs.
Banyatworakul et al., 2021 [20]	L-PRF	Canine periodontal ligament cells	1, 3 and 7 days	Eluate	Proliferation; migration; in vitro mineralization.	PRF derived from Thai buffalo blood promoted the proliferation, migration, and increased mineral deposition in vitro of canine periodontal ligament cells.
Bi et al., 2020 [21]	L-PRF	Stem cells from the apical papilla (SCAP)	1, 3 and 5 days	Eluate	Proliferation; migration; in vitro mineralization; ERK; pERK; ALP; DMP-1.	PRF improved the proliferation, migration, and the osteo-/odontogenic differentiation of SCAPs by activating the ERK pathway.
Blatt et al., 2021 [22]	A-PRF and iPRF	Human osteoblasts (HOBs)	24 h	Co-culture	Cell viability; proliferation; migration; ALP; Col-I; BMP2; Runx2.	The combination of PRF with bone substitute materials increased the viability, early proliferation, and migration potential of human osteoblasts via Runx2 alkaline phosphatase, collagen, and BMP2.
Chang, Tsai, and Chang, 2010 [23]	L-PRF	Human osteosarcoma osteoblast-like cells (U2OS)	1, 3 and 5 days	Co-culture	Proliferation; p-ERK, RANKL; OPG.	PRF stimulated osteoblast proliferation with positive regulation of the expression of p-ERK and increased the secretion of OPG.
Chen et al., 2015 [24]	L-PRF	Canine dental pulp stem cells (DPSCs)	7, 14 and 21 days	Co-culture	Proliferation; ALP activity; ALP; DSPP; DMP 1; BSP.	PRF not only provides a well-organized scaffold for cell adhesion and migration but also induces DPSC proliferation and differentiation markers.
Cheng et al., 2022 [25]	L-PRF	Rabbit bone marrow mesenchymal stem cells (BMSCs)	Up to 28 days	Co-culture	Mineralization; adipogenic differentiation; aggrecan, Col-II; Sox9; b-catenin; P-GSK3b; CaMKII; PKC.	Co-culture with PRF reversed the activation of Wnt/Ca^{2+} signaling in BMSCs under hydrostatic pressure, with increased expression of chondrogenic differentiation markers.
Chi et al., 2019 [26]	Decellularized PRF	Bone marrow stem cells	every 24 h for 9 days	Cultured on PRF	Adhesion; proliferation; Col I; ALP; OPN; OCN; Runx-2.	Decellularized PRF combined with chitosan/gelatin scaffolds accelerate the attachment, proliferation, and osteogenesis-related marker expression of bone marrow stem cells.
Clipet et al., 2012 [27]	L-PRF	Human osteosarcoma osteoblast-like cells (Saos-2)	1 and 2 days	Eluate	Cytotoxicity; proliferation; Cell Cycle; cbfa1, Col1, OCN; OPN	Exposure to a PRF-conditioned medium increased the cell viability, proliferation, and expression of the late and early markers of osteogenesis.

Table 3. Cont.

Publication	PRF Protocol	Mineralizing Cell Type	Exposure Time	Exposure Method	Biological Parameters	Results
Dohan Ehrenfest et al., 2010 [28]	L-PRF	Human bone mesenchymal stem cells (BMSCs)	7, 14, 21 and 28 days	Co-culture	Cytotoxicity; proliferation; ALP activity; mineralization; morphology (SEM).	Increased proliferation and differentiation of BMSC when exposed to Choukroun's PRF.
Dohle et al., 2018 [29]	iPRF	Primary osteoblasts (pOBs)	1 and 7 days	Cultured on PRF	VEGF; ICAM-1; ALP.	The expression of E-selectin, ICAM-1, VEGF, and ALP was significantly higher in the co-culture of primary osteoblasts and outgrowth endothelial cells cultured in PRF in vitro, in addition to improving the angiogenesis process.
Douglas et al., 2012 [30]	L-PRF	Human osteosarcoma osteoblast-like cells (Saos-2)	3, 5 and 7 days	Co-culture	Cytocompatibility; migration.	PRF functionalized with ALP and induced to mineralization was not cytotoxic and promoted colonization by human osteoblasts.
Duan et al., 2018 [31]	L-PRF	Rat periodontal ligament stem cells (PDLSCs)	1, 2, 3, 4, 7 and 14 days	Cultured on PRF	Proliferation; BSP; OCN; Runx2; ALP activity.	PRF enhanced cell proliferation and the expression of osteogenic markers in rat PDLSCs.
Ehrenfest et al., 2009 [32]	L-PRF	Human maxillofacial osteoblasts	7, 14, 21 and 28 days	Co-culture	Proliferation; mineralization; ALP activity.	PRF stimulates the proliferation of several very different cell types, and the effects on osteoblastic differentiation are highly significant.
Esmaeilnejad et al., 2023 [33]	A-PRF and L-PRF	Human osteosarcoma osteoblast-like cells (MG-63)	24 and 72 h	Eluate	Proliferation; mineralization.	L-PRF increased proliferation, while A-PRF increased the in vitro mineralization of MG-63 cells.
Fernandez-Medina et al., 2019 [34]	A-PRF and I-PRF	Primary human osteoblasts	24 and 72 h	Eluate	Proliferation; migration; mineralization; cytokine release.	Cell viability and migration assays have demonstrated a detrimental effect when the concentration was ≥60. i-PRF demonstrated superior induction of mineralization. A negative impact of A-PRF was demonstrated at high concentrations.
Gassling et al., 2009 [35]	L-PRF	Human osteoblasts (HOBs) and osteosarcoma (Saos-2)	10 days	Co-culture	PDGF; IGF; TGF-Beta.	PRF exposure led to an increased secretion of growth factors by osteoblasts.
Gassling et al., 2010 [36]	L-PRF	Human periosteal cells	10 min, 1 h and 1 day.	Eluate	Cell viability; proliferation.	PRF appears to be superior to collagen (Bio-Gide) as a scaffold for human periosteal cell proliferation.
Gassling et al., 2013 [37]	Mg-enhanced and enzymatically mineralized PRF	Human osteosarcoma osteoblast-like cells (Saos-2)	1, 3 and 7 days	Co-culture	Cell viability; proliferation; morphology.	The enzymatic mineralization of PRF did not affect osteoblast viability and the proliferation on the membrane.
Gassling et al., 2013 [38]	L-PRF	Human osteoblasts	1, 5, 7 and 36 days	Eluate	Cell viability; proliferation; ALP activity.	The PRF membrane supports the proliferation of human osteoblast cells, in addition to being an adequate support for the cultivation of human osteoblasts in vitro.

Table 3. Cont.

Publication	PRF Protocol	Mineralizing Cell Type	Exposure Time	Exposure Method	Biological Parameters	Results
Girija and Kavitha, 2020 [39]	PRF (undefined protocol)	Dental pulp cells	2 h, overnight	Eluate	IL-6; IL-8; DMP-1, DSPP, STRO-1; mineralization.	The addition of bioactive radiopacifiers into PRF has a synergistic effect on the stimulation of odontoblastic differentiation of HDPCs, inducing mineralization.
He et al., 2009 [40]	L-PRF	Rat calvaria osteoblasts	1, 7, 14, 21 and 28 days	Exudates	Proliferation; mineralization; ALP activity; cytokine release.	PRF released autologous growth factors gradually and expressed stronger and more durable effects on the proliferation and differentiation of rat osteoblasts than PRP in vitro.
Hong, Chen, and Jiang, 2018 [41]	Freeze-dried L-PRF	Apical papilla (SCAPs)	7 and 14 days	Membrane dissolved in 10 mL of DMEM	Proliferation; migration; morphology; differentiation (CD45, CD90, and CD146), mineralization; ALP, BSP; DMP-1; DSPP.	Freeze-dried PRF promotes the proliferation, migration, and differentiation of SCAPs
Huang et al., 2010 [42]	L-PRF	Dental pulp cells (DPCs)	0, 1, 3 and 5 days	Co-culture	Viability; proliferation; OPG; ALP activity.	PRF stimulates cell proliferation and the differentiation of DPCs by upregulating OPG and ALP expression.
Irastorza et al., 2019 [43]	L-PRF	Pulp stem cells	4 days	Co-culture	Mineralization; ALP activity; ALP; Col-1; Osteonectin; Runx2, OSX.	Osteoblastic differentiation from human pulp stem cells was achieved with a combination of biomimetic rough titanium surfaces (BASTMs) with autologous plasma-derived fibrin-clot membranes.
Isobe et al., 2017 [44]	L-PRF from stored (frozen) blood	Human periosteal cells	3 days	Eluate	Proliferation.	The quality of PRF clots prepared from stored whole blood samples is not significantly reduced and induced similar proliferation of periosteal cells as fresh PRF.
Ji et al., 2015 [45]	L-PRF	Periodontal ligament stem cells and bone marrow mesenchymal stem cells	1, 2, 3, 4, 5, 6 and 7 days	Transwell inserts	Migration; proliferation; BSP; OCN; OPN; Col-III.	The association of PRF and TDM (treated dentin matrix) induced cell differentiation according to different markers.
Kang et al., 2011 [46]	L-PRF	Human alveolar bone marrow stem cells (hABMSCs)	0, 0.5, 3, 6, and 12 h. 1, 7, 14, 21, 28 and 35 days	Eluate	Proliferation; mineralization; migration; MMP9 activity.	PRF increased the proliferation, aggregation, activation of MMP9, and mineralization by decreasing the migration of the hABMSCs.
Kardos et al., 2018 [47]	Fresh, frozen, and freeze-dried L-PRF	Mesenchymal stem cells	1, 7 and 14 days	Co-culture	Viability; proliferation; adhesion.	Preserved PRF membranes presented the same biological properties as fresh samples.
Kim et al., 2017 [48]	L-PRF	Human primary osteoblasts	1, 2, 3 and 7 days	Co-culture	Proliferation; ALP activity.	PRF presented significantly higher data on DNA quantification, synthesis and proliferation, differentiation, and bone generation of osteoblasts, PDGFs, and TGF-b.

Table 3. Cont.

Publication	PRF Protocol	Mineralizing Cell Type	Exposure Time	Exposure Method	Biological Parameters	Results
Kim et al., 2017 [49]	L-PRF	Human dental pulp cells (HDPCs)	1, 2 and 3 days	Eluate	Viability; IL-1b; IL-6, and IL-8; VCAM-1, DSP; DMP-1; ALP activity; mineralization.	PRF presents odontogenic capacity in inflamed HDPCs.
Koyanagi et al., 2022 [50]	Arterial blood-derived PRF (Ar-PRF) and venous blood-derived PRF (Ve-PRF)	Primary rabbit osteoblasts	1, 3 and 5 days	Eluate	Viability; Col-1; OCN; mineralization.	Exposed osteoblasts presented greater differentiation potential, including higher osteocalcin expression and mineralization with no difference between Ar and Ve-PRF.
Kosmidis et al., 2023 [51]	A-PRF, i-PRF, and L-PRF	Human osteosarcoma osteoblast-like cells (U2OS)	Up to 28 days	Eluate	Mineralization; ALP activity; ALP; OCN; ON; ICAM-1; Runx2; Col 1a.	The three PRF preparations increased the osteogenic potential of U2OS cells. A-PRF presented the highest effect on mineralization, and i-PRF had the highest potential for early cell differentiation.
Kyyak et al., 2020 [52]	i-PRF	Human osteoblasts (HOBs)	3, 7 and 10 days	Eluate	Viability; migration; proliferation; ALP; BMP-2; OCN.	i-PRF in combination with allogenic biomaterials enhances human osteoblast activity compared to xenogenic bone substitute material + i-PRF.
Kyyak et al., 2021 [53]	i-PRF	Human osteoblasts (HOBs)	3, 7 and 10 days	Eluate	Viability; migration; proliferation; ALP; BMP-2; OCN.	The combination of four bovine bone substitute materials with i-PRF improved all cellular parameters, ALP and BMP-2 expression at earlier stages, and osteonectin expression at later stages.
Li et al., 2013 [54]	L-PRF	Dental follicle (DF), alveolar bone (AB), and periodontal ligament (PDL)	7, 14 and 21 days	Co-culture	Proliferation; migration; mineralization; ALP; MGP; Runx2.	PRF induced an increase in the early osteoblast transcription factor Runx2 and a reduction in the mineralization inhibitor MGP.
Li et al., 2014 [55]	Lyophilized PRF	Rat alveolar bone cells	7, 14 and 21 days	Co-culture	Mineralization; proliferation; ALP; Runx2.	Lyophilized PRF caused greater proliferation and elevation in the Runx2 expression in alveolar bone cells compared to fresh PRF and a more than 10-fold rise of ALP and in vitro mineralization.
Li et al., 2018 [56]	L-PRF	Human periodontal ligament stem cells (hPDLCs)	21 days	Exudates	Adhesion; proliferation; mineralization; ALP activity; ALP; OCN; OSX; Runx2.	PRF exudate enhances hPDLC adhesion and proliferation and induces the differentiation of hPDLCs into mineralized tissue formation cells.
Li et al., 2018 [57]	L-PRF	Human periodontal ligament cells (PDLSCs)	1, 2, 3, 7 and 14 days	Co-culture	Proliferation; Runx2; MAPK; ERK1/2; pERK1/2; JNK1/2/3; pJNK1/2/3; P38; OSX; OCN; ALP activity.	PRF and IGF-1 can promote the osteogenic differentiation of PDLSCs and enhance their osteogenic mineralization through the regulation of the MAPK pathway.

55

Table 3. Cont.

Publication	PRF Protocol	Mineralizing Cell Type	Exposure Time	Exposure Method	Biological Parameters	Results
Liu et al., 2022 [59]	Lyophilized L-PRF, crosslinked with genipin	Pulp stem cells from human exfoliated deciduous teeth (SHEDs)	Up to 14 days	Eluate	Proliferation; mineralization; Runx2; Col 1; OCN.	Genipin crosslinked L-PRF induced cell proliferation and enhanced the expression of key genes in osteogenesis.
Liang et al., 2021 [58]	A-PRFe	Adipose-derived stem cells (ASCs)	7 days	Eluate	Roliferation; mineralization; adipogenesis; ALP, OPN; OCN; Runx2.	A-PRF stimulated ASC proliferation and adipogenic and osteogenic differentiation in a dose-dependent manner.
Liu et al., 2019 [60]	Fresh/lyophilized PRF	Bone mesenchymal stem cells (BMSCs)	1–7 days	Eluate	Proliferation; mineralization.	Fresh/lyophilized PRF (1:1) increased BMSC proliferation and in vitro mineralization.
Lo Monaco et al., 2020 [61]	L-PRF	Dental pulp stem cells (DPSCs)	24, 48 and 72 h	Eluate	Chondrogenic differentiation; TIMP-1; proliferation.	L-PRF induced differential chondrogenesis on DPSCs.
Marchetti et al., 2020 [62]	L-PRF	Periodontal ligament fibroblasts	24 h, 72 h and 7 days	Eluate	Proliferation; viability; morphology.	L-PRF stimulated the onset of the growth of the periodontal ligament fibroblasts.
Moradian et al., 2017 [63]	L-PRF	Bone marrow mesenchymal stem cells (BMMSCs)	1, 5, 7, 9 and 12 days	Cultured on PRF	Proliferation; adhesion.	PRF significantly induced BMMSC proliferation. Scanning electron microscopy showed that BMMSCs tightly adhered to the fibrin scaffold after seeding.
Nguyen et al., 2022 [64]	A-PRF	Human periodontal ligament stem cells (hPDLSCs)	1 h, 6 h, 24 h, 3 days, 5 days and 7 days	Exudates	Proliferation; migration.	A-PRF in combination with xenogenic bone induced hPDLSC migration or proliferation, depending on the exudate concentration.
Nie et al., 2020 [65]	Lyophilized L-PRF	MC3T3-E1 murine preosteoblasts	1, 3 and 5 days	Eluate	Proliferation; mineralization; OCN; OPN.	Eluates from lyophilized PRF added as a component for electrospinning preparation enhanced the proliferation, mineralization, and expression of the OCN and OPN of MEC3T3-E1 cells.
Nugraha et al., 2018a [66]	L-PRF	Rat gingival mesenchymal stem cells (GMSCs)	7, 14 and 21 days	Cultured on PRF	ALP; OC.	PRF induced increased ALP and OCN expression on GMSCs.
Nugraha et al., 2018b [67]	L-PRF	Rat gingival somatic cells (GSCs)	7, 14 and 21 days	Cultured on PRF	BSP-1.	PRF increases and stimulates GSC BSP-1 expression.
Nugraha et al., 2018c [68]	L-PRF	Rat gingival stromal progenitor cells (GSPCs)	7, 14 and 21 days	Cultured on PRF	Cbfa-1; sox9.	GSPCs cultured in PRF possessed a potential osteogenic differentiation ability, as predicted by the cbfa-1/sox9 expression ratio.
Nugraha et al., 2019 [69]	L-PRF	Rat gingival mesenchymal stem cells (GMSCs)	7, 14 and 21 days	Cultured on PRF	Aggrecan.	Platelet-rich fibrin increases the aggrecan expression of GMSCs during osteogenic differentiation.
Rastegar et al., 2021 [70]	L-PRF	Human osteosarcoma osteoblast-like cells (MG-63)	3 days	Co-culture	ALP activity; mineralization.	PRF loaded into PCL/chitosan core-shell fibers promoted in vitro mineralization and increased ALP activity.

Table 3. Cont.

Publication	PRF Protocol	Mineralizing Cell Type	Exposure Time	Exposure Method	Biological Parameters	Results
Shah et al., 2021 [71]	i-PRF	Human osteosarcoma osteoblast-like cells (MG-63)	1, 7, 14 and 21 days	Co-culture	Proliferation; ALP activity; mineralization.	Coating titanium discs with i-PRF causes increased proliferation, alkaline phosphatase production, and mineralization at days 1, 7, 14, and 21.
Song et al., 2018 [72]	L-PRF	Rabbit bone marrow-derived mesenchymal stem cells (BMSCs)	7 days	Eluate	Adhesion; proliferation; ALP; Col-1; OPN; Runx2.	Printed scaffolds of BCP/PVA associated with PRF promoted the adhesion, proliferation, and differentiation of BMSCs.
Steller et al., 2019 [73]	L-PRF	Human osteoblasts (HOBs)	72 h	Eluate	Proliferation; migration; viability.	The use of PRF improves the behavior of osteoblasts treated with zoledronic acid.
Steller et al., 2019 [74]	PRF	Human primary osteoblasts	24 h	Eluate	Adhesion; viability; morphology.	Zoledronic acid decreased osteoblast adhesion on implant surfaces. PRF increased the primary adhesion of zoledronic acid-treated osteoblasts on implant surfaces in vitro.
Sui et al., 2023 [75]	3D-printed L-PRF composite scaffolds	MC3T3-E1 murine preosteoblasts	1 to 3 days	Cultured on a PRF composite scaffold	Proliferation.	The proliferation of preosteoblasts into the scaffolds increased with the release of GFs, indicating that L-PRF remains bioactive after 3D printing.
Thanasrisuebwong et al., 2020 [76]	Subfractioned (red and yellow) i-PRF	Periodontal ligament stem cells	0, 3 and 5 days	Eluate	Proliferation; migration; mineralization; ALP activity.	The factors released from the red i-PRF had a greater effect on cell proliferation and cell migration, while yellow i-PRF stimulated earlier osteogenic differentiation of periodontal ligament stem cells.
Verboket et al., 2019 [77]	High (208 g) and low (60 g) RCF PRF	Bone marrow mononuclear cells (BMCs)	2, 7 and 14 days	Eluate	Viability; apoptosis; VEGFA; ICAM3; MMP2; MMP7; MMP9; TGF-β1; BCL2; BAX; ALP; COL-1; FGF2; SPP1.	PRF produced with low RCF significantly increased mediator contents and stimulatory effects on BMC with regard to the gene expression of MMPs and metabolic activity/viability.
Wang et al., 2015 [78]	L-PRF	Rabbit mesenchymal stem cells (MSCs)	1, 2, 3, 4, 5, 6, 7, 8 and 14 days	Eluate	Proliferation; ALP; BMP2; OCN; OPN; Col-1.	PRF significantly stimulated MSC proliferation and osteogenesis in vitro.
Wang et al., 2018 [79]	i-PRF	Human primary osteoblasts	1, 3, 5, 7 and 14 days	Co-culture	Proliferation; migration; adhesion; mineralization; ALP activity; ALP; Col-1; OC.	i-PRF was able to influence osteoblast behavior, including migration, proliferation, and differentiation, at higher levels than PRP.
Wang et al., 2022 [80]	i-PRF	Human bone marrow stem cells (hBMSCs)	1 to 7 days	Eluate	Proliferation; survival; migration; mineralization; Col 1; OCN; OPN; Runx2, ERK 1/2; p-ERK.	i-PRF improved the proliferation and migration of hBMSCs, with an increased expression of osteogenic markers, mineralization, and activation of the ERK pathway.

Table 3. Cont.

Publication	PRF Protocol	Mineralizing Cell Type	Exposure Time	Exposure Method	Biological Parameters	Results
Wang et al. 2022 [81]	L-PRF	Rabbit mesenchymal stem cells from the Schneiderian membrane (SM-MSCs)	1 to 14 days	Eluate	Proliferation; migration; mineralization; ALP activity; ALP; Col 1; Run×2; ERK 1/2; p-ERK.	PRF stimulated proliferation, migration, and osteogenic differentiation of SM-MSCs, with the upregulation of the ERK 1/2 signaling pathway.
Wong et al., 2021 [7]	Large-pore PRF (LPPRF)	MC3T3-E1 preosteoblasts	6 days	Eluate	Proliferation; migration; mineralization.	Large-pore LPPRF combined with a Mg ring increased preoteoblast proliferation, migration, and in vitro calcium deposition.
Wong et al., 2021 [82]	L-PRF	Rabbit primary osteoblasts	3 and 6 days	Eluate	Viability; ALP activity; Col-1; OPN; ALP.	L-PRF positively affected primary osteoblast behavior and induced bone formation when associated with TCP.
Woo et al. 2016 [83]	L-PRF	Human dental pulp cells (HDPCs)	12 h. 1, 2 and 7 days	Eluate	Viability; ALP activity; DSP; DMP1; BMP 2/4; pSmad1/5/8.	A combination of MTA and PRF synergistically stimulated odontoblastic differentiation of HDPCs by the modulation of the BMP/Smad pathway.
Wu et al. 2012 [84]	L-PRF	Human osteosarcoma osteoblast-like cells (U2OS)	2 h. 1, 3 and 5 days	Co-culture	Adhesion; proliferation p-Akt; HSP47; LOX.	PRF increased cell attachment and proliferation by the Akt pathway and matrix synthesis via HSP47 and LOX accumulation.
Yu et al. 2016 [85]	L-PRF	Canine deciduous and permanent dental pulp cells (DPCs)	1, 4, 7 and 11 days	Co-culture	Cytotoxicity; proliferation; ALP activity; mineralization; Col-1; OCN; OPN; Run×2, ALP.	PRF stimulated the proliferation and differentiation of both deciduous and permanent DPCs, and deciduous pulp cells were more responsive to the effects of PRF.
Yu et al., 2023 [86]	H-PRF	Human osteoblasts (hFOBs)	3 days	Transwell inserts	Migration.	The culture medium from H-PRF bone blocks markedly promoted the migration of osteoblasts.
Zhang et al., 2019 [87]	L-PRF	Dental pulp stem cells (DPSCs)	1, 3, 5 and 7 days	Eluate	Migration; morphology; ALP activity; mineralization (SEM); OPN; Col-1; ALP.	Multifunctional triple-layered scaffolds combined with PRF significantly increased ALP activity and the expression of differentiation markers on DPSCs.
Zhang et al., 2023 [88]	i-PRF	Human dental pulp stem cells (hDPSCs)	Up to 21 days	Eluate	Proliferation; mineralization; ALP activity; Run×2; DSPP; DMP1; BSP; Notch 1; Jagged 1; Hes 1.	I-PRF induced a dose-dependent increase in the proliferation of hDPSCs and the expression of osteo-/odontoblastic differentiation markers, as well as key proteins in the Notch signaling.
Zhao et al., 2013 [89]	L-PRF	Periodontal ligament stem cells (PDLSCs)	7, 14 and 21 days	Co-culture	Proliferation; mineralization (SEM); ALP activity; BSP; OCN; Col-I; CP23.	PRF induced proliferation in PDLSCs while suppressing the osteoblastic differentiation of PDLSCs by decreasing ALP activity and the gene expression of BSP and OCN while upregulating the mRNA expression levels of Col-I and CP23 during the testing period.

Table 3. Cont.

Publication	PRF Protocol	Mineralizing Cell Type	Exposure Time	Exposure Method	Biological Parameters	Results
Zheng et al., 2015 [90]	Lyophilized PRF	Human osteosarcoma osteoblast-like cells (MG63)	1, 3 and 5 days	Co-culture	Viability; adhesion; proliferation.	A combination of hydrogel and a nanostructured scaffold loaded with PRF improved the adhesion and proliferation of MG63 cells compared to the controls.
Zheng et al., 2020 [91]	i-PRF	Human periodontal ligament cells (hPDLCs)	1, 3 and 5 days	Eluate	Migration; proliferation; ALP activity; mineralization; Runx2; Col-1; OCN; IL-1β; TNF-α and p65 (in the presence of LPS).	Liquid PRF promoted hPDLC proliferation and differentiation and attenuated the inflammatory state induced by LPS.

The name of a protein indicates the assessment of its expression. L-PRF: fibrin rich in platelets and leukocytes produced by Choukrun's protocol; i-PRF: liquid, injectable PRF; A-PRF: advanced PRF, produced with intermediary centrifugation forces; H-PRF: produced through horizontal centrifugation. RCF: relative centrifugal force; ALP: alkaline phosphatase; OPN: osteopontin; OPG: osteoprotegerin; DMP-1: dentin matrix protein 1; DSPP: dentin sialophosphoprotein; DSP: dentin sialoprotein; SPP: sialophosphoprotein; BSP: bone sialoprotein; OCN: osteocalcin; Col-1: collagen type I; OSX: osterix; MMP: matrix metalloproteinase; VCAM-1: vascular cell adhesion molecule 1; BMP-2: bone morphogenetic protein 2; MGP: matrix Gla protein; LOX: lysyl oxidase; LPS: lipopolysaccharide; P-GSK3b: phosphorylated glycogen synthase kinase-3-beta.

Regarding the cell types employed in the studies, several different models were identified from diverse mineralizing tissues of both human and animal origin. More than half of the studies (n = 44, 58%) employed human cells, while the other half investigated cells from animal sources (42%), including cells from rabbits, canines, and murine models. None of the selected studies performed a comparison between human or animal cells in order to provide direct evidence of different responses to PRF between these origins. All studies that performed assessments of cell viability and proliferation after exposure of either human or animal cells to PRF presented similar descriptive results, even with incomparable size effects, as the methodological settings were very heterogeneous (the tables include records of studies without any data). Furthermore, very similar regulatory pathways are reported as activated by exposure to PRF, including the Cbfa-1/Runx2, MAPK, and Wnt signaling pathways, regardless of the human or animal origin of cells, as will be further described and discussed in the next section of this review. Nevertheless, it is important to notice that data resulting from human cells are usually considered more relevant and representative of human physiology and pathology than animal cells, which may have different molecular and cellular mechanisms, responses, and interactions. Furthermore, their obtention may reduce ethical and practical issues associated with the use of animals for research, such as animal welfare, availability, cost, and regulatory approval.

Several of the selected studies utilized primary cells, such as osteoblasts, dental pulp stem cells (hDPSCs), periodontal ligament cells (cPDLs), and bone marrow stem cells (BMSCs) (Table 4). Primary cells are isolated directly from living tissues or organs and offer several advantages over immortalized cell lines. They retain the physiological functions of their tissue of origin, such as gene expression, metabolism, and responsiveness to stimuli. They provide a more realistic model system, making them more suitable for studying complex biological processes. However, immortalized cell lines, which have been modified to proliferate indefinitely in culture, offer some benefits over primary cells. They are more homogeneous and consistent, easier to maintain and manipulate, and more readily available and cost-effective. Some of the selected studies utilized immortalized cell lines, including the well-established preosteoblasts from rat calvaria MC3T3-E1 and the human osteosarcoma cell lines Saos-2, MG-63, and U2OS (Table 4).

The majority of the selected articles investigated cells in monoculture. A single exception is the study by Dohle et al. [29], which employed a co-culture of outgrowth endothelial cells (OECs) and primary osteoblasts (pOBs) exposed together to injectable PRF. The authors presented evidence that i-PRF may have a positive effect on wound healing processes and the angiogenic activation of endothelial cells, as the expression of E-selectin, ICAM-1, VEGF, and ALP was significantly higher in the exposed cells. OECs are a subpopulation of endothelial progenitor cells (EPCs) that have high proliferative and angiogenic potential, which have been already shown to interact with osteoblasts in a positive manner, enhancing osteogenic differentiation and increased mineralization. Additionally, osteoblasts secrete IL-8, which enhances the migration, survival, and expression of angiogenic factors and matrix metalloproteinases [92]. In this context, identifying that PRF may enhance these interactions may provide an interesting tool for bone tissue engineering.

Table 4. The main data extracted from the studies with PRF associated with other materials and/or compounds.

References	Associated Material	Relevance	Results
Al-Maawi, 2021 [17]	OsteoporeTM (OP), a commercially available PCL mesh	Combination of differently centrifuged PRF matrices with a polymeric resorbable scaffold to influence their biological properties on bone regeneration.	The presented results suggest that PRF produced according to the low-speed centrifugation concept exhibits autologous blood cells and growth factors and seems to have a significant effect on osteogenesis, showing promising results to support bone regeneration.
Chi, 2019 [26]	Chitosan/gelatin (C/G)	Test whether decellularized PRF (DPRF) maintains its bioactive effects to improve chitosan/gelatin (C/G) base scaffolds, which display appropriate biocompatibility and mechanical properties but lack biological activity to promote soft and hard tissue repair.	C/G/DPRF scaffolds accelerated attachment, proliferation, and osteogenesis-related marker expression of bone marrow stem cells. In vivo, C/G/DPRF scaffolds led to enhanced bone healing and defect closure in a rat calvarial defect model. Thus, it was concluded that DPRF remains bioactive, and the prepared C/G/DPRF scaffold is a promising material for bone regeneration.
Douglas, 2012 [30]; Gassling, 2013 [37]	Calcium glycerophosphate (CaGP) and ALP	Induce the mineralization of PRF membranes to achieve mechanical reinforcement of the gel and stability as a barrier membrane in guided bone regeneration.	The mineralization was confirmed, and WST test results showed that cell proliferation was inferior on PRF after the addition of ALP, confirming its properties as a barrier.
Girija and Kavitha, 2020 [39]	Bioactive radiopacifiers—nanohydroxyapatite (nHA) and dentin chips (DCs)	Combine bioactive radiopacifiers, nanohydroxyapatite (nHA) and dentin chips (DC), to PRF, aiming to produce a traceable material for endodontic procedures while still inducing adequate biological responses.	The results suggest that the addition of bioactive radiopacifiers into PRF has a synergistic effect on the stimulation of odontoblastic differentiation of HDPCs, inducing mineralization.
Ji B, 2015 [45]	Treated dentin matrix (TDM)	Associate endogenous stem cells, PRF, and TDM in the local microenvironment to contribute to the regeneration of periodontal tissues around the tooth root.	The study confirmed the role of PRF as a bioactive agent with TDM as an inductive scaffold for cells of the tooth socket microenvironment involved in endogenous tooth root regeneration.
Kyyak, 2020 [52]	Allogenic (ABSM) and xenogenic bone substitute material (XBSM)	The comparison of allogenic and xenogenic bone substitutes with i-PRF for the production of the more bioactive composite material for bone treatment.	i-PRF in combination with ABSM enhances HOB activity compared to XBSM-i-PRF or untreated BSM in vitro. Therefore, the addition of i-PRF to ABSM and—to a lower extent—XBSM may influence osteoblast activity in vivo in an interesting way for bone therapy.
Kyyak, 2021 [52]	Cerabone R (CB), Bio-Oss R (BO), Creos Xenogain R (CX), and MinerOSS R X (MO)	Four bovine bone substitute materials (XBSMs) were associated with i-PRF and aimed to increase their osteoinductive properties.	XBSM sintered under high temperatures showed increased HOB viability and metabolic activity throughout the whole period compared to XBSM manufactured at lower temperatures. Overall, the combination of XBSM with i-PRF improved all cellular parameters related to osteogenesis.

Table 4. *Cont.*

References	Associated Material	Relevance	Results
Nguyen, 2022 [64]	Xenogenic bone substitute material (XBSM)	Advanced platelet-rich fibrin (A-PRF) and xenogenic bone substitute material (XBSM) were associated and aimed to increase periodontal tissue regeneration.	The PRF-XBSM mixture continuously released growth factors over 7 days and enhanced human ligament stem cell proliferation and migration.
Nie, 2020 [65]	Polyvinyl alcohol/sodium alginate	The addition of lyophilized PRF as a component for electrospinning preparations to increase the proliferation and osteogenesis of osteogenic precursor cells for bioengineering purposes.	The resulting material presented adequate physicochemical properties and was able to increase osteogenic markers on bone cells.
Rastegar, 2021 [70]	PCL/chitosan	Platelet-rich fibrin (PRF)-loaded PCL/chitosan (PCL/CS-PRF) core-shell nanofibrous scaffold was made through a coaxial electrospinning method. The goal was to evaluate the effect of CS-RPF in the core layer of the nanofibrous on the osteogenic differentiation of human mesenchymal stem cells (HMSCs).	The formation of Ca-P on the surface of the scaffold immersed in a simulated body fluid solution indicated the suitable osteoconductivity of the PCL/CS-PRF core-shell nanofibrous scaffold. Due to the higher hydrophilicity and porosity of the PCL/CS-PRF core-shell nanofibrous scaffold compared to the PCL/CS scaffold, better bone cell growth on the surface of the PCL/CS-PRF scaffold was observed.
Song, 2018 [72]	Nano-biphasic calcium phosphate (BCP) and polyvinyl alcohol (PVA)	The low-temperature 3D printing of BCP/PVA/PRF scaffolds would preserve the biological activity of PRF and provide an innovative biomaterial for restoring segmental bone defects.	The biological activity of PRF was retained during the 3D printing process, and the presence of PRF in the biocompatible microenvironment of the scaffold provided cell binding sites and promoted the adhesion, proliferation, and the differentiation of BMSCs.
Steller, 2019 [73]	Zoledronic acid	An investigation of the effects or bone cells treated with bisphosphonates as a potential mitigator of osteonecrosis associated with treatments with these drugs.	The negative effects of ZA on osteoblast survival and behavior (proliferation, morphology, adhesion to implant surface) were especially reduced using PRF, indicating that the autologous material may have positive effects in the therapy of bisphosphonate-related osteonecrosis of the kaw.
Sui et al., 2023 [75]	Chitosan (CS)-hydroxyapatite (HAP) scaffolds	A study aiming to identify if the 3D printing of a CS-HAP-PRF would compromise the biological properties of the platelet aggregate.	Based on the presented experimental results, it is possible to infer that the 2.5% P-C-H scaffold exhibits remarkable biological activity. And, therefore, it is not negatively affected by 3D printing.
Woo, 2016 [83]	Mineral trioxide aggregate (MTA)	Combined PRF as a bioactive matrix and MTA as a root-filling material beneficial for the endodontic management of an open apex.	The combination of MTA and PRF was proven as an odontogenic inducer in human dental pulp cells (HDPCs) in vitro.

Table 4. Cont.

References	Associated Material	Relevance	Results
Wong, 2021 [7]	Magnesium rings	The freeze-drying enlarges the pores of PRF to engineer large-pore PRF (LPPRF), a type of PRF that has expanded pores for cell migration. Biodegradable Mg rings were used to provide stability to these pores and release Mg ions during degradation, with the potential to enhance osteoconduction and osteoinduction.	The results revealed that cell migration was more extensive when LPPRF was used rather than PRF. Moreover, the Mg ions released from the Mg rings significantly enhanced the calcium deposition by preosteoblasts, evidencing in vitro osteoinduction.
Wong, 2021 [82]	Tricalcium phosphate (TCP)	The development of a composite biomaterial combining the osteoconductive TCP incorporated with bioactive PRF for bio-synergistic bone regeneration.	The in vitro results showed that PRF plus TCP had excellent biosafety and was favorable for increasing osteoblast activity related to bone repair.
Zhang, 2019 [87]	Polycaprolactone, chitosan, and hydroxyapatite	Polycaprolactone/gelatin (PG) nanofiber films by electrospinning chitosan/poly (γ-glutamic acid)/hydroxyapatite (CPH) hydrogels were formed by electrostatic interaction and lyophilization to exert osteoconduction, and platelet-rich fibrin (PRF) was added to promote bone induction through the release of growth factors.	This study provided evidence that the composite biomaterial positively affects dental pulp stem cells, with great potential for endodontics and wider applications, such as calvarial repair and oral alveolar bone regeneration.
Zheng, 2015 [90]	Copolymer poly-polyethylene glycol (PEG)-PLGA (PLGA-PEG-PLGA)	A combination of PRF with PLGA and nano-hydroxyapatite (nHA/PLGA) might produce a scaffold with high porosity, controlled pore size to better mimic natural bone, and improved osteogenic ability.	The resulting scaffold provided a good substrate for osteoblast proliferation with sustained-release growth factors, producing a promising therapeutic agent for local applications in bone tissue engineering.

Five studies investigated more than one cell type with the same methodology, even though not in co-culture, providing data that allowed us to identify some cell type-specific differences in the response to PRF preparations. The study by Dohan Ehrenfest et al. [28] was one of the first identified assessing different responses to L-PRF by exposing gingival fibroblasts, dermal prekeratinocytes, preadipocytes, and maxillofacial osteoblasts. The results showed that PRF continually stimulates proliferation in all studied cell types, but this stimulation was stronger and dose-dependent in osteoblasts, while it was observed only on day 14 with fibroblasts. Adipocytes and prekeratinocytes also differed by presenting increased metabolic activity (as detected by mitochondrial activity) and were probably related to different regulations of metabolism in these cells. Clipet et al. [27] also compared human osteoblasts (Saos-2), fibroblasts (MRC5), and epithelial (KB) cell lines. Similar to the findings of Dohan et al., while PRF increased the proliferation of all cell types, the effects were more evident in osteoblasts at shorter experimental times. Gassling et al. [35], 2009, also compared the exposure of human osteoblasts, human fibroblasts, and human osteoblast-derived osteosarcoma cells (Saos-2) to PRF, assessing their effects not on proliferation but on the induction of the release of growth factors by these cells. While growth factors could be detected in all of the samples, fibroblasts secreted lower levels of PDGF-AB, PDGF-BB, IGF-I, and TGF-ß1 than osteoblasts, especially those derived from osteossarcoma, suggesting increased paracrine activation by PRF in transformed cells. A similar pattern was also observed in the study by Kardos et al. [47], 2018, where mesenchymal stem cells presented higher rates of proliferation when exposed to fresh or lyophilized PRF samples compared to gingival fibroblasts. However, a recent study by Al-Maawi et al. [18], 2022, comparing different centrifugation protocols for PRF production, including L-PRF and H-PRF, reported relatively higher effects on the viability, proliferation, and adhesion of primary human dermal fibroblasts compared to osteoblasts. The very different methodologies employed impair the comparisons of these studies, but it is possible that the size of the effects of PRF on fibroblasts may be influenced by their tissue of origin, as fibroblasts from different anatomical sites may have distinct phenotypic and functional characteristics.

In the selected studies, different biological markers were observed that point to the molecular effects of PRF in cell differentiation and mineralization events (Table 2), depending on the cell type, including the expression and secretion of alkaline phosphatase, sialoproteins and sialophosphoproteins, type 1 collagen, osteocalcin, ostepontin, bone morphogenetic protein-2 (BMP-2), and the regulation of the transcription factors osterix and Runx2, which will be further discussed below.

Table 4 shows that a considerable proportion of the selected studies (n = 19, 25%) investigated the association of PRF with other compounds or materials in order to produce bioactive composites for different applications, which is a trend in the development of advanced, smart materials. These associations, which will be further discussed, include polymers (polycaprolactone meshes, chitosan/gelatin, polyvinyl alcohol/sodium alginate composites, PEG/PLGA copolymers), cements (MTA), calcium phosphates (nHA radiopacifiers, BCP, TCP), and allogenic or xenogeneic materials, including dentin chips and bovine bone substitutes. The myriad of methodologies and proposals impair the comparison of the relative performance of these materials between studies, and only a few of them included intra-study comparisons. Most of the studies indicated that the associations contribute to achieving the specific expected outcome, with increased cell response to PRF-containing composites, either by increased attachment, proliferation, or differentiation. As an exception, the study by Kyyak et al. [52] presented comparative evidence that the association of i-PRF with a xenogenic bone substitute material (XBSM) is less bioactive, promoting lower osteoblastic activity than allogenic bone substitute material (ABSM) associated with i-PRF. Nevertheless, further studies by Kyyak et al. [53] indicated that sintering XBSM samples under high temperatures could increase osteoblast viability and metabolic activity. Furthermore, Nguyen et al. [64] described that XBSM associated with other PRF types (A-PRF) enhanced human ligament stem cell proliferation and migration, even without sintering.

4. Discussion

4.1. Protocols for PRF Production and Preservation

As indicated in Table 3, apart from the classical Choukrun's L-PRF, other production protocols were also identified in the selected studies. These platelet concentrates differ not only in their preparation methods but also in mechanical properties, degradation rates, and growth factor release profiles, resulting in possible differences in the response of mineralizing cells after exposure. In this regard, a few studies compared such differences, with interesting findings that will be discussed below.

The study by Marchetti et al. [62] compared L-PRF with two other autologous biomaterials: concentrated growth factors (CGFs) and autologous platelet gel (APG). The authors reported stronger stimulation of the proliferation of human periodontal ligament fibroblasts (HPLFs) by CGFs compared to L-PRF and correlated these effects with the different secretion profiles of growth factors by these materials.

Verboket et al. [77] used the low-speed centrifugation concept, reducing the centrifugal force in the production of L-PRF to produce a membrane with a higher concentration of cells and growth factors. The study compared the protocols of PRF medium-RCF (1300 RPM for 8 min) and PRF low-RCF (700 RPM for 3 min). Although there was significant heterogeneity between the protocols to produce platelet aggregates and experimental design, the positive effects observed on proliferation, differentiation, and mineralization were rather similar between the protocols.

Fernandez-Medina et al. [34] compared the biological activity of A-PRF and i-PRF, along with two PRP protocols. After 21 days, i-PRF induced superior mineralization by human primary osteoblasts compared to the other materials, while A-PRF presented a negative impact at high concentrations, which was related to increased cytotoxicity. Despite its low content in growth factors, the author concluded that i-PRF was the best candidate for bone tissue engineering applications and was probably related to the prolonged release of BMP-2 by this material. Esmaeilnejad et al. [33] also investigated the effects of A-PRF, this time compared to classic L-PRF, on the cellular activity of MG-63 osteosarcoma-derived osteoblasts. Their findings indicate that L-PRF induced higher proliferation than A-PRF, while the latter was only capable of inducing in vitro mineralization at the employed experimental conditions, suggesting positive but very different effects of these materials. The study by Kosmidis et al. [50], on the other hand, investigated the effects of A-PRF, L-PRF, and i-PRF on the osteogenesis of the human osteoblast-like U2OS cell line. Similar to the findings by Esmaeilnejad et al. [33], A-PRF induced more mineralization and calcium production. i-PRF induced more ALP activity, suggesting it has the potential to enhance early cell differentiation.

Lourenço et al. [13] suggested using swing-out rotors instead of fixed-angle centrifugation to produce a product similar to L-PRF. According to some authors, the process known as H-PRF (platelet-rich fibrin produced through horizontal centrifugation) allows for a greater number of live cells and growth factors to be distributed more evenly in the final product. Al-Maawi et al. [18] compared the effects of PRF products produced by fixed-angle and horizontal centrifugation over osteoblast behavior, identifying very similar effects on proliferation and viability, with increased cell adhesion in the fixed-angle group. These results indicate that very similar materials may be produced with different centrifuge types, as long as the g-force is standardized.

The study by Li Q et al. [55] included physical modifications in the PRF protocol to increase shelf life, such as freeze-drying membranes. Their results indicated that the proliferation and migration of periodontal progenitors were increased with exposure to lyophilized PRF compared to fresh PRF, which was probably due to increased porosity and the release of growth factors from the processed membranes. Kardos et al. [47] also analyzed PRF membranes in different presentations (fresh, frozen, and freeze-dried) compared different centrifugation protocols (1700 RCF in 5 min and 8 min) and the use of modified tubes (single-syringe closed system—hypACT Inject Auto). Living cells were observed only in fresh PRF membranes, while freezing induced, as expected, the disruption of leukocytes embedded in the PRF membrane. However, MSCs were reported as proliferating even faster over freeze-thawed PRF than over fresh samples, suggesting the adequacy of such a procedure.

Liu et al. [59] proposed the combination of fresh and lyophilized PRF at different ratios, tailored for different delivery rates of GFs in tissue healing. Their findings indicate a significant increase in proliferation and differentiation of BMSCs exposed to eluates of different combinations, with the best results achieved a fresh/lyophilized PRF ratio of 1:1. A subsequent study by the same group [60] proposed the use of a natural crosslinker agent, genipin, derived from gardenia flowers, to increase the stability and controlled release of growth factors by lyophilized PRF. Genipin-modified lyophilized PRF presented better biomechanical properties, slower biodegradation, and sustained release of growth factors, promoting the proliferation of pulp stem cells from human exfoliated deciduous teeth (SHEDs).

Isobe et al. [44] added the anticoagulant formulation acid citrate dextrose solution-A (ACD-A) in blood samples, with the objective of enabling its storage for later production of PRF. Its coagulation was obtained by the addition of $CaCl_2$ (showing similarities with the protocol of PRP production), without a significant reduction in its bioactivity. This method tends to improve the flexibility of successful PRF preparations, and the quality of membranes prepared from whole blood samples were stored for up to 2 days.

4.2. Association of PRF and Other Materials/Compounds

Several of the selected studies investigated the association of PRF with other agents, including biomaterials, scaffolds, bioactive compounds, and ions, as described in Table 4. Irastorza et al. [43] investigated the use of L-PRF as a biomimetic coat of titanium implant surfaces, aiming for improved osteointegration. When combined with hDPSCs (human dental pulp stem cells), the material induced both proliferation and osteogenic differentiation of stem cells. The study by Steller et al. [73] also assessed the use of PRF coating over titanium implants, this time to reverse the negative effects of a bisphosphonate (zoledronic acid) over osteoblast attachment to the implant surfaces. Indeed, zoledronic acid led to a decrease in osteoblast adherence onto the implant surface, but it was reversed by a previous coating with L-PRF, suggesting that PRF may contribute to bone apposition in dental patients undergoing bisphosphonate treatment. Furthermore, L-PRF acted directly on the viability, migration, and proliferation of osteoblasts and fibroblasts treated with zoledronic acid [74].

Song et al. [72] explored the effectiveness of 3D-printed biphasic calcium phosphate/PVA scaffolds combined with PRF using a straightforward low-temperature method. These scaffolds demonstrated impressive biological activity and biocompatibility in vitro. When implanted into critical bone defects in a rabbit's radius, the inclusion of PRF encouraged proper bone regeneration and repair by providing osteoconductive and osteoinductive stimuli [72]. Similarly, Sui et al. [75] proposed the production of 3D-printed L-PRF scaffolds composed of chitosan (CS)–hydroxyapatite (HAP) associated with lyophilized PRF. MC3T3-E1 murine preosteoblasts presented increased proliferation over the composite scaffold after association with PRF. The proliferation of preosteoblasts into the scaffolds increased with the release of GFs, indicating that L-PRF remains bioactive even after 3D printing. Zhang et al. [86] fabricated a complex, multifunctional triple-layered composite scaffold including polycaprolactone/gelatin (PG) nanofiber films made by electrospinning, chitosan/poly (γ-glutamic acid)/hydroxyapatite (CPH) hydrogels, and platelet-rich fibrin (PRF). The resulting scaffold presented induced the proliferation of both fibroblasts and bone mesenchymal stem cells (BMSCs) and also induced osteogenic differentiation in the latter. Other calcium phosphates, such as tricalcium phosphate (TCP), also presented interesting outcomes after association with PRF, as reported by Wong et al. [81], where the composite presented a controlled release of bioactive factors with the increase in osteoblast attachment, cell proliferation, migration, and ECM formation.

Dentin, known for its bone-inducing properties, fuses and is gradually replaced by bone when grafted into it. This is likely due to its osteoinductive properties, biocompatibility, and BMP content [93]. In a study by Ji et al. [45], after seven days of coculture with PRF and a treated dentin matrix, BMSCs exhibited increased expression of BSP and OPN mRNA, while PDLSCs showed higher expressions of BSP, OPN, and OCN. Mahendran et al. (2019) [94] combined PRF with dentin chips and nanohydroxyapatite to enhance radiopacity, creating a biocompatible structure that promoted cell proliferation as a mitogen. Girija and Kavitha [39] compared the combination of PRF with 50 wt% of radiopacifier nanohydroxyapatite (nHA) or with 50 wt% dentin chips and their effects on odontoblastic differentiation. While both materials increased the expression of dentin sialophosphoprotein (DSP) and dentin matrix protein-1 (DMP-1), there were two important extracellular matrix proteins involved in the differentiation and mineralization of human dental pulp cells (HDPCs), and exposure to PRF + 50 wt% nHA induced more mineralization nodules in these cells.

Zheng et al. [88] found that when developing a combination of PRF with a polypolyethylene glycol (PEG)-PLGA copolymer, the hydrogel was evenly distributed on the inner surface of the PRF scaffolds. The hydrogel did not impact the inherently high porosity of the PRF scaffolds. A system containing nHA/PLGA/Gel/PRF allowed for a slow and sustained release of PRF-derived growth factors, leading to increased adhesion and the proliferation of MG63 human osteoblasts.

HDPCs treated with mineral trioxide aggregate (MTA) and PRF extracts exhibited a significantly increased expression of dentin sialoprotein and dentin matrix protein-1 along with enhanced ALP activity and mineralization compared to MTA or PRF treatment alone. The MTA and PRF extracts together activated bone morphogenic proteins (BMPs), while the BMP inhibitor LDN193189 diminished dentin sialophosphoprotein and dentin matrix protein-1 expression, ALP activity, and mineralization enhanced by MTA and PRF treatment [83].

In the study by Blatt et al. [22], four different bone substitute materials (allogeneic, alloplastic, and two of xenogeneic origin) were associated with a combination of A-PRF and i-PRF. The addition of PRF increased cell proliferation and migration for all bone substitutes, but only the allogeneic and alloplastic materials significantly increased Runx2 expression in human osteoblasts. On the other hand, bone morphogenic protein was expressed significantly higher when xenogeneic material was combined with PRF, suggesting that the biofunctionalization of bone substitutes with PRF might improve their performance, even for materials of different origins.

4.3. Cell-Type Related Effects of PRF

PRF possesses significant proliferative potential due to its fibrin structure, which contains live leukocytes and activated platelets. This promotes the continuous release of growth factors such as FGFs, PDGFs, TGF-beta1, and VEGFs. These factors act through specific signaling pathways, including MAPK and PI3K/Akt, which modulate gene expression and osteoblast proliferation and survival [94].

Gingival stromal progenitor cells (GSPCs) are a population of mesenchymal stem cells derived from the gingival connective tissue that have been shown to possess multipotent differentiation capacity, including osteogenic, adipogenic, and chondrogenic lineages. The study by Nugraha et al. [67] investigated the effects of PRF on the osteogenic differentiation of GSPCs, identifying a role of the Cbfa1/Sox9 expression ratio in this process, as it positively correlated with the osteogenic markers and the mineralization of GSPCs. Later, another study by this group [69] showed that PRF also increased the expression of aggrecan, a chondrogenic differentiation marker that has a significant role in the early stage of osteogenic differentiation of gingival stem cells, which may contribute to accelerating bone remodeling with an increased expression of alkaline phosphatase and osteocalcin [67,68].

Bone marrow stem cells (BMSCs) are multipotent progenitor cells with regenerative potential for various tissues, including bones [95]. In the selected studies, these cells exhibited increased proliferation when combined with PRF, irrespective of direct or indirect exposure [12,28,30,38,47,60]. These results not only provide evidence for the potential clinical success of PRF but also lay the foundation for its further use in bone tissue engineering. Although BMSCs are widely used in cell therapy, one of the main challenges is ensuring their efficient migration and homing to target tissues following systemic or local administration. The proliferative effects of PRF on BMSCs, combined with their other properties, such as biocompatibility, biodegradability, mechanical strength, porosity, and potential for vascularization [96], could help overcome the limitations of conventional injection-based delivery of BMSC single-cell suspensions and enhance their retention and engraftment in injured tissues. The results by Cheng et al. [25] regarding the exposure of BMSCs to L-PRF also provided some insights into its effects when combined with environmental factors, such as exposure to hydrostatic pressure, a mechanical stimulus that plays an important role in bone formation. In this sense, the co-culture of BMSCs with L-PRF reversed the activation of Wnt/Ca^{2+} signaling in BMSCs under hydrostatic pressure, with an increased expression of chondrogenic differentiation markers, suggesting a modulation of the differentiation pathways by the released growth factors from PRF.

Human adipose stem cells (hASCs) are a type of mesenchymal stem cell (MSC) that can be isolated from adipose tissue and have the potential to differentiate into various cell types, including osteoblasts. This complex process involves multiple factors such as growth factors, signaling pathways, transcription factors, and epigenetic modifications [97]. hASCs are attractive for regenerative medicine applications because they are autologous, abundant, and easily accessible. However, various factors like age, disease, and culture conditions can influence the proliferation and differentiation capacities of hASCs. Consequently, enhancing hASC proliferation is crucial for their clinical use. Human ASCs exhibited increased proliferation when exposed to different concentrations of PRF eluates [54]. Platelet-derived growth factor (PDGF-BB), one of the main growth factors secreted by PRF, has been shown to be a potent mitogen for hASCs [97]. It induces multiple signaling pathways such as ERK1/2, PI3K/Akt, and JNK, which regulate various cellular processes, including cell cycle progression through the expression of cyclins D1 and E. Previous studies have demonstrated that hASC proliferation may be blocked by inhibitors of the PDGF receptor tyrosine kinase, ERK1/2, and Akt, but not by a p38 inhibitor. These results suggest that the proliferation of hASCs through platelet concentrates, like PRF, may be mediated by the PDGF-BB-induced activation of ERK1/2, PI3K/Akt, and JNK signaling pathways.

Apical papilla stem cells (SCAPs) are mesenchymal stem cells found at the root tip of developing teeth. They play a crucial role in root formation and dentin–pulp complex regeneration. SCAPs secrete various bioactive factors that can modulate their microenvironment and influence tissue repair and regeneration [86], including some involved in forming bone-like tissue. The present search revealed that SCAPs exhibited increased proliferation when exposed to PRF eluates [23,37]. These findings are promising for developing stem cell-based bone therapies combining PRF and SCAPs, with the feasibility of transplantation in treating bone defects already demonstrated in animal models.

Another type of mesenchymal stem cell investigated in association with PRF is one that resides in the periodontal ligament, a connective tissue that anchors the tooth to the alveolar bone. Periodontal ligament stem cells (PDLSCs) have demonstrated osteogenic potential, meaning they can differentiate into osteoblasts and produce the bone matrix, playing a vital role in periodontal tissue regeneration and bone repair [98]. These cells exhibited proliferation when co-cultured with PRF [68,80] or after exposure to eluates [70,80]. These effects may contribute to the reported success in improving the regenerative potential and healing of PDL tissues presented by PRF in cases of late dental replantation or intraosseous defects.

Dental pulp stem cells (DPSCs) are also mesenchymal stem cells present in the dental pulp tissue of human teeth and have the potential to differentiate into osteoblasts, odontoblasts, adipocytes, and neural cells. DPSCs have been shown to promote wound healing, bone regeneration, nerve regeneration, and pulp regeneration in animal models and clinical trials. DPSCs offer a promising source of autologous stem cells that can be used for tissue engineering and the cell therapy of dental and oral diseases. In this sense, several selected studies assessed the exposure or association of DPSCs with PRF. Huang et al. [42] showed that L-PRF increases the proliferation and differentiation of human DPSCs [38]. The study by Bagio et al. [19] evidenced that A-PRF induces an increase in the expression of VEGF-A by these cells, which is an important factor in the angiogenesis process in dental pulp regeneration. More recently, Zhang et al. [87] have shown that i-PRF eluates induce a dose-dependent increase in the proliferation of hDPSCs and the expression of osteo-/odontoblastic differentiation markers and key proteins in the Notch signaling. This is a key pathway that regulates the fate and function of DPSCs, modulating the balance between self-renewal and differentiation, along with their angiogenic properties for tissue regeneration and repair. Lo Monaco et al. [61] exploited these effects by proposing the association of DPSCs with L-PRF for the treatment of osteoarthritis, as these cells can undergo chondrogenic differentiation and secrete growth factors associated with tissue repair. Indeed, the association with PRF promoted in vitro chondrogenesis and stimulated the survival of articular chondrocytes.

Osteoblasts are bone-forming cells that secrete extracellular matrix proteins supporting bone tissue formation and mineralization. These cells are derived from various progenitor populations, such as mesenchymal stromal/stem cells (MSCs), with their differentiation influenced by molecular mechanisms including signaling pathways, transcription factors, and epigenetic events [11]. Osteoblasts produce and respond to the main growth factors stimulating bone formation and are typically released by PRF and its derivatives. The present search found evidence that primary human osteoblasts and murine MC3T3-E1 preosteoblasts exhibit strong proliferative responses to PRF [12,22,33,35,43,45,48,49,76,80]. However, it is important to note that human osteosarcoma cell lines SaOS, MG63, and U2OS also showed consistent proliferative behavior after exposure to PRF [17,23,27,29,55,60,61,72,77,83]. This finding warrants further assessment and should be considered by clinicians for its potential risk of stimulating cancer cell growth and dissemination by creating a favorable niche for tumor development.

Due to the good cell response to PRF, some authors proposed the use of this material as a scaffold for bone cell therapy. It includes the proposal by Gassling et al. [35,38] for the use of PRF for periosteal tissue engineering, who reported an increased proliferation of periosteal cells [35] and human osteoblasts [38] over PRF compared to collagen scaffolds (Bio-Gides). As expected, PRF also promoted increased expression of osteogenic markers in osteoblasts compared to commercial collagen scaffolds.

In summary, the in vitro evidence from the selected studies highlights a robust effect on the proliferation of different cell types as an essential aspect of the clinical potential of PRF in treating bone and other mineralized tissues.

4.4. The Molecular Effects of PRF on Differentiation and Mineralization

Bone regeneration is a complex process involving the interaction of cells, growth factors, and the extracellular matrix. Clinical studies have described PRF as effective in oral and maxillofacial bone regeneration, increasing the amount of bone formation following procedures such as sinus floor elevation [99]. The molecular effects of PRF on the differentiation and mineralization of bone cells may involve various intracellular signaling pathways, as evidenced by the selected studies in this review and the summary in Figure 3.

The mitogen-activated protein kinase (MAPK) pathway is a cell signaling route that regulates numerous biological processes, including cell differentiation. Among the MAPKs, ERK1/2 plays a crucial role in osteoblast differentiation by regulating the expression of osteogenesis-related genes [90]. The phosphorylation of ERK was increased by exposure to PRF in the osteosarcoma-derived osteoblast cell line U2OS [23,100]. Consequently, the expression of osteoprotegerin (OPG) was upregulated by PRF, while the expression of the receptor activator of NFkB ligand (RANKL) was not significantly altered. These results suggest that PRF could inhibit osteolytic activity by modulating osteoclastogenesis through the control of the OPG/RANKL ratio in osteoblasts [23,100].

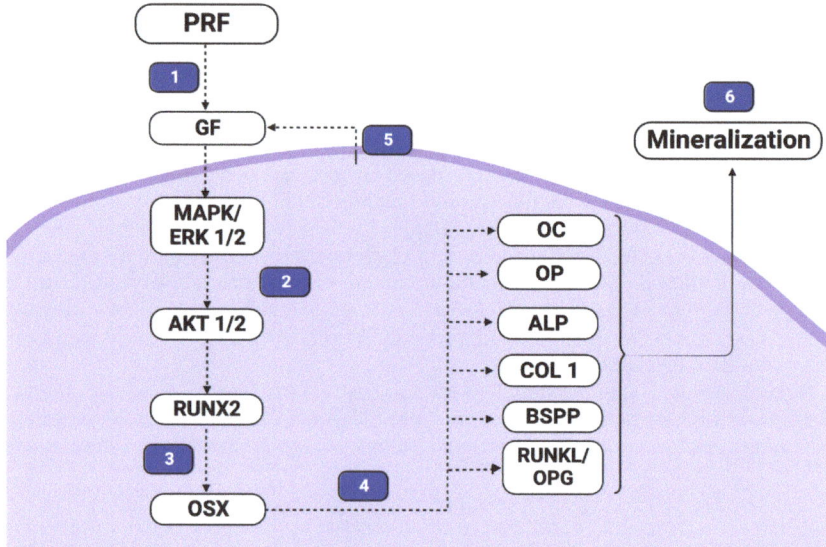

Figure 3. Main biological events involved in the response of mineralizing cells to PRF, according to the literature evidence. Several growth factors and important mediators are released in the medium by PRF (1), many of which are able to activate mitogen-induced signaling pathways (2), which are known to modulate the expression of transcription factors, such as Runx2 and osterix, directly involved on bone cell differentiation (3). These transcription factors are responsible for the altered expression and secretion of different proteins responsible for the formation of the mineralized matrix and the control of osteoclastogenesis (4). Furthermore, exposure to PRF may induce increased secretion of growth factors, such as BMP-2, VEGF, or IGF (5), indicating that exposed cells may also be activated by paracrine regulation in response to PRF. All of these processes result in increased nodule formation and, therefore, biological mineralization (6). In the figure, an arrow indicates activation/stimulation, while a perpendicular bar indicates inhibition/suppression.

The Runt-related transcription factor 2 (Runx2) is a key transcription factor that regulates the expression of genes involved in osteoblast differentiation and function. Research has demonstrated that various members of the MAPK family, including ERK1/2 and p38, can phosphorylate Runx2 at specific serine residues, enhancing its transcriptional activity and promoting osteogenic gene expression [101]. As a result, ERK1/2 and Runx2 are connected by a positive feedback loop that stimulates osteoblast differentiation and bone formation. In selected studies, a significant increase in the expression and/or phosphorylation of Runx2 was detected after exposure to platelet-rich fibrin (PRF) in different cell types [30,51–53,66,74,86]. The studies by Wang et al. [80,81] confirmed, with both human bone marrow and rabbit mesenchymal stem cells, that exposure to PRF preparations increases proliferation, the expression of osteogenic markers, and in vitro mineralization concomitant to the upregulation of the ERK 1/2 signaling pathway.

Additional evidence of these regulatory pathways comes from investigations of osterix (Osx), a zinc-finger transcription factor essential for osteoblast differentiation and bone formation in bone homeostasis [102]. Osx is a downstream target of Runx2 and regulates several target genes involved in osteoblast differentiation, such as Col5a1, Col5a3, and connexin43 (Cx43). Osx is controlled by multiple signaling pathways, including BMP, Wnt, FGF, and ERK1/2, which modulate its transcriptional activity and stability [103].

Data from a study by Li et al. [56] suggest that osterix levels significantly increase in periodontal ligament stem cells treated with PRF and IGF-1 at 14 days compared to the control group ($p < 0.01$). Furthermore, by the third day of exposure, the expression of genes controlled by Osx was upregulated in the PRF-exposed group. These findings imply that these transcription factors contribute to the stimulation of osteoblast differentiation by PRF, potentially through the activation of MAPKs in response to growth factors released by this autologous biomaterial.

The overexpression of Osx and Runx2 after exposure to PRF could potentially impact several essential proteins for osteoblast maturation and mineralization, whose expression is regulated by these factors, including collagen type-I a1 (Col1a1), osteonectin, osteopontin, bone sialoprotein, and osteocalcin. Osteocalcin is responsible for fixing calcium and hydroxyapatite in the extracellular matrix, contributing to the effective mineralization that occurs in bone tissue [104]. Molecular analyses through real-time PCR have shown a significant increase in RNA expression for osteocalcin in various mineralizing cells exposed to PRF [26,43,63,68,73,79]. These findings were reinforced by a functional assessment by western blotting, indicating increased levels of this protein in periodontal ligament stem cells, which is associated with increased bone formation in a rat in vivo model [30].

Different studies have reported that PRF also induces increased expression of dentin sialoprotein (DSP) and dentin sialophosphoprotein (DSPP) [24,77], which are enhanced in the presence of lipopolysaccharide [47]. The results by Hong et al. [41] suggest that this effect is dependent on the duration of exposure, as the expression level of DSPP was downregulated after incubation in PRF for 7 days and then significantly increased after 14 days of incubation. Bone sialoprotein (BSP) is also reported to increase when cells are exposed to PRF, primarily around 14 to 21 days [24,30,39,43,63]. Only human periodontal ligament stem cells had DSPP downregulated when co-cultured with PRF over extended experimental periods [81]. These results are important since this non-collagenous protein plays a crucial role in the biomineralization of hard tissues, such as bones and teeth, inducing the formation and growth of hydroxyapatite crystals in the extracellular matrix [104].

Osteopontin is another phosphorylated glycoprotein secreted into the mineralizing extracellular matrix by osteoblasts during bone development. Although osteopontin is an osteogenic marker that does not affect the cellular development of osteoblasts in vitro, it impacts the mineralization of bone tissue [105]. Various studies have shown that this osteogenic marker is present and highly expressed after exposure to PRF in osteoblasts [20], dental pulp cells [79], and mesenchymal stem cells (MSCs) [73]. Real-time PCR revealed that bone marrow-derived mesenchymal stem cells (BMSCs) cultured on printed BCP/PVA/PRF scaffolds expressed significantly higher levels of osteopontin on days 7 and 14 compared to those cultured on other scaffolds ($p < 0.05$) [66]. Verboket et al. [66] observed a higher expression in bone marrow cells exposed to a medium and low RCF PRF, indicating that these protocols did not affect the expected effects of the material on the expression of matrix proteins.

The increase in collagen gene expression induced by PRF was reported in several studies [27,69,75,78,79], typically around the 14th to the 21st day of exposure. Zhao et al. [88] observed slight upregulation by PRF in a dose-dependent manner after 14 or 21 days of culture ($p < 0.01$). In contrast, Ji B et al. [45] and Verboket et al. [77] did not observe a significant difference in the expression of Col-III, the primary type of collagen in bones, between the control group and the test group.

ICAM-1 (intercellular adhesion molecule 1) is a protein that mediates cell–cell interactions and plays a role in inflammation and immune responses. ICAM-1 is expressed by various cell types, including osteoblasts, and it may have different effects depending on the context [98]. In healthy individuals, ICAM-1 may facilitate osteoblast contact with lymphocytes, enhancing mineralization and bone formation through the downregulation of TGF-β1 (transforming growth factor beta 1), a negative regulator of osteogenesis. In pathological conditions, such as osteoarthritis and osteoporosis, ICAM-1 expression by osteoblasts may be increased by proinflammatory cytokines and contribute to bone resorption and loss of bone mass. ICAM-1-positive osteoblasts can adhere to osteoclast precursors and stimulate their differentiation and activation through the osteoclastogenic factor RANKL [106]. Moreover, ICAM-1-positive osteoblasts may have impaired proliferation and differentiation potential due to cell cycle arrest [99]. When exposed to both regular and low-speed PRF, Kang et al. [46] and Verboket et al. [77], respectively, observed a high expression of ICAM-1 in mesenchymal stem cells, including in the presence of lipopolysaccharide to stimulate inflammation. On the other hand, Dohle et al. [29] reported that PRF appears to have no effect on the expression of the ICAM-1 protein by exposed primary human osteoblasts. This is an important finding since PRF is described as releasing considerable amounts of proinflammatory cytokines [13,107].

Alkaline phosphatase (ALP) is located on the outer surface of the cell membrane of osteoblasts. ALP is an early marker of osteoblast differentiation that indicates the transition of osteoprogenitor stem cells to immature preosteoblasts [102]. It plays an essential role in osteoid formation and mineralization and is recognized as a nonspecific marker of bone formation and osteoblast activity. ALP also regulates RUNX2, a master transcription factor in osteoblasts, through a positive feedback loop that modulates osteoblast differentiation. The present review identified several different studies assessing the effects of exposure to PRF on the expression of ALP, with increased levels evidenced from 14 to 21 days of culture [25,26,29,39,52,56,64,83,85]. The study by Woo et al. [83] observed that the effects of PRF associated with MTA on ALP and the in vitro mineralization of human dental pulp cells were impaired by pretreatment with a BMP inhibitor (LDN193189), indicating the participation of specific growth factors in the effects of PRF on ALP.

Osteoblast and bone cell activity are regulated by various growth factors, many of which are released by platelet-rich fibrin (PRF) membranes. Examples of these growth factors include transforming growth factor-beta (TGF-beta) and fibroblast growth factors (FGFs). Osteoblasts themselves can produce and release growth factors that regulate the differentiation and activity of other bone cells, such as osteoclasts and osteocytes. These factors include RANKL/OPG, M-CSF, VEGFs, PDGFs, and BMPs [12]. These growth factors can act in paracrine or endocrine manners, influencing bone and systemic metabolism by promoting or inhibiting the differentiation and function of various bone cells. When exposed to PRF, osteoblasts engage in a complex cellular communication system involving both the exposure and secretion of growth factors that impact bone tissue, as evidenced by selected studies.

TGF-beta, a member of the TGF-beta superfamily of cytokines, regulates numerous cellular processes such as proliferation, differentiation, migration, and apoptosis. TGF-beta plays a significant role in bone formation and remodeling by influencing the balance between bone-forming cells (osteoblasts) and bone-resorbing cells (osteoclasts) [108]. TGF-beta stimulates osteoblastic differentiation and activity by activating canonical and non-canonical signaling pathways and increasing the expression of osteogenic genes like Runx2, osterix, and collagen I in osteoblasts. Conversely, TGF-beta inhibits osteoclastogenesis and osteoclastic activity by modulating the interaction between osteoblasts and osteoclasts through OPG/RANKL, BMPs, and Wnt proteins, thereby affecting both aspects of the bone remodeling cycle.

Studies have shown that osteoblasts exposed to PRF demonstrate increased production of TGF-beta1. For instance, Saos-2 osteosarcoma-derived osteoblasts exposed to PRF exhibited significantly higher TGF-beta1 production [105]. Rat calvaria osteoblasts exposed to PRF showed a time-dependent increase in TGF-beta1 production [48]. Human alveolar bone marrow stem cells treated with PRF extracts exhibited increased TGF-beta1 levels at 24 h [46]. A study by Kim et al. [49] compared the release of TGF-beta1 associated with PRF in osteoblast cultures exposed to PRF membranes produced by different protocols. The results indicated that the secreted levels of the growth factor were significantly higher in low-RCF PRF than in medium-RCF PRF ($p < 0.05$) [76]. However, lyophilized PRF samples only slightly increased the release rate of TGF-beta1 in another osteosarcoma cell line, MG63 [85].

Bone morphogenetic protein 2 (BMP-2) is a multifunctional protein belonging to the TGF-beta superfamily. It plays a crucial role in bone formation by stimulating the differentiation of mesenchymal stem cells (MSCs) into osteoblasts. Osteoblasts and osteocytes constitutively secrete BMP-2, which has been used as a therapy for bone fractures and diseases, such as osteoporosis, due to its osteogenic potential [14]. Rabbit mesenchymal stem cells exposed to PRF demonstrated a significant upregulation of BMP-2 mRNA expression, reaching levels that stimulate in vitro osteogenic differentiation [96]. Combining 1 mg/mL MTA with 1.25% PRF extracts increased BMP-2 expression in human dental pulp cells compared to PRF extracts alone, while MTA treatment alone showed no release [83]. BMP-2 expression was also higher in the co-cultures of i-PRF and primary osteoblasts [29].

Saos-2 cells exposed to PRF exhibited noticeably higher peaks of insulin-like growth factor-1 (IGF-1), especially compared to fibroblast cultures [105]. Human alveolar bone marrow stem cells exposed to PRF extracts showed a high expression of IGF-1 [107], similar to MG63 osteosarcoma cells and primary osteoblasts [66,76]. These findings are significant since IGF-1 plays a crucial role in regulating osteoblast function and development [108]. IGF-1 initiates a complex signaling pathway involving the PI3-K/PDK-1/Akt and Ras/Raf/MAPK pathways, which stimulate cell function and/or survival. IGF-1 also influences osteoclastogenesis by regulating RANKL and RANK expression.

The available data suggest that most of PRF's effects on bone and mineralizing cells may be attributed to the release of specific biological mediators that activate signaling pathways related to cell proliferation, survival, and differentiation. Investigating the release of growth factors, cytokines, and chemokines by PRF membranes could help understand these effects. However, only a few selected studies have detected such release in their in vitro assessments. Zhao Y-H et al. [88] observed a time-dependent decrease in VEGFs, IGF-1, and EGF release from PRF membranes within five days. In contrast, Dohle et al. [29] found the highest concentration of VEGFs in osteoblast supernatants mixed with PRF cultured for seven days, confirmed by relative gene expression of VEGFs after 24 h of osteoblast monocultures. Isobe et al. [44] observed that PDGF-BB concentration was significantly reduced in extracts from PRF membranes made from stored blood compared to fresh samples, indicating a potential drawback of long storage. Zheng et al. [89] observed a sustained release of PDGF, IGF-I, and TGF-B1 for up to four weeks when combining nHA/PLGA/gel with lyophilized PRF, which positively affected MG63 cell mineralization. Studies evaluating platelet-derived growth factor (PDGF AA, AB, or BB) reported variations in the day of the highest in vitro release [27,38,43], ranging from the 1st to the 14th days of exposure. This suggests that the choice of extraction time may impact the observed effects of PRF treatment.

5. Final Considerations

Due to the considerable relevance of the theme for regenerative medicine and dentistry, several narrative and systematic reviews have been published issuing the clinical and biological effects of PRF. Many of these reviews are focused on the level of evidence supporting the use of PRF in regenerative dentistry and oral and maxillofacial surgery by assessing randomized clinical trials [2], including data indicating that PRF significantly improves bone tissue regeneration [109,110], regardless of recent reviews on preclinical studies that failed to identify such effects on animal models [111]. Despite any clinical controversies, only a few literature reviews visited the molecular and cellular evidence of PRF effects and are usually restricted to smaller groups of in vitro studies focusing on specific protocols, such as i-PRF [112]. An exception is the interesting review by Strauss et al. [113], who assessed in vitro evidence of the biological effects of PRF in cells from different tissues published up to 2018. However, unlike the present review, that study was not focused on bone and mineralized tissues and had a limited reach, as it was based on data retrieved from a single database (Medline). Therefore, more than an update on the literature, the present scoping review represents the most comprehensive mapping of the available evidence supporting the molecular mechanisms that set the basis of the PRF effects in the behavior of the cells of bones and mineralized tissues.

While this approach provided valuable insights, it also introduced some limitations. By focusing exclusively on PRF, we ensured the feasibility and comparability of this review but may have overlooked data on other similar platelet aggregates or protocols, such as Concentrated Growth Factors (CGFs). Additionally, the scope of this review may be limited by the interpretation or reporting of the data, as some studies may have omitted important information necessary for a comprehensive understanding of the results. Nevertheless, it is possible to state, through the raised data, that the literature consistently provides in vitro evidence that PRF, produced by different protocols or in combination with other biomaterials, influences the proliferation, differentiation, and mineralization of cells from bone and mineralized tissue. These effects involve well-known pathways of cell survival, the activation of transcription factors (Runx2, OSX), and the increased expression of various proteins, including osteopontin, osteocalcin, collagen, ALP, BSPs, RANKL/OPG, and growth factors like TGF-beta, PDGF, and BMP2. Different studies have associated these effects with specific growth factors released by PRF, suggesting that this is an important factor to consider in the development and improvement of these autologous biomaterials for the treatment of mineralized tissues, such as bones.

PRF is widely used in regenerative medicine and dentistry, and in vitro models represent only a small aspect of wound healing and bone regeneration. As such, it is not possible to guarantee that the reported results can be directly extrapolated to clinical settings. On the other hand, improved in vitro proliferation, differentiation, and mineralization of osteoblasts may represent interesting evidence in support of enhanced regenerative activity, osteoinductive properties, or enhanced osseointegration. Therefore, by gathering and analyzing information related to PRF and mineralizing cells, we can gain a better understanding of the mechanisms behind PRF's impact on bone regeneration and optimize its properties and applications. This includes determining optimal concentrations, exploring associations with other bone graft materials or drugs, and developing new production protocols to improve clinical outcomes of this promising autologous material.

Author Contributions: Conceptualization, C.F.M. and G.G.A.; methodology, R.d.L.B., C.F.M. and G.G.A., formal analysis, R.d.L.B., C.F.M. and G.G.A.; investigation, R.d.L.B., E.S.L., J.V.d.A.d.S. and N.R.S.R.; writing—original draft preparation, R.d.L.B., E.S.L. and G.G.A.; writing—review and editing, C.F.M. and G.G.A.; supervision, C.F.M. and G.G.A. All authors have read and agreed to the published version of the manuscript.

Funding: This research received no external funding.

Institutional Review Board Statement: Not applicable.

Informed Consent Statement: Not applicable.

Data Availability Statement: No new data were created.

Acknowledgments: The authors wish to express their gratitude for the financial support provided to PPBi by CAPES, CNPq, and FAPERJ. Additionally, we would like to extend our thanks to Suelen Sartoretto for her assistance with the illustrations.

Conflicts of Interest: The authors declare no conflict of interest.

References

1. Dimitriou, R.; Jones, E.; McGonagle, D.; Giannoudis, P.V. Bone regeneration: Current concepts and future directions. *BMC Med.* **2011**, *9*, 66. [CrossRef]
2. Miron, R.J.; Zucchelli, G.; Pikos, M.A.; Salama, M.; Lee, S.; Guillemette, V.; Fujioka-Kobayashi, M.; Bishara, M.; Zhang, Y.; Wang, H.L.; et al. Use of platelet-rich fibrin in regenerative dentistry: A systematic review. *Clin. Oral Investig.* **2017**, *21*, 1913–1927. [CrossRef] [PubMed]

3. Choukroun, J.; Diss, A.; Simonpieri, A.; Girard, M.-O.; Schoeffler, C.; Dohan, S.L.; Dohan, A.J.; Mouhyi, J.; Dohan, D.M. Platelet-rich fibrin (PRF): A second-generation platelet concentrate. Part IV: Clinical effects on tissue healing. *Oral Surg. Oral Med. Oral Pathol. Oral Radiol. Endod.* **2006**, *101*, e56–e60. [CrossRef] [PubMed]
4. Choukroun, J.; Diss, A.; Simonpieri, A.; Girard, M.-O.; Schoeffler, C.; Dohan, S.L.; Dohan, A.J.; Mouhyi, J.; Dohan, D.M. Platelet-rich fibrin (PRF): A second-generation platelet concentrate. Part V: Histologic evaluations of PRF effects on bone allograft maturation in sinus lift. *Oral Surg. Oral Med. Oral Pathol. Oral Radiol. Endod.* **2006**, *101*, 299–303. [CrossRef]
5. Dohan, D.M.; Choukroun, J.; Diss, A.; Dohan, S.L.; Dohan, A.J.; Mouhyi, J.; Gogly, B. Platelet-rich fibrin (PRF): A second-generation platelet concentrate. Part III: Leucocyte activation: A new feature for platelet concentrates? *Oral Surg. Oral Med. Oral Pathol. Oral Radiol. Endod.* **2006**, *101*, e51–e55. [CrossRef]
6. Dohan, D.M.; Choukroun, J.; Diss, A.; Dohan, S.L.; Dohan, A.J.; Mouhyi, J.; Gogly, B. Platelet-rich fibrin (PRF): A second-generation platelet concentrate. Part I: Technological concepts and evolution. *Oral Surg. Oral Med. Oral Pathol. Oral Radiol. Endod.* **2006**, *101*, e37–e44. [CrossRef] [PubMed]
7. Wong, C.C.; Yeh, Y.Y.; Chen, C.H.; Manga, Y.B.; Jheng, P.R.; Lu, C.X.; Chuang, E.Y. Effectiveness of treating segmental bone defects with a synergistic co-delivery approach with platelet-rich fibrin and tricalcium phosphate. *Mater. Sci. Eng. C Mater. Biol. Appl.* **2021**, *129*, 112364. [CrossRef] [PubMed]
8. Borie, E.; Olivi, D.G.; Orsi, I.A.; Garlet, K.; Weber, B.; Beltrán, V.; Fuentes, R. Platelet-rich fibrin application in dentistry: A literature review. *Int. J. Clin. Exp. Med.* **2015**, *8*, 7922.
9. Patel, G.K.; Gaekwad, S.S.; Gujjari, S.K.; SC, V.K. Platelet-Rich Fibrin in Regeneration of Intrabony Defects: A Randomized Controlled Trial. *J. Periodontol.* **2017**, *88*, 1192–1199. [CrossRef]
10. Shivashankar, V.Y.; Johns, D.A.; Vidyanath, S.; Sam, G. Combination of platelet rich fibrin, hydroxyapatite and PRF membrane in the management of large inflammatory periapical lesion. *J. Conserv. Dent. JCD* **2013**, *16*, 261–264. [CrossRef]
11. Chen, Q.; Shou, P.; Zheng, C.; Jiang, M.; Cao, G.; Yang, Q.; Cao, J.; Xie, N.; Velletri, T.; Zhang, X. Fate decision of mesenchymal stem cells: Adipocytes or osteoblasts? *Cell Death Differ.* **2016**, *23*, 1128–1139. [CrossRef] [PubMed]
12. Han, Y.; You, X.; Xing, W.; Zhang, Z.; Zou, W. Paracrine and endocrine actions of bone—The functions of secretory proteins from osteoblasts, osteocytes, and osteoclasts. *Bone Res.* **2018**, *6*, 16. [CrossRef] [PubMed]
13. Lourenço, E.S.; Mourão, C.; Leite, P.E.C.; Granjeiro, J.M.; Calasans-Maia, M.D.; Alves, G.G. The in vitro release of cytokines and growth factors from fibrin membranes produced through horizontal centrifugation. *J. Biomed. Mater. Res. Part A* **2018**, *106*, 1373–1380. [CrossRef] [PubMed]
14. Zou, M.L.; Chen, Z.H.; Teng, Y.Y.; Liu, S.Y.; Jia, Y.; Zhang, K.W.; Sun, Z.L.; Wu, J.J.; Yuan, Z.D.; Feng, Y.; et al. The Smad Dependent TGF-β and BMP Signaling Pathway in Bone Remodeling and Therapies. *Front. Mol. Biosci.* **2021**, *8*, 593310. [CrossRef]
15. McGowan, J.; Straus, S.; Moher, D.; Langlois, E.V.; O'Brien, K.K.; Horsley, T.; Aldcroft, A.; Zarin, W.; Garitty, C.M.; Hempel, S.; et al. Reporting scoping reviews-PRISMA ScR extension. *J. Clin. Epidemiol.* **2020**, *123*, 177–179. [CrossRef]
16. Schneider, K.; Schwarz, M.; Burkholder, I.; Kopp-Schneider, A.; Edler, L.; Kinsner-Ovaskainen, A.; Hartung, T.; Hoffmann, S. "ToxRTool", a new tool to assess the reliability of toxicological data. *Toxicol. Lett.* **2009**, *189*, 138–144. [CrossRef] [PubMed]
17. Al-Maawi, S.; Dohle, E.; Lim, J.; Weigl, P.; Teoh, S.H.; Sader, R.; Ghanaati, S. Biologization of Pcl-mesh using platelet rich fibrin (Prf) enhances its regenerative potential in vitro. *Int. J. Mol. Sci.* **2021**, *22*, 2159. [CrossRef]
18. Al-Maawi, S.; Dohle, E.; Kretschmer, W.; Rutkowski, J.; Sader, R.; Ghanaati, S. A standardized g-force allows the preparation of similar platelet-rich fibrin qualities regardless of rotor angle. *Tissue Eng. Part A* **2022**, *28*, 353–365. [CrossRef]
19. Bagio, D.A.; Julianto, I.; Margono, A.; Suprastiwi, E. Increased VEGF-A Expression of Human Dental Pulp Stem Cells (hDPSCs) Cultured with Advanced Platelet Rich Fibrin (A-PRF). *Open Dent. J.* **2021**, *15*. [CrossRef]
20. Banyatworakul, P.; Osathanon, T.; Chumprasert, S.; Pavasant, P.; Pirarat, N. Responses of canine periodontal ligament cells to bubaline blood derived platelet rich fibrin in vitro. *Sci. Rep.* **2021**, *11*, 11409. [CrossRef]
21. Bi, J.; Liu, Y.; Liu, X.-M.; Lei, S.; Chen, X. Platelet-rich Fibrin Improves the Osteo-/Odontogenic Differentiation of Stem Cells from Apical Papilla via the Extracellular Signal–regulated Protein Kinase Signaling Pathway. *J. Endod.* **2020**, *46*, 648–654. [CrossRef] [PubMed]
22. Blatt, S.; Thiem, D.G.; Kyyak, S.; Pabst, A.; Al-Nawas, B.; Kämmerer, P.W. Possible implications for improved osteogenesis? The combination of platelet-rich fibrin with different bone substitute materials. *Front. Bioeng. Biotechnol.* **2021**, *9*, 640053. [CrossRef]
23. Chang, I.C.; Tsai, C.H.; Chang, Y.C. Platelet-rich fibrin modulates the expression of extracellular signal-regulated protein kinase and osteoprotegerin in human osteoblasts. *J. Biomed. Mater. Res. Part A* **2010**, *95*, 327–332. [CrossRef] [PubMed]
24. Chen, Y.-J.; Zhao, Y.-H.; Zhao, Y.-J.; Liu, N.-X.; Lv, X.; Li, Q.; Chen, F.-M.; Zhang, M. Potential dental pulp revascularization and odonto-/osteogenic capacity of a novel transplant combined with dental pulp stem cells and platelet-rich fibrin. *Cell Tissue Res.* **2015**, *361*, 439–455. [CrossRef] [PubMed]
25. Cheng, B.; Feng, F.; Shi, F.; Huang, J.; Zhang, S.; Quan, Y.; Tu, T.; Liu, Y.; Wang, J.; Zhao, Y. Distinctive roles of Wnt signaling in chondrogenic differentiation of BMSCs under coupling of pressure and platelet-rich fibrin. *Tissue Eng. Regen. Med.* **2022**, *19*, 823–837. [CrossRef]
26. Chi, H.; Song, X.; Song, C.; Zhao, W.; Chen, G.; Jiang, A.; Wang, X.; Yu, T.; Zheng, L.; Yan, J. Chitosan-gelatin scaffolds incorporating decellularized platelet-rich fibrin promote bone regeneration. *ACS Biomater. Sci. Eng.* **2019**, *5*, 5305–5315. [CrossRef]

27. Clipet, F.; Tricot, S.; Alno, N.; Massot, M.; Solhi, H.; Cathelineau, G.; Perez, F.; De Mello, G.; Pellen-Mussi, P. In vitro effects of Choukroun's platelet-rich fibrin conditioned medium on 3 different cell lines implicated in dental implantology. *Implant. Dent.* **2012**, *21*, 51–56. [CrossRef]
28. Ehrenfest, D.M.D.; Doglioli, P.; de Peppo, G.M.; Del Corso, M.; Charrier, J.-B. Choukroun's platelet-rich fibrin (PRF) stimulates in vitro proliferation and differentiation of human oral bone mesenchymal stem cell in a dose-dependent way. *Arch. Oral Biol.* **2010**, *55*, 185–194. [CrossRef]
29. Dohle, E.; El Bagdadi, K.; Sader, R.; Choukroun, J.; James Kirkpatrick, C.; Ghanaati, S. Platelet-rich fibrin-based matrices to improve angiogenesis in an in vitro co-culture model for bone tissue engineering. *J. Tissue Eng. Regen. Med.* **2018**, *12*, 598–610. [CrossRef]
30. Douglas, T.E.; Gassling, V.; Declercq, H.A.; Purcz, N.; Pamula, E.; Haugen, H.J.; Chasan, S.; de Mulder, E.L.; Jansen, J.A.; Leeuwenburgh, S.C. Enzymatically induced mineralization of platelet-rich fibrin. *J. Biomed. Mater. Res. Part A* **2012**, *100*, 1335–1346. [CrossRef]
31. Duan, X.; Lin, Z.; Lin, X.; Wang, Z.; Wu, Y.; Ji, M.; Lu, W.; Wang, X.; Zhang, D. Study of platelet-rich fibrin combined with rat periodontal ligament stem cells in periodontal tissue regeneration. *J. Cell. Mol. Med.* **2018**, *22*, 1047–1055. [CrossRef] [PubMed]
32. Ehrenfest, D.M.D.; Diss, A.; Odin, G.; Doglioli, P.; Hippolyte, M.-P.; Charrier, J.-B. In vitro effects of Choukroun's PRF (platelet-rich fibrin) on human gingival fibroblasts, dermal prekeratinocytes, preadipocytes, and maxillofacial osteoblasts in primary cultures. *Oral Surg. Oral Med. Oral Pathol. Oral Radiol. Endod.* **2009**, *108*, 341–352. [CrossRef] [PubMed]
33. Esmaeilnejad, A.; Ardakani, M.T.; Shokri, M.; Khou, N.H.; Kamani, M. Comparative evaluation of the effect of two platelet concentrates (a-PRF and L-PRF) on the cellular activity of pre-osteoblastic MG-63 cell line: An in vitro study. *J. Dent.* **2023**, *24*, 235.
34. Fernández-Medina, T.; Vaquette, C.; Ivanovski, S. Systematic comparison of the effect of four clinical-grade platelet rich hemoderivatives on osteoblast behaviour. *Int. J. Mol. Sci.* **2019**, *20*, 6243. [CrossRef] [PubMed]
35. Gassling, V.L.; Açil, Y.; Springer, I.N.; Hubert, N.; Wiltfang, J. Platelet-rich plasma and platelet-rich fibrin in human cell culture. *Oral Surg. Oral Med. Oral Pathol. Oral Radiol. Endod.* **2009**, *108*, 48–55. [CrossRef]
36. Gassling, V.; Douglas, T.; Warnke, P.H.; Açil, Y.; Wiltfang, J.; Becker, S.T. Platelet-rich fibrin membranes as scaffolds for periosteal tissue engineering. *Clin. Oral Implant. Res.* **2010**, *21*, 543–549. [CrossRef]
37. Gassling, V.; Douglas, T.E.; Purcz, N.; Schaubroeck, D.; Balcaen, L.; Bliznuk, V.; Declercq, H.A.; Vanhaecke, F.; Dubruel, P. Magnesium-enhanced enzymatically mineralized platelet-rich fibrin for bone regeneration applications. *Biomed. Mater.* **2013**, *8*, 055001. [CrossRef]
38. Gassling, V.; Hedderich, J.; Açil, Y.; Purcz, N.; Wiltfang, J.; Douglas, T. Comparison of platelet rich fibrin and collagen as osteoblast-seeded scaffolds for bone tissue engineering applications. *Clin. Oral Implant. Res.* **2013**, *24*, 320–328. [CrossRef]
39. Girija, K.; Kavitha, M. Comparative evaluation of platelet-rich fibrin, platelet-rich fibrin+ 50 wt% nanohydroxyapatite, platelet-rich fibrin+ 50 wt% dentin chips on odontoblastic differentiation-An in vitro study-part 2. *J. Conserv. Dent. JCD* **2020**, *23*, 354. [CrossRef]
40. He, L.; Lin, Y.; Hu, X.; Zhang, Y.; Wu, H. A comparative study of platelet-rich fibrin (PRF) and platelet-rich plasma (PRP) on the effect of proliferation and differentiation of rat osteoblasts in vitro. *Oral Surg. Oral Med. Oral Pathol. Oral Radiol. Endod.* **2009**, *108*, 707–713. [CrossRef]
41. Hong, S.; Chen, W.; Jiang, B. A Comparative Evaluation of Concentrated Growth Factor and Platelet-rich Fibrin on the Proliferation, Migration, and Differentiation of Human Stem Cells of the Apical Papilla. *J. Endod.* **2018**, *44*, 977–983. [CrossRef] [PubMed]
42. Huang, F.M.; Yang, S.F.; Zhao, J.H.; Chang, Y.C. Platelet-rich fibrin increases proliferation and differentiation of human dental pulp cells. *J. Endod.* **2010**, *36*, 1628–1632. [CrossRef] [PubMed]
43. Irastorza, I.; Luzuriaga, J.; Martinez-Conde, R.; Ibarretxe, G.; Unda, F. Adhesion, integration and osteogenesis of human dental pulp stem cells on biomimetic implant surfaces combined with plasma derived products. *Eur. Cells Mater.* **2019**, *38*, 201–214. [CrossRef]
44. Isobe, K.; Suzuki, M.; Watanabe, T.; Kitamura, Y.; Suzuki, T.; Kawabata, H.; Nakamura, M.; Okudera, T.; Okudera, H.; Uematsu, K.; et al. Platelet-rich fibrin prepared from stored whole-blood samples. *Int. J. Implant Dent.* **2017**, *3*, 6. [CrossRef]
45. Ji, B.; Sheng, L.; Chen, G.; Guo, S.; Xie, L.; Yang, B.; Guo, W.; Tian, W. The combination use of platelet-rich fibrin and treated dentin matrix for tooth root regeneration by cell homing. *Tissue Eng. Part A* **2015**, *21*, 26–34. [CrossRef] [PubMed]
46. Kang, Y.H.; Jeon, S.H.; Park, J.Y.; Chung, J.H.; Choung, Y.H.; Choung, H.W.; Kim, E.S.; Choung, P.H. Platelet-rich fibrin is a Bioscaffold and reservoir of growth factors for tissue regeneration. *Tissue Eng. Part A* **2011**, *17*, 349–359. [CrossRef]
47. Kardos, D.; Hornyák, I.; Simon, M.; Hinsenkamp, A.; Marschall, B.; Várdai, R.; Kállay-Menyhárd, A.; Pinke, B.; Mészáros, L.; Kuten, O.; et al. Biological and Mechanical Properties of Platelet-Rich Fibrin Membranes after Thermal Manipulation and Preparation in a Single-Syringe Closed System. *Int. J. Mol. Sci.* **2018**, *19*, 3433. [CrossRef]
48. Kim, J.; Ha, Y.; Kang, N.H. Effects of Growth Factors From Platelet-Rich Fibrin on the Bone Regeneration. *J. Craniofacial Surg.* **2017**, *28*, 860–865. [CrossRef]
49. Kim, J.H.; Woo, S.M.; Choi, N.K.; Kim, W.J.; Kim, S.M.; Jung, J.Y. Effect of Platelet-rich Fibrin on Odontoblastic Differentiation in Human Dental Pulp Cells Exposed to Lipopolysaccharide. *J. Endod.* **2017**, *43*, 433–438. [CrossRef]
50. Kosmidis, K.; Ehsan, K.; Pitzurra, L.; Loos, B.; Jansen, I. An in vitro study into three different PRF preparations for osteogenesis potential. *J. Periodontal Res.* **2023**, *58*, 483–492. [CrossRef]

51. Koyanagi, M.; Fujioka-Kobayashi, M.; Yoneyama, Y.; Inada, R.; Satomi, T. Regenerative Potential of Solid Bone Marrow Aspirate Concentrate Compared with Platelet-Rich Fibrin. *Tissue Eng. Part A* **2022**, *28*, 749–759. [CrossRef] [PubMed]
52. Kyyak, S.; Blatt, S.; Pabst, A.; Thiem, D.; Al-Nawas, B.; Kämmerer, P.W. Combination of an allogenic and a xenogenic bone substitute material with injectable platelet-rich fibrin—A comparative in vitro study. *J. Biomater. Appl.* **2020**, *35*, 83–96. [CrossRef] [PubMed]
53. Kyyak, S.; Blatt, S.; Schiegnitz, E.; Heimes, D.; Staedt, H.; Thiem, D.G.E.; Sagheb, K.; Al-Nawas, B.; Kämmerer, P.W. Activation of Human Osteoblasts via Different Bovine Bone Substitute Materials With and Without Injectable Platelet Rich Fibrin in vitro. *Front. Bioeng. Biotechnol.* **2021**, *9*, 599224. [CrossRef]
54. Li, Q.; Pan, S.; Dangaria, S.J.; Gopinathan, G.; Kolokythas, A.; Chu, S.; Geng, Y.; Zhou, Y.; Luan, X. Platelet-rich fibrin promotes periodontal regeneration and enhances alveolar bone augmentation. *BioMed Res. Int.* **2013**, *2013*, 638043. [CrossRef]
55. Li, Q.; Reed, D.A.; Min, L.; Gopinathan, G.; Li, S.; Dangaria, S.J.; Li, L.; Geng, Y.; Galang, M.T.; Gajendrareddy, P.; et al. Lyophilized platelet-rich fibrin (PRF) promotes craniofacial bone regeneration through Runx2. *Int. J. Mol. Sci.* **2014**, *15*, 8509–8525. [CrossRef] [PubMed]
56. Li, X.; Yang, H.; Zhang, Z.; Yan, Z.; Lv, H.; Zhang, Y.; Wu, B. Platelet-rich fibrin exudate promotes the proliferation and osteogenic differentiation of human periodontal ligament cells in vitro. *Mol. Med. Rep.* **2018**, *18*, 4477–4485. [CrossRef] [PubMed]
57. Li, X.; Yao, J.; Wu, J.; Du, X.; Jing, W.; Liu, L. Roles of PRF and IGF-1 in promoting alveolar osteoblast growth and proliferation and molecular mechanism. *Int. J. Clin. Exp. Pathol.* **2018**, *11*, 3294–3301.
58. Liang, Z.; Huang, D.; Nong, W.; Mo, J.; Zhu, D.; Wang, M.; Chen, M.; Wei, C.; Li, H. Advanced-platelet-rich fibrin extract promotes adipogenic and osteogenic differentiation of human adipose-derived stem cells in a dose-dependent manner in vitro. *Tissue Cell* **2021**, *71*, 101506. [CrossRef]
59. Liu, Z.; Jin, H.; Xie, Q.; Jiang, Z.; Guo, S.; Li, Y.; Zhang, B. Controlled Release Strategies for the Combination of Fresh and Lyophilized Platelet-Rich Fibrin on Bone Tissue Regeneration. *BioMed Res. Int.* **2019**, *2019*, 4923767. [CrossRef] [PubMed]
60. Liu, X.; Yin, M.; Li, Y.; Wang, J.; Da, J.; Liu, Z.; Zhang, K.; Liu, L.; Zhang, W.; Wang, P. Genipin modified lyophilized platelet-rich fibrin scaffold for sustained release of growth factors to promote bone regeneration. *Front. Physiol.* **2022**, *13*, 1007692. [CrossRef]
61. Lo Monaco, M.; Gervois, P.; Beaumont, J.; Clegg, P.; Bronckaers, A.; Vandeweerd, J.M.; Lambrichts, I. Therapeutic Potential of Dental Pulp Stem Cells and Leukocyte- and Platelet-Rich Fibrin for Osteoarthritis. *Cells* **2020**, *9*, 980. [CrossRef]
62. Marchetti, E.; Mancini, L.; Bernardi, S.; Bianchi, S.; Cristiano, L.; Torge, D.; Marzo, G.; Macchiarelli, G. Evaluation of Different Autologous Platelet Concentrate Biomaterials: Morphological and Biological Comparisons and Considerations. *Materials* **2020**, *13*, 2282. [CrossRef]
63. Moradian, H.; Rafiee, A.; Ayatollahi, M. Design and Fabrication of a Novel Transplant Combined with Human Bone Marrow Mesenchymal Stem Cells and Platelet-rich Fibrin: New Horizons for Periodontal Tissue Regeneration after Dental Trauma. *Iran. J. Pharm. Res.* **2017**, *16*, 1370–1378.
64. Nguyen, M.; Nguyen, T.T.; Tran, H.L.B.; Tran, D.N.; Ngo, L.T.Q.; Huynh, N.C. Effects of advanced platelet-rich fibrin combined with xenogenic bone on human periodontal ligament stem cells. *Clin. Exp. Dent. Res.* **2022**, *8*, 875–882. [CrossRef]
65. Nie, J.; Zhang, S.; Wu, P.; Liu, Y.; Su, Y. Electrospinning With Lyophilized Platelet-Rich Fibrin Has the Potential to Enhance the Proliferation and Osteogenesis of MC3T3-E1 Cells. *Front. Bioeng. Biotechnol.* **2020**, *8*, 595579. [CrossRef]
66. Nugraha, A.P.; Narmada, I.B.; Ernawati, D.S.; Dinaryanti, A.; Hendrianto, E.; Ihsan, I.S.; Riawan, W.; Rantam, F.A. Osteogenic potential of gingival stromal progenitor cells cultured in platelet rich fibrin is predicted by core-binding factor subunit-α1/Sox9 expression ratio (in vitro). *F1000Research* **2018**, *7*, 1134. [CrossRef]
67. Nugraha, A.P.; Narmada, I.B.; Ernawati, D.S.; Dinaryanti, A.; Hendrianto, E.; Ihsan, I.S.; Riawan, W.; Rantam, F.A. In vitro bone sialoprotein-I expression in combined gingival stromal progenitor cells and platelet rich fibrin during osteogenic differentiation. *Trop. J. Pharm. Res.* **2018**, *17*, 2341–2345. [CrossRef]
68. Nugraha, A.P.; Narmada, I.B.; Ernawati, D.S.; Dinaryanti, A.; Hendrianto, E.; Riawan, W.; Rantam, F.A. Bone alkaline phosphatase and osteocalcin expression of rat's Gingival mesenchymal stem cells cultured in platelet-rich fibrin for bone remodeling (in vitro study). *Eur. J. Dent.* **2018**, *12*, 566–573. [CrossRef]
69. Nugraha, A.; Narmada, I.B.; Ernawati, D.S.; Dınaryantı, A.; Hendrianto, E.; Ihsan, I.; Riawan, W.; Rantam, F. The Aggrecan Expression Post Platelet Rich Fibrin Administration in Gingival Medicinal Signaling Cells in Wistar Rats (*Rattus novergicus*) During the Early Osteogenic Differentiation (In Vitro). *Kafkas Univ. Vet. Fak. Derg.* **2019**, *25*, 421–425.
70. Rastegar, A.; Mahmoodi, M.; Mirjalili, M.; Nasirizadeh, N. Platelet-rich fibrin-loaded PCL/chitosan core-shell fibers scaffold for enhanced osteogenic differentiation of mesenchymal stem cells. *Carbohydr. Polym.* **2021**, *269*, 118351. [CrossRef]
71. Shah, R.; Thomas, R.; Gowda, T.M.; Baron, T.K.A.; Vemanaradhya, G.G.; Bhagat, S. In Vitro Evaluation of Osteoblast Response to the Effect of Injectable Platelet-rich Fibrin Coating on Titanium Disks. *J. Contemp. Dent. Pract.* **2021**, *22*, 107–110. [CrossRef] [PubMed]
72. Song, Y.; Lin, K.; He, S.; Wang, C.; Zhang, S.; Li, D.; Wang, J.; Cao, T.; Bi, L.; Pei, G. Nano-biphasic calcium phosphate/polyvinyl alcohol composites with enhanced bioactivity for bone repair via low-temperature three-dimensional printing and loading with platelet-rich fibrin. *Int. J. Nanomed.* **2018**, *13*, 505–523. [CrossRef] [PubMed]
73. Steller, D.; Herbst, N.; Pries, R.; Juhl, D.; Hakim, S.G. Positive impact of Platelet-rich plasma and Platelet-rich fibrin on viability, migration and proliferation of osteoblasts and fibroblasts treated with zoledronic acid. *Sci. Rep.* **2019**, *9*, 8310. [CrossRef]

74. Steller, D.; Herbst, N.; Pries, R.; Juhl, D.; Klinger, M.; Hakim, S.G. Impacts of platelet-rich fibrin and platelet-rich plasma on primary osteoblast adhesion onto titanium implants in a bisphosphonate in vitro model. *J. Oral Pathol. Med.* **2019**, *48*, 943–950. [CrossRef] [PubMed]
75. Sui, X.; Zhang, H.; Yao, J.; Yang, L.; Zhang, X.; Li, L.; Wang, J.; Li, M.; Liu, Z. 3D printing of 'green'thermo-sensitive chitosan-hydroxyapatite bone scaffold based on lyophilized platelet-rich fibrin. *Biomed. Mater.* **2023**, *18*, 025022. [CrossRef] [PubMed]
76. Thanasrisuebwong, P.; Kiattavorncharoen, S.; Surarit, R.; Phruksaniyom, C.; Ruangsawasdi, N. Red and Yellow Injectable Platelet-Rich Fibrin Demonstrated Differential Effects on Periodontal Ligament Stem Cell Proliferation, Migration, and Osteogenic Differentiation. *Int. J. Mol. Sci.* **2020**, *21*, 5153. [CrossRef] [PubMed]
77. Verboket, R.; Herrera-Vizcaíno, C.; Thorwart, K.; Booms, P.; Bellen, M.; Al-Maawi, S.; Sader, R.; Marzi, I.; Henrich, D.; Ghanaati, S. Influence of concentration and preparation of platelet rich fibrin on human bone marrow mononuclear cells (in vitro). *Platelets* **2019**, *30*, 861–870. [CrossRef]
78. Wang, Z.; Weng, Y.; Lu, S.; Zong, C.; Qiu, J.; Liu, Y.; Liu, B. Osteoblastic mesenchymal stem cell sheet combined with Choukroun platelet-rich fibrin induces bone formation at an ectopic site. *J. Biomed. Mater. Res. Part B Appl. Biomater.* **2015**, *103*, 1204–1216. [CrossRef]
79. Wang, X.; Zhang, Y.; Choukroun, J.; Ghanaati, S.; Miron, R.J. Effects of an injectable platelet-rich fibrin on osteoblast behavior and bone tissue formation in comparison to platelet-rich plasma. *Platelets* **2018**, *29*, 48–55. [CrossRef]
80. Wang, J.; Sun, Y.; Liu, Y.; Yu, J.; Sun, X.; Wang, L.; Zhou, Y. Effects of platelet-rich fibrin on osteogenic differentiation of Schneiderian membrane derived mesenchymal stem cells and bone formation in maxillary sinus. *Cell Commun. Signal.* **2022**, *20*, 88. [CrossRef]
81. Wang, J.; Li, W.; He, X.; Li, S.; Pan, H.; Yin, L. Injectable platelet-rich fibrin positively regulates osteogenic differentiation of stem cells from implant hole via the ERK1/2 pathway. *Platelets* **2023**, *34*, 2159020. [CrossRef] [PubMed]
82. Wong, P.C.; Wang, C.Y.; Jang, J.S.; Lee, C.H.; Wu, J.L. Large-Pore Platelet-Rich Fibrin with a Mg Ring to Allow MC3T3-E1 Preosteoblast Migration and to Improve Osteogenic Ability for Bone Defect Repair. *Int. J. Mol. Sci.* **2021**, *22*, 4022. [CrossRef] [PubMed]
83. Woo, S.M.; Kim, W.J.; Lim, H.S.; Choi, N.K.; Kim, S.H.; Kim, S.M.; Jung, J.Y. Combination of Mineral Trioxide Aggregate and Platelet-rich Fibrin Promotes the Odontoblastic Differentiation and Mineralization of Human Dental Pulp Cells via BMP/Smad Signaling Pathway. *J. Endod.* **2016**, *42*, 82–88. [CrossRef]
84. Wu, C.L.; Lee, S.S.; Tsai, C.H.; Lu, K.H.; Zhao, J.H.; Chang, Y.C. Platelet-rich fibrin increases cell attachment, proliferation and collagen-related protein expression of human osteoblasts. *Aust. Dent. J.* **2012**, *57*, 207–212. [CrossRef] [PubMed]
85. Yu, J.; Zhao, W.; Lu, J.; Hao, Y.; Lv, C.; Cao, C.; Zou, D. Platelet-rich fibrin as a scaffold in combination with either deciduous or permanent dental pulp cells for bone tissue engineering. *Int. J. Clin. Exp. Med.* **2016**, *9*, 15177–15184.
86. Yu, S.; Bd, Y.T.; Bd, Y.W.; Bd, M.F.; BMed, S.L.; BMed, G.T.; BMed, Z.Y.; Miron, R.J.; Zhang, Y.; Yang, Z.; et al. Early tissue and healing responses after maxillary sinus augmentation using horizontal platelet rich fibrin bone blocks. *BMC Oral Health* **2023**, *23*, 589. [CrossRef]
87. Zhang, L.; Dong, Y.; Xue, Y.; Shi, J.; Zhang, X.; Liu, Y.; Midgley, A.C.; Wang, S. Multifunctional Triple-Layered Composite Scaffolds Combining Platelet-Rich Fibrin Promote Bone Regeneration. *ACS Biomater. Sci. Eng.* **2019**, *5*, 6691–6702. [CrossRef]
88. Zhang, J.; Wu, J.; Lin, X.; Liu, X. Platelet-rich Fibrin Promotes the Proliferation and Osteo-/odontoblastic Differentiation of Human Dental Pulp Stem Cells. *Curr. Stem Cell Res. Ther.* **2023**, *18*, 560–567. [CrossRef]
89. Zhao, Y.H.; Zhang, M.; Liu, N.X.; Lv, X.; Zhang, J.; Chen, F.M.; Chen, Y.J. The combined use of cell sheet fragments of periodontal ligament stem cells and platelet-rich fibrin granules for avulsed tooth reimplantation. *Biomaterials* **2013**, *34*, 5506–5520. [CrossRef]
90. Zheng, L.; Wang, L.; Qin, J.; Sun, X.; Yang, T.; Ni, Y.; Zhou, Y. New Biodegradable Implant Material Containing Hydrogel with Growth Factors of Lyophilized PRF in Combination with an nHA/PLGA Scaffold. *J. Hard Tissue Biol.* **2015**, *24*, 54–60. [CrossRef]
91. Zheng, S.; Zhang, X.; Zhao, Q.; Chai, J.; Zhang, Y. Liquid platelet-rich fibrin promotes the regenerative potential of human periodontal ligament cells. *Oral Dis.* **2020**, *26*, 1755–1763. [CrossRef] [PubMed]
92. Fuchs, S.; Dohle, E.; Kolbe, M.; Kirkpatrick, C.J. Outgrowth endothelial cells: Sources, characteristics and potential applications in tissue engineering and regenerative medicine. In *Bioreactor Systems for Tissue Engineering II*; Advances in Biochemical Engineering/Biotechnology; Springer: Berlin/Heidelberg, Germany, 2010; Volume 123, pp. 201–217. [CrossRef]
93. Niu, B.; Li, B.; Gu, Y.; Shen, X.; Liu, Y.; Chen, L. In vitro evaluation of electrospun silk fibroin/nano-hydroxyapatite/BMP-2 scaffolds for bone regeneration. *J. Biomater. Sci. Polym. Ed.* **2017**, *28*, 257–270. [CrossRef] [PubMed]
94. Mahendran, K.; Kottuppallil, G.; Sekar, V. Comparative evaluation of radiopacity and cytotoxicity of platelet-rich fibrin, platelet-rich fibrin + 50wt% nano-hydroxyapatite, platelet-rich fibrin + 50wt% dentin chips: An in vitro study. *J. Conserv. Dent. JCD* **2019**, *22*, 28–33.
95. Chen, G.; Deng, C.; Li, Y.-P. TGF-β and BMP signaling in osteoblast differentiation and bone formation. *Int. J. Biol. Sci.* **2012**, *8*, 272. [CrossRef] [PubMed]
96. Polymeri, A.; Giannobile, W.V.; Kaigler, D. Bone Marrow Stromal Stem Cells in Tissue Engineering and Regenerative Medicine. *Horm. Metab. Res.* **2016**, *48*, 700–713. [CrossRef]
97. Canceill, T.; Jourdan, G.; Kémoun, P.; Guissard, C.; Monsef, Y.A.; Bourdens, M.; Chaput, B.; Cavalie, S.; Casteilla, L.; Planat-Bénard, V.; et al. Characterization and Safety Profile of a New Combined Advanced Therapeutic Medical Product Platelet Lysate-Based Fibrin Hydrogel for Mesenchymal Stromal Cell Local Delivery in Regenerative Medicine. *Int. J. Mol. Sci.* **2023**, *24*, 2206. [CrossRef]

98. Zanetti, A.S.; Sabliov, C.; Gimble, J.M.; Hayes, D.J. Human adipose-derived stem cells and three-dimensional scaffold constructs: A review of the biomaterials and models currently used for bone regeneration. *J. Biomed. Mater. Res. Part B Appl. Biomater.* **2013**, *101*, 187–199. [CrossRef]
99. Lai, F.; Kakudo, N.; Morimoto, N.; Taketani, S.; Hara, T.; Ogawa, T.; Kusumoto, K. Platelet-rich plasma enhances the proliferation of human adipose stem cells through multiple signaling pathways. *Stem Cell Res. Ther.* **2018**, *9*, 107. [CrossRef]
100. Lei, F.; Li, M.; Lin, T.; Zhou, H.; Wang, F.; Su, X. Treatment of inflammatory bone loss in periodontitis by stem cell-derived exosomes. *Acta Biomater.* **2022**, *141*, 333–343. [CrossRef]
101. Cho, Y.S.; Hwang, K.G.; Jun, S.H.; Tallarico, M.; Kwon, A.M.; Park, C.J. Radiologic comparative analysis between saline and platelet-rich fibrin filling after hydraulic transcrestal sinus lifting without adjunctive bone graft: A randomized controlled trial. *Clin. Oral Implant. Res.* **2020**, *31*, 1087–1093. [CrossRef]
102. Chang, Y.C.; Zhao, J.H. Effects of platelet-rich fibrin on human periodontal ligament fibroblasts and application for periodontal infrabony defects. *Aust. Dent. J.* **2011**, *56*, 365–371. [CrossRef] [PubMed]
103. Jo, S.; Lee, J.K.; Han, J.; Lee, B.; Kang, S.; Hwang, K.T.; Park, Y.S.; Kim, T.H. Identification and characterization of human bone-derived cells. *Biochem. Biophys. Res. Commun.* **2018**, *495*, 1257–1263. [CrossRef] [PubMed]
104. Liu, Q.; Li, M.; Wang, S.; Xiao, Z.; Xiong, Y.; Wang, G. Recent Advances of Osterix Transcription Factor in Osteoblast Differentiation and Bone Formation. *Front. Cell Dev. Biol.* **2020**, *8*, 601224. [CrossRef] [PubMed]
105. Liu, M.M.; Li, W.T.; Xia, X.M.; Wang, F.; MacDougall, M.; Chen, S. Dentine sialophosphoprotein signal in dentineogenesis and dentine regeneration. *Eur. Cells Mater.* **2021**, *42*, 43–62. [CrossRef]
106. Wang, Z.; Han, L.; Sun, T.; Wang, W.; Li, X.; Wu, B. Preparation and effect of lyophilized platelet-rich fibrin on the osteogenic potential of bone marrow mesenchymal stem cells in vitro and in vivo. *Heliyon* **2019**, *5*, e02739. [CrossRef]
107. Tanaka, Y.; Nakayamada, S.; Okada, Y. Osteoblasts and osteoclasts in bone remodeling and inflammation. *Curr. Drug Targets-Inflamm. Allergy* **2005**, *4*, 325–328. [CrossRef]
108. Lourenço, E.S.; Alves, G.G.; de Lima Barbosa, R.; Spiegel, C.N.; de Mello-Machado, R.C.; Al-Maawi, S.; Ghanaati, S.; de Almeida Barros Mourão, C.F. Effects of rotor angle and time after centrifugation on the biological in vitro properties of platelet rich fibrin membranes. *J. Biomed. Mater. Res. Part B Appl. Biomater.* **2021**, *109*, 60–68. [CrossRef]
109. Jann, J.; Gascon, S.; Roux, S.; Faucheux, N. Influence of the TGF-β Superfamily on Osteoclasts/Osteoblasts Balance in Physiological and Pathological Bone Conditions. *Int. J. Mol. Sci.* **2020**, *21*, 7597. [CrossRef]
110. Ghanaati, S.; Herrera-Vizcaino, C.; Al-Maawi, S.; Lorenz, J.; Miron, R.J.; Nelson, K.; Schwarz, F.; Choukroun, J.; Sader, R. Fifteen years of platelet rich fibrin in dentistry and oromaxillofacial surgery: How high is the level of scientific evidence? *J. Oral Implantol.* **2018**, *44*, 471–492. [CrossRef]
111. Reis, N.T.d.A.; João Lucas Carvalho, P.; Paranhos, L.R.; Bernardino, I.d.M.; Moura, C.C.G.; Irie, M.S.; Soares, P.B.F. Use of platelet-rich fibrin for bone repair: A systematic review and meta-analysis of preclinical studies. *Braz. Oral Res.* **2022**, *36*. [CrossRef]
112. Farshidfar, N.; Jafarpour, D.; Firoozi, P.; Sahmeddini, S.; Hamedani, S.; de Souza, R.F.; Tayebi, L. The application of injectable platelet-rich fibrin in regenerative dentistry: A systematic scoping review of In vitro and In vivo studies. *Jpn. Dent. Sci. Rev.* **2022**, *58*, 89–123. [CrossRef] [PubMed]
113. Strauss, F.-J.; Nasirzade, J.; Kargarpoor, Z.; Stähli, A.; Gruber, R. Effect of platelet-rich fibrin on cell proliferation, migration, differentiation, inflammation, and osteoclastogenesis: A systematic review of in vitro studies. *Clin. Oral Investig.* **2020**, *24*, 569–584. [CrossRef] [PubMed]

Disclaimer/Publisher's Note: The statements, opinions and data contained in all publications are solely those of the individual author(s) and contributor(s) and not of MDPI and/or the editor(s). MDPI and/or the editor(s) disclaim responsibility for any injury to people or property resulting from any ideas, methods, instructions or products referred to in the content.

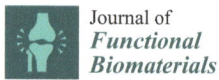

Review

Decellularization Techniques for Tissue Engineering: Towards Replicating Native Extracellular Matrix Architecture in Liver Regeneration

Ishita Allu [1,†], Ajay Kumar Sahi [2,†], Meghana Koppadi [1], Shravanya Gundu [1,*] and Alina Sionkowska [3,4,*]

1. Department of Biomedical Engineering, University College of Engineering (UCE), Osmania University, Hyderabad 500007, India; saiishitaallu@gmail.com (I.A.); kmeghana203@gmail.com (M.K.)
2. School of Medicine, McGowan Institute for Regenerative Medicine, University of Pittsburgh, Pittsburgh, PA 15219, USA; ajaysahi15@gmail.com
3. Faculty of Chemistry, Nicolaus Copernicus University in Torun, Jurija Gagarina 11, 87-100 Torun, Poland
4. Faculty of Health Sciences, Calisia University, Nowy Świat 4, 62-800 Kalisz, Poland
* Correspondence: shravanya.g@uceou.edu (S.G.); alinas@umk.pl (A.S.)
† These authors contributed equally to this work.

Abstract: The process of tissue regeneration requires the utilization of a scaffold, which serves as a structural framework facilitating cellular adhesion, proliferation, and migration within a physical environment. The primary aim of scaffolds in tissue engineering is to mimic the structural and functional properties of the extracellular matrix (ECM) in the target tissue. The construction of scaffolds that accurately mimic the architecture of the extracellular matrix (ECM) is a challenging task, primarily due to the intricate structural nature and complex composition of the ECM. The technique of decellularization has gained significant attention in the field of tissue regeneration because of its ability to produce natural scaffolds by removing cellular and genetic components from the extracellular matrix (ECM) while preserving its structural integrity. The present study aims to investigate the various decellularization techniques employed for the purpose of isolating the extracellular matrix (ECM) from its native tissue. Additionally, a comprehensive comparison of these methods will be presented, highlighting their respective advantages and disadvantages. The primary objective of this study is to gain a comprehensive understanding of the anatomical and functional features of the native liver, as well as the prevalence and impact of liver diseases. Additionally, this study aims to identify the limitations and difficulties associated with existing therapeutic methods for liver diseases. Furthermore, the study explores the potential of tissue engineering techniques in addressing these challenges and enhancing liver performance. By investigating these aspects, this research field aims to contribute to the advancement of liver disease treatment and management.

Keywords: decellularization; liver; tissue engineering; extracellular matrix; scaffold

1. Introduction

The field of tissue engineering has led to a considerable breakthrough in hepatic decellularization. This has made it possible to generate functioning liver tissues, which may have implications in transplantation as well as tissue regeneration. Decellularization corresponds to the precise removal of donor liver cells, resulting in an acellular scaffold that preserves the complicated three-dimensional architecture and extracellular matrix composition of the organ [1–3]. This scaffold can then be repopulated with patient-specific hepatocytes or hepatic stem cells, which could facilitate the construction of bioengineered hepatic structures [4,5]. This novel strategy has the potential to address the organ donor shortage and advance the understanding of issues pertaining to the liver, such as the causes of various disorders and the corresponding therapeutic solutions [4,6,7].

2. Anatomy of the Liver

The liver is the largest internal organ in the human body, accounting for about 2% of the total body weight of an average adult. It is a wedge-shaped organ located just beneath the diaphragm in the right hypochondrium, extending into the epigastric region to reach the left hypochondriac region in the abdominal cavity [8]. Hepatic tissue consists of two cell types: parenchymal cells called hepatocytes and cholangiocytes (biliary epithelial cells) and non-parenchymal cells encompassing Pit cells, Kupffer cells, hepatic stellate/fat-storing cells, and sinusoidal endothelial cells [9]. One of the primary roles of hepatocytes is the secretion of proteins into the blood (albumin and clotting factors). Cholangiocytes line the biliary tree's ducts and interact with the hepatocytes via the canals of Hering. Cholangiocytes create 30% of total bile flow and significantly interact with bicarbonate and other molecules. Hepatic stellate cells are a storehouse for Vitamin A. Kupffer cells are specialized macrophages capable of phagocytizing foreign materials, generating pro-inflammatory cytokines, and presenting antigens. Located beneath the endothelial cells and fibroblasts are the Pit cells, which account for a small proportion of the non-parenchymal cell population and are natural killer cells [10,11]. The parenchymal cell population is estimated to be around 80% of the hepatic tissue volume, while non-parenchymal cells account for approximately 6.3% (2.8% endothelial cells, 2.1% Kupffer cells, and 1.4% stellate cells) [12].

Being a highly vascular organ, the liver receives about 25% of the total cardiac output and has a unique angioarchitecture with a dual blood supply from two afferent vessels. The hepatic artery, arising from the celiac trunk, is responsible for 25–30% of the liver's blood supply, which is rich in oxygen. Contributing to the remaining 70–75% of blood flow is the portal vein, formed by the junction of the splenic vein and the superior mesenteric vein. Portal blood is enriched with monosaccharides and amino acids absorbed by the intestine from the splanchnic circulation, but it also contains bile salts, bilirubin, and GI hormones [8,13]. Toxins and metabolic waste are brought into the liver by the portal blood for detoxification before this blood enters the systemic circulation.

The liver is divided, rather unequally, into two parts called lobes: a larger right lobe and a smaller left lobe. Topographically, the falciform ligament demarcates the right lobe from the left, but from a functional standpoint, this division is inaccurate. The medial part of the left lobe is anatomically placed to the right of the falciform ligament, centered on the anterior branches of the left portal vein [8,9]. Each hepatic lobe consists of numerous lobules, which are the structural and functional units of the liver tissue. Figure 1 shows the gross structure of the liver and its lobular architecture. Each lobule is constructed around a central vein with rows of hepatocytes arranged in cellular plates radiating outwards, forming a roughly hexagonal pattern. The lobules are surrounded by multiple portal triads, which consist of a branch of the portal vein, a branch of the hepatic artery, and a tributary of the bile duct [14]. Hepatic plates are typically two cells thick and are separated by small bile canaliculi, which empty into bile ducts in the fibrous septa that separate adjacent liver lobules. The fibrous septa also contain small portal venules that receive blood from the portal vein. Hepatic cells are constantly in contact with portal venous blood. Interlobular septa contain hepatic arterioles, which feed arterial blood to the tissues between the lobules. Adjacent plates are divided by sinusoids, which are blood passages lined with endothelial cells and contain the Kupffer cells [15]. The branches of the hepatic artery and portal vein open into the sinusoids, while the sinusoids open into the central vein. Ultimately, the central vein drains into the vena cava via the hepatic vein. Large pores in the endothelium lining allow plasma substances to reach the space of Disse, which interact with lymphatic vessels in the septa. The lymphatics drain excess fluid from these areas, and plasma proteins can also diffuse into them [16,17].

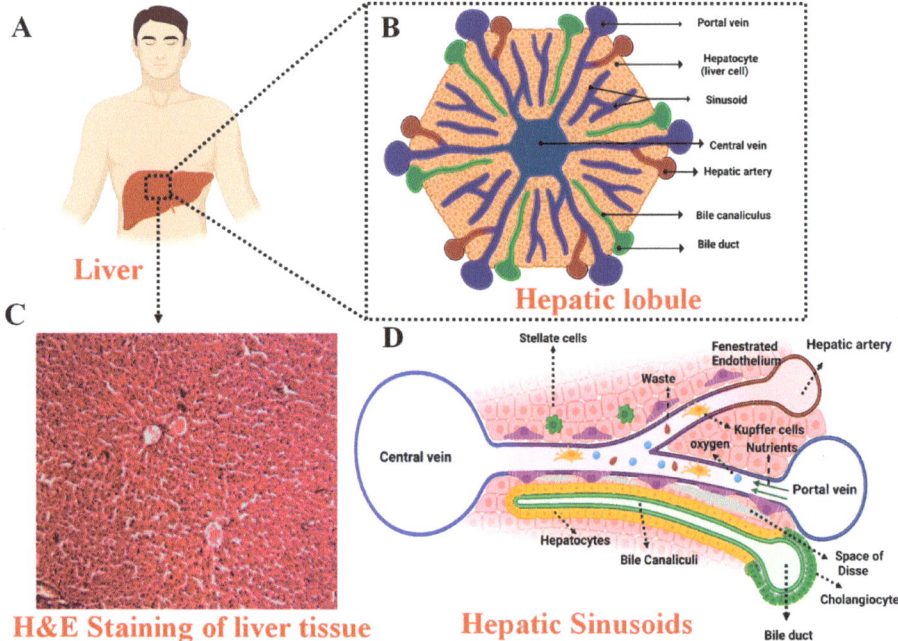

Figure 1. Liver architecture: (**A**) Illustration of the Macroscopic Liver Structure (**B**) Detailed Description of Liver's Lobular Architecture, encompassing vascular and biliary elements (**C**) Microscopic histological examination of liver tissue staining (**D**) composition and architecture of the Liver Lobule structure [10].

A remarkable feature of the hepatic tissue is its regenerative capability in that the organ can be restored completely even after significant tissue loss from partial hepatectomy, where two-thirds of the liver tissue is lost or after an acute liver injury as long as it is not aggravated by inflammation or viral infection [16]. After excision, the remaining liver expands in mass upon the replication of hepatocytes, facilitated by the hepatocyte growth factor (HGF), to compensate for the lost tissue. Once the original volume and size of the liver are restored, the hepatocytes cease to replicate and revert to their usual dormant state [18].

3. Functions of the Liver

The liver's functions encompass a wide range of metabolic, detoxification, regulatory, and synthesis processes, which are crucial for maintaining the body's homeostasis [19].

3.1. Metabolic Functions

Through glycogenesis, the liver regulates glucose in the body by converting and storing it in the form of glycogen. Certain aspects of lipid metabolism occur mainly in the liver, such as the synthesis of cholesterol, essential lipoproteins, and triglycerides and the oxidation of fatty acids via β-oxidation, generating energy for cellular processes. The liver also governs protein metabolism by synthesizing albumin, clotting factors, and globulins. It also participates in the deamination of amino acids and removes toxic ammonia through the urea cycle [20].

3.2. Bile Production

Bile is a fluid composed mainly of water, bile salts, electrolytes, phospholipids, bilirubin, and bile salts, among other substances. Produced by the hepatocytes, it helps excrete material that the kidneys do not eliminate and aids in the absorption and digestion of lipids. Bile is secreted into the bile canaliculi, where it travels to the larger ducts to end up in the duodenum or stored in the gallbladder. In the duodenum, it undergoes enterohepatic circulation, where it performs its job in the bowel, and the bile components are expelled in the feces [21]. The by-products after detoxification of drugs such as penicillin, sulfonamides, erythromycin, and more are excreted from the body through bile [13,22].

3.3. Bilirubin Metabolism

Hemolysis represents the intricate process wherein red blood cells (RBCs), having fulfilled their remarkable lifespan of 120 days, undergo breakdown. This degradation occurs at multiple locations, including the spleen, bone marrow, and liver [13]. Heme is broken down into biliverdin, which is reduced to unconjugated bilirubin. The unconjugated bilirubin is carried through albumin into the liver via the circulatory system. To become hydrophilic, unconjugated bilirubin is conjugated via the uridine diphosphate glucuronyltransferase (UGT) system in a phase II process. The newly conjugated bilirubin is subsequently released into the bile canaliculi or dissolves in the circulation, where it is filtered for elimination by the kidneys [23,24].

3.4. Other Functions

The liver regulates the synthesis of clotting factors and almost all the plasma proteins of the body, such as albumin, protein C, and protein S, to name a few. Additionally, the liver performs modification and excretion of hormones such as estrogenic, thyroxine, cortisol, and aldosterone. The liver is also an important site of the body's immune system and immune-mediated damage induced by malignant, infectious, and autoimmune stimuli [16,22].

4. Prevalence of Liver Diseases

Accounting for over 4% of deaths worldwide, liver diseases are the eleventh leading cause of mortality and the fifteenth leading cause of disability-adjusted life-years (DALYs) [25]. Notably, out of the two million deaths attributed to liver-to-liver dysfunction, two-thirds afflict men. Liver disease has the greatest impact on the young, as it stands 12th top cause of DALY's among individuals aged 25 to 49 years [26,27]. Cirrhosis is the most prevalent chronic liver disease, characterized by the hepatic tissue being replaced by dense scar tissue. This condition arises from recurring liver injury, necrosis, and inflammation, with culprits including hepatitis B and C, alcoholism, and non-alcoholic fatty liver disease (NAFLD) [11]. The consumption of alcohol elevates the risk of liver disease-related mortality by a staggering 260-fold, cardiovascular mortality by 3.2-fold, and cancer mortality by 5.1-fold. Notably, the number of deaths linked to NAFLD has witnessed a twofold increase over the past three decades. In 2020, viral Hepatitis B and Hepatitis C caused about 1.1'million deaths. The global prevalence of acute and chronic liver diseases is expected to increase significantly in the future [28].

To date, the ultimate remedy for addressing chronic liver diseases, particularly end-stage liver disease, is orthotopic transplantation. In 2020, a total of 129,681 solid organs were successfully transplanted across the globe, with liver transplants accounting for 25.1% of these cases [27]. However, there is still a huge discrepancy between the number of patients awaiting liver transplantation and that of donors, and a substantial number of people die while still on the waiting list. Furthermore, patients undergoing liver transplantation are highly susceptible to post-surgical complications such as infections, while the long-term effects include cardiovascular events, malignancies, and metabolic complications associated with immunosuppressive therapy. Strategic pre-transplant work-up and post-operative management are required in order to minimize the incidence of such complications, but it is a highly challenging task [26,27,29]. These limitations associated with organ transplantation necessitated the need for alternative therapeutic approaches such as cell therapy, bioartificial liver devices, organ-on-chip technology, and the bioengineering of hepatic tissue in vitro using primary or stem cells seeded into three-dimensional scaffolds [30].

Over the past few years, significant progress has been made toward the utilization of tissue engineering and regenerative medicine principles to restore liver functionality. Liver tissue engineering aims to produce functional liver tissue seeded with hepatic cells, followed by successful implantation into a patient with chronic liver disease [31]. Key variables that must be optimized for a successful hepatic tissue graft include selecting the optimal cellular sources, using the appropriate biomaterials for the scaffold, and locating suitable implantation sites [32]. For fabricating scaffolds mimicking vasculature and complex microarchitecture of the liver, bottom-up approaches such as 3D bioprinting, bio-microelectromechanical systems ("bioMEMS"), and 3D molding have shown promising results. However, it is challenging to accurately engineer macro-scale liver tissues using bottom-up approaches because of their inability to recreate the liver-specific extracellular matrix, its components, the controlled distribution, interconnectivity, and geometry of the pores [10,30].

5. Decellularized Extracellular Matrix Scaffolds

Decellularized ECM scaffolds have attracted the attention of researchers because of their biocompatibility properties, reduced risk of rejection due to the immune response, and similar mechanical and chemical properties to that of the native tissue or organ [33]. Such scaffolds are prepared using the decellularization technique, which involves the removal of the cellular or nuclear components while preserving the structural and functional proteins of the ECM. Cellular components and antigens are removed to prevent recognition by the immune system and cause an inflammatory response [34]. The proteins are preserved as they aid in cell adhesion, proliferation, and differentiation and also provide a natural environment for the stimulation of cell growth and, therefore, serve as an ideal material in tissue engineering [35–38].

The first successful account of liver decellularization was reported in 2004 when the researchers specifically explored a decellularized, porcine, liver-derived biomatrix as a bioresorbable scaffold for primary hepatocytes [39]. The research field has since demonstrated that decellularization is a relatively superior method for acquiring natural scaffolds compared to previous techniques, as it effectively preserves the native extracellular matrix (ECM) of the decellularized tissue [32,40]. Liver decellularization aims to preserve the major ECM components, including laminin, fibronectin, collagen type I, III, and IV, and proteoglycans.

Hepatic ECM

Most organs comprise comparable ECM components, although the concentrations and ratios differ [41]. The ECM is composed of two structures that are morphologically and biochemically different. They include the basement membrane and the interstitial matrix [42]. The basement membrane forms thin acellular layers that connect the epithelium to the interstitial matrix. The liver is characterized by a less dense basement membrane facilitating easier diffusion between plasma and the organ [41,43]. It is primarily composed of laminin, heparan sulfate proteoglycan (Perlecan), and collagen IV [5,44,45]. However, it is found to be absent in the parenchyma and sinusoids of healthy livers [5,44,46–48]. The interstitial matrix of the liver is primarily composed of collagen and fibronectin. The principal collagen types identified are Type I and Type III [5,47,49]. Figure 2 indicates the principal components of the liver ECM.

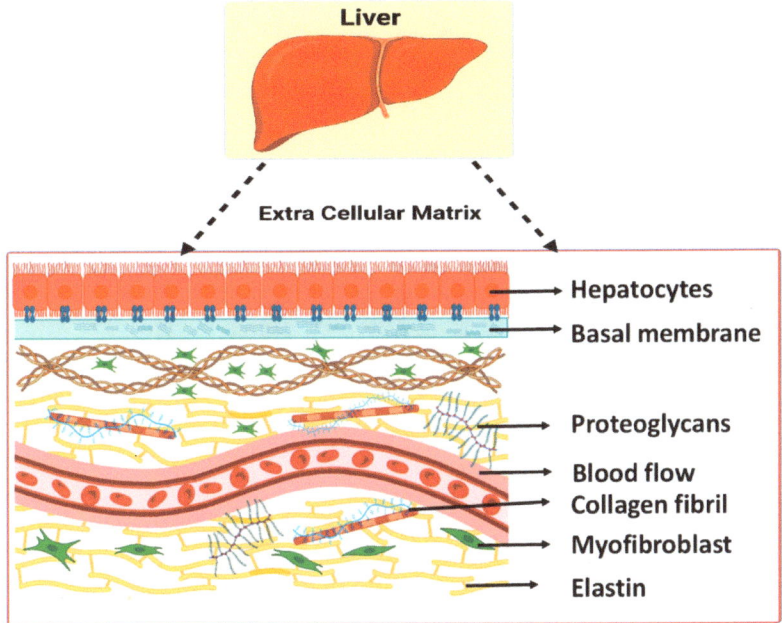

Figure 2. Schematic illustration of the major components of the hepatic ECM [50].

The liver ECM, accounting for 16% of the volume of the tissue, plays a vital role in cell-matrix adhesion, creating the milieu essential for hepatocyte growth, regulating tissue development, and the polarization of cells. ECM proteins trigger intracellular signaling by interacting with cell adhesion molecules such as integrins. These molecules play an important role in regulating cell differentiation, proliferation, migration, and gene expression [51,52]. Hence, it is crucial that the engineered scaffolds effectively mimic the innate microenvironment that supports the aforementioned phenomenon without eliciting immune-mediated rejection.

Decellularization can be achieved by various physical, chemical, or enzymatic methods, and the resultant ECM scaffold is sterilized before implantation [53]. The sterilization technique depends on the application considered, and it is performed either using irradiation or exposure to certain chemical agents such as ethylene oxide, hydrogen peroxide, etc. [54]. Subsequently, cells are embedded into the decellularized ECM, which serves as a scaffolding to support the implanted cells, and this process is known as recellularization [55]. In this review, we will focus on various decellularization procedures and provide a detailed analysis of the most effective approach for decellularizing liver tissue.

6. General Decellularization Techniques

As previously stated, decellularization can be achieved either by chemical, physical, or enzymatic means. Chemical and enzymatic methods are most often used to produce decellularized matrices. The physical approach is used to complement the chemical and enzymatic techniques, as it might have a damaging effect on the matrix. However, chemical techniques may also produce a chemical reaction that might alter the chemical composition of the ECM. Therefore, choosing the right decellularization protocol is necessary based on the application [56,57]. Figure 3 outlines the numerous approaches for developing decellularized extracellular matrix scaffolds.

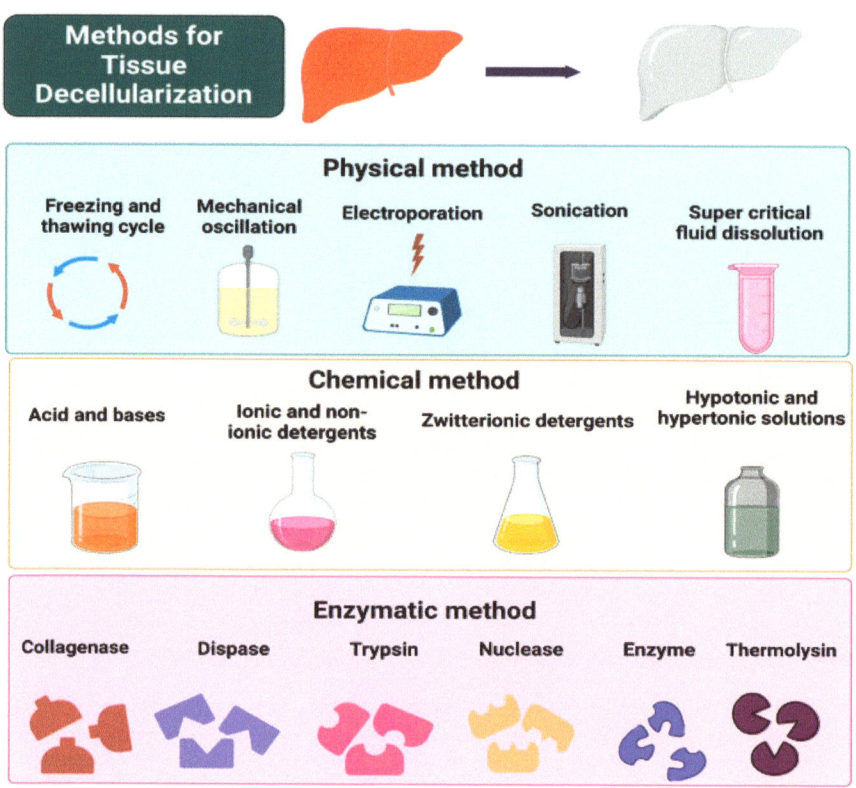

Figure 3. Various decellularization processes for the fabrication of acellular matrices [56,57].

6.1. Chemical Methods

Chemical decellularizing agents can be categorized into surfactants, acids, and bases, of which surfactants are the most commonly employed chemical agents to achieve decellularization [58].

6.1.1. Surfactants

Surfactants can be ionic, non-ionic, or Zwitter-ionic based on their charge [58]. Ionic surfactants work by solubilizing the cytoplasmic components of cells and disrupting the nucleic acids [59]. Sodium dodecyl sulfate (SDS) is the most commonly used ionic agent. They were effective in the complete removal of cellular content. They also facilitated the elimination of about 90% of host DNA. However, they also had detrimental effects on some of the structural and signaling proteins in the ECM [56,58].

Non-ionic surfactants were relatively less strident than ionic decellularizing agents [58]. They cause disruption of the DNA-protein, lipid–lipid, and lipid–protein interactions [59]. The most commonly used non-ionic surfactant is Triton X-100. It was effective in preserving the structural proteins and thereby maintained the integrity and mechanical properties of the tissue [7,58]. However, it was inefficient in completely removing the cellular components from the ECM [59]. It was observed that when employed in conjunction with ammonium hydroxide, DNA elimination occurred to a large extent while the mechanical characteristics of the tissue were also retained [58].

Zwitterionic surfactants exhibit the properties of both ionic and non-ionic surfactants [59]. 3-[(3-cholamidopropyl)-dimethylammonio]-1-propanesulfonate (CHAPS) is generally used. Due to the non-denaturing properties of CHAPS, it is highly efficient in preserving the structural proteins of the ECM, such as collagen and elastin [58,60]. Vacuum-assisted decellularization (VAD) improves the ability of chemical agents to reach the target tissues and thereby enhances the overall efficacy of the procedure [61]. This response could be accounted for by the potential of negative pressures to drive reagents into tissue structures [7,62]. By coupling a vacuum pump to a container housing, the chemical solution, it is possible to create the negative pressures that serve as the driving force of the reagents [62,63]. However, this is not necessarily a decellularization technique but acts as a facilitator and reduces the overall treatment time [64]. Additionally, as indicated by certain research studies, this approach was able to diminish the genetic material within the tissue with no adverse effects on the structural ECM proteins [64,65]. Nevertheless, it is recommended to maintain optimal vacuum duration and pressures because certain studies have indicated disruption of collagen fibrils and increased porosity under prolonged exposure to sub-atmospheric pressures, which corresponds to decreased mechanical properties [33,64,66].

6.1.2. Acids and Bases

Acids cause the dissociation of nuclear DNA from ECM by disrupting nucleic acids and solubilizing cytoplasmic contents [59]. On treatment with peracetic acid, it was observed that the cells were not effectively removed, and the mechanical properties of the tissue, such as stiffness, elastic modulus, and yield stress, were altered. It was observed that the mechanical properties were enhanced, and therefore, this treatment cannot be used for tissues where compliance and expandability are required. Peracetic acid was highly corrosive and oxidizing in nature and, therefore, more often used as a sterilizing agent than as a decellularizing agent [58]. Acetic acid caused the removal of collagen and thereby reduced the overall mechanical strength of ECM; however, it did not affect the sulfated glycosaminoglycans [67].

Treatment with an alkaline solution such as calcium hydroxide was efficient in the removal of cellular and genetic material and also maintained the structural integrity of the tissue. However, the addition of an alkaline solution resulted in swelling of the structure due to the induction of a negative charge on collagen in the tissue, and this swelling caused a reduction in the glycosaminoglycans and, thereby, its viscosity [58]. In addition to the above-mentioned protocols, chelating agents such as ethylene glycol tetraacetic acid (EGTA) and ethylenediaminetetraacetic acid (EDTA) can also be used in decellularization through binding to divalent metal cations and thereby disrupting cell adhesion to ECM [59,68]. Alcohols such as methanol and ethanol can also cause decellularization by dehydration, that is, by replacing the intra-cellular water and therefore disrupting the cell and reducing the content of genetic material in the cell.

6.2. Enzymatic Methods

Enzymatic decellularization is often used in conjunction with other methods to assist in the complete removal and degradation of cellular components and nuclear material, respectively, from the ECM. Commonly used enzymatic agents include nucleases, trypsin, collagenase, lipase, dispase, etc. Enzymatic agents such as DNases and RNases function by catalyzing the hydrolysis of deoxyribonucleotide and ribonucleotide chains. Trypsin is the most frequently used proteolytic enzyme to achieve decellularization. It has specific activity on peptides and can have an undesirable effect on ECM components such as collagen, elastin, and GAGs [69]. Therefore, it is usually employed in concert with chelating agents like EDTA and EGTA to prevent undesirable damage to the structural proteins in ECM [58,69]. Collagenase and dispase are scarcely used as they have a direct effect on collagen fibers and may affect the ECM ultrastructure. Furthermore, they do not cause the complete removal of cellular components from the ECM. Therefore, enzymatic agents are generally employed in conjunction with other protocols to achieve effective decellularization [69]. For instance, when SDS, Triton X-100, and peracetic acid/ethanol were used in combination with DNase, it resulted in the effective elimination of cells and genetic material from the ECM while preserving the structural proteins. Thereby, the decellularized matrix displayed similar mechanical properties to that of the native specimen, with its vasculature, ultrastructure, and neural channels intact. The treatment time is of utmost importance and must be carefully monitored since shorter treatment periods may cause ineffective cell removal, while a longer treatment time may result in reduced GAG, collagen, and elastin content [58].

6.3. Physical Methods

Physical techniques are not solely employed to achieve decellularization but are used in conjunction with other chemical or enzymatic methods [56]. Some of the techniques that are discussed in this article include freeze–thawing, mechanical loading, hydrostatic pressure, ultrasonication, electroporation, perfusion, and supercritical fluid treatment [61].

6.3.1. Freeze–Thawing

This technique involves cell lysis by alteration of the temperatures between freezing temperatures of about $-80\ °C$ and thawing temperatures of about $37\ °C$. The temperatures to be maintained and the number of cycles to be performed may vary based on the application. For instance, the decellularization of fibroblast cell sheets required three cycles, while lumbar vertebrae cells required only one. The studies reported that collagen and elastin were preserved, but about 88% of the DNA content was also maintained in the fibroblast cells [58]. This proves that freeze–thawing cannot be performed solely as it is not effective in removing the genetic material and, therefore, generally used in assistance with other techniques. A study reported that freeze–thawing, along with using Triton X-100 and sodium dodecyl sulfate detergents on large tendon cells, resulted in about a 20% decrease in DNA content [61]. Thereby, this technique was efficient in preserving the structural proteins; however, it is necessary that it is complemented with certain chemical actions to facilitate effective decellularization.

6.3.2. Mechanical Loading

In this technique, some mechanical stress is applied to the tissues to induce cell lysis. This method typically entails scraping with a sharp instrument to remove the surface cellular components. Given that the underlying components are susceptible to the mechanical force exerted, the amount of force applied should be precise enough [56,61].

6.3.3. Hydrostatic Pressure

This method involves the application of high hydrostatic pressures (HHP) to the tissues to destroy the cell membranes. In some studies, an HHP of about 980 MPa was applied to the porcine cornea for 10 min. It was observed that this treatment had been effective in removing the cell contents; however, it failed to eliminate the nuclear remnants. Therefore, this treatment technique was paired with DNase to completely remove the DNA remnants and thereby prevent immune rejection [58,70]. Several investigations also demonstrated that pressures above 320 MPa increased enthalpy, destabilizing collagen [71]. Very high hydrostatic pressures applied for long durations also pose the problem of denaturing the ECM proteins and altering the mechanical properties of the tissue [58,72]. Therefore, some researchers have performed super cooling pre-treatment before HHP application to weaken the cell membrane and prevent denaturing of tissue structures so that moderately high hydrostatic pressure may suffice to cause effective decellularization [71].

6.3.4. Ultrasonication

High-frequency ultrasonic waves are used to achieve cell isolation by disrupting the inter-molecular bonds and thus lysing the cell membrane. Low-frequency ultrasonic waves can produce some undesirable mechanical effects, such as cavitation, which is associated with bubble formation that may have a damaging effect on the structural and mechanical properties of the tissue [61,73]. Factors such as temperature, presence of dissolved matter, and frequency of ultrasound waves also affect ultrasound cavitation [74]. This treatment technique is collectively used with chemical agents such as SDS and CHAPS to achieve effective decellularization and retain the structural proteins intact. One of the advantages of this procedure is reduced treatment time while achieving high efficiency in the removal of cellular and nuclear material [75].

6.3.5. Electroporation

This technique involves applying microsecond electrical pulses through tissue and destabilizing the cell membrane potential, thereby forming nano-sized pores in the cell membrane and ultimately causing cell apoptosis. Choosing the right electrical parameters is crucial so that no thermal damage is caused to the other structures in the tissue. This decellularization procedure must be carried out in vivo to prevent an immunological response. Due to its non-thermal nature, it is observed that there is no denaturing of the collagen and elastin molecules within the tissue, and the mechanical properties of the matrix remain unaltered [61,76].

6.3.6. Perfusion

Perfusion involves the infusion of chemical agents through the vasculature, which facilitates the removal of cellular and nuclear material. This treatment procedure also preserves the ECM composition and architecture. However, the flow rate must be supervised and controlled as it may damage the capillaries and other vessels [61,72].

6.3.7. Supercritical Fluid Treatment

Supercritical fluid possesses the properties of a normal liquid and a gas; that is, it has a density similar to that of a liquid and a high diffusing capacity similar to a gas [61,77]. In a study involving the decellularization of the optic nerve, it was discovered that the DNA content was reduced by 40% while the GAGs and other structural proteins remained unaltered [77]. Generally, supercritical CO_2 is used because of its ability to be rapidly removed from the tissue in addition to its non-toxic and non-flammable properties [61,72].

Therefore, it is evident that a variety of procedures may be employed to ensure that the tissue is completely decellularized. A comparison of different methods and the most common applications pertaining to each is illustrated in Table 1 (A–C).

Table 1. (A) A comparative study of the various decellularization procedures using physical methods and their applicability to various tissues. (B) A comparative study of the various decellularization procedures using enzymatic methods and their applicability to various tissues. (C) A comparative study of the various decellularization procedures using chemical methods and their applicability to distinct tissues.

Technique	Mechanism of Action	Effects	Advantages	Limitations	Applications	References
(A)						
Freeze–thawing	denatured proteins, resulting in cell necrosis.	eliminated cellular contents completely. retained structural proteins.	adequate cell removal. intact basement membrane.	inefficient removal of genetic material. Ice crystal formation may disrupt the ECM ultrastructure.	tendon, porcine carotid artery, porcine renal tissue.	[78–82]
Mechanical Loading	application of physical force caused cell lysis.	removed the surface cellular components of the tissue or the whole organ.	minimal disruption to the ECM architecture.	only suitable for tissues with sufficient mechanical hardness and a less dense ECM. applying force must be performed with the utmost caution to prevent damage to interior structures.	small intestine, urinary bladder	[56,61]

Table 1. Cont.

Technique	Mechanism of Action	Effects	Advantages	Limitations	Applications	References
(A)						
Hydrostatic pressure	high hydrostatic pressure caused cell membrane disruption resulting in cell death.	effectively removed cellular and nuclear content.	biomechanical properties of decellularized grafts remain unaltered. relatively short treatment time.	ultra-high pressures can result in protein denaturation.	blood vessels, uterine tissue, and corneal tissue.	[70,71,83]
Ultrasonication	caused cell membrane disruption due to induced shear stresses by cavitation.	effective removal of about 90% of cellular content. preserved structural proteins of cells.	retained the ECM microstructure. short treatment time.	demand perfect control over sonication power.	umbilical artery, aorta	[75,84–86]
Electroporation	distortion of the cell membrane occurred following the application of pulsed electric fields.	efficient cell removal. ECM remained intact.	porosity can be controlled by adjusting the electrical parameters. intact basement membrane.	relatively smaller electrodes limit the tissue surface area decellularized. not preferable for cardiac applications.	porcine liver, skin tissue.	[61,76,87,88]
Perfusion	eliminated the cell remnants by allowing a constant flow of decellularizing agents through the tissue.	solubilized cellular and nuclear material. Preserved structural proteins.	generation of biocompatible, non-toxic decellularized scaffolds. maintained ECM ultrastructure.	size shrinkage occurred following the procedure.	porcine renal tissue, heart, and lung tissue.	[89–92]
Supercritical fluid	A relatively inert gas, carbon dioxide at low temperature and pressure conditions facilitated the removal of cellular components.	effectively removed cellular and immunogenic agents. cause tissue dehydration.	preserved the structural integrity of ECM proteins. easily achievable treatment conditions with relatively brief treatment times.	tissue dehydration results in increased scaffold brittleness.	bovine neural tissue, porcine cartilage, adipose tissue, and bovine dermis.	[77,93–96]
(B)						
Nucleases (DNases and RNases)	disintegrated nucleic acid sequences by cleaving the phosphodiester bonds.	eliminated cellular remnants. retained collagen and elastin	retained the biomechanical properties of the original tissue.	ineffective in the complete removal of nuclear material. Induced immunological response	neural tissue, trachea, adipose tissue, intervertebral discs, porcine heart valves	[7,58,59,67,97,98]
Proteases (Trypsin, collagenase and dispase)	cleaved peptide bonds selectively.	detached cells from the tissue. removed matrix proteins such as collagen, elastin, laminins, etc.	efficient in complete cell removal in soft tissues. impedes cell conglomeration.	disrupted the ECM integrity. reduced biomechanical strength of decellularized scaffolds. Ineffective in complete cell removal.	porcine cornea, heart valves, and the dermis.	[7,67–69,97,99,100]
(C)						
Surfactants						
Ionic (SDS)	solubilized the cell and nucleic materials Denatured proteins	effectively removed cellular and nuclear material. distorted the structural and signaling proteins.	allowed for complete cell removal and about 90% of host DNA.	disrupted the ECM. decreased GAGs and growth factors. cytotoxic and required an extensive wash process.	porcine cornea, porcine myocardium, porcine kidney, human vein, etc.	[58,59]

Table 1. *Cont.*

Technique	Mechanism of Action	Effects	Advantages	Limitations	Applications	References
(C)						
Non-ionic (Triton X-100)	disrupted DNA-protein, lipid-protein, and lipid-lipid interactions	partially efficient in removing genetic material. Retained elastin.	less harsh than SDS and, therefore, caused less damage to the structural integrity of ECM.	less effective than SDS in removing cells and nuclear material. should be used in conjunction with Ammonium Hydroxide to facilitate complete cell removal.	bovine pericardium, porcine kidney, etc.	[58,59,101]
Zwitterionic (CHAPS)	solubilized cell and nuclear membranes Exhibited properties of both ionic and non-ionic surfactants	preserved structural proteins. Effectively removed about 95% of nuclear constituents.	superior cell removal. substantial preservation of ECM architecture.	disrupted the integrity of the basement membrane of ECM	vasculature, neural tissue.	[59,60,102]
Acids and Bases	hydrolyzed cytoplasmic constituents of cell	reduced collagen, GAG content, and growth factors.	treatment with an alkaline solution allowed for the complete removal of cellular and nuclear material. acid-mediated decellularization was effective in eliminating residuary genetic constituents.	effects on ECM were found to be strident disrupting the peptide bonds and reducing the overall mechanical properties.	small intestine submucosa, urinary bladder matrix, and dermis samples.	[53,56,58,67, 102,103]

7. Suggested Methodology for Optimal Results in Liver Tissue Decellularization

Among the many techniques listed previously, perfusion-based decellularization is reportedly the most popular approach to decellularizing the liver. This technique involves the delivery of chemical and enzymatic agents such as Triton X-100, SDS, EDTA, and others into the portal or hepatic vein in order to efficiently remove cells and create acellular ECM scaffolds [104–107]. Certain studies have suggested that the process of freezing–thawing may minimize the quantities of decellularization reagents required; nonetheless, cryoprotectants are recommended to prevent any possible damage to the ECM microstructure [5].

Hepatic artery and portal vein cannulations were most frequently performed on rat or porcine livers [108–111]. A cold NaCl solution and heparin were perfused via the vascular system to remove any remaining blood from the liver [108,110]. The organ was then stored at a temperature of about $-80\ °C$ until the decellularization procedure commenced. Prior to starting the procedure, the cryopreserved liver was thawed at a temperature of about $4\ °C$ [108,110,111].

Following this, several studies demonstrated the use of chemical agents such as Triton X-100 or SDS or a combination of both perfused via the hepatic artery or portal vein [6,110–113]. This was typically carried out iteratively, with the specific chemical detergent being administered initially and continuous perfusion being maintained for around 2 h. The organ was also perfused with distilled water mid-cycle to remove any residual agent and prepare for the next perfusion cycle [110,111]. Finally, the liver was flushed with deionized water and phosphate-buffered saline (PBS) to remove the remnant detergents [110–113]. A schematic representation of liver decellularization by perfusion is shown in Figure 4.

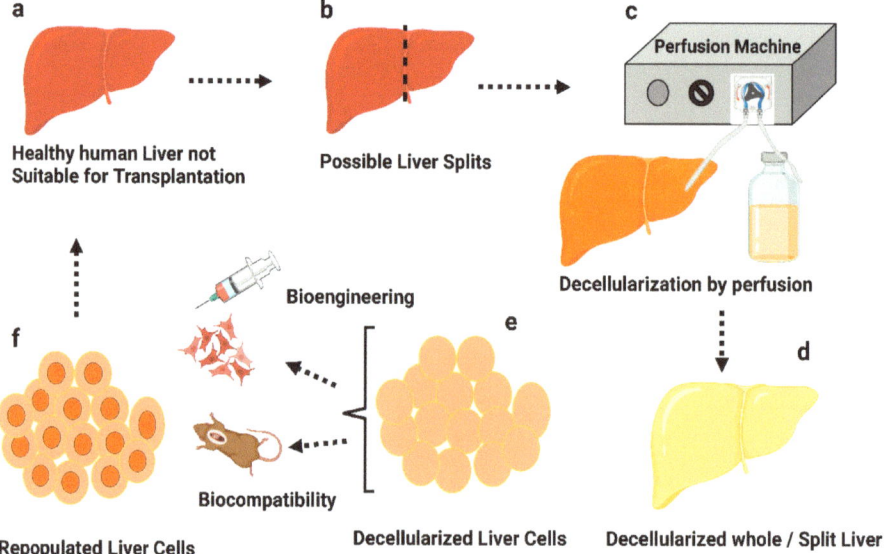

Figure 4. Schematic representation of perfusion-induced liver decellularization. Human livers unfit for transplantation are surgically separated into left lobes or utilized whole (**a**,**b**). Perfusion enables lobes or whole organs to become cannulated and decellularized (**c**) after decellularization the liver cells are dissected by scalpel (**d**).The studies of biocompatibility and bioengineering were analyzed using 3-d techniques (**e**,**f**) [107].

Perfusion-based decellularization has the advantage of pressure-controlled or flow rate-controlled infusion, allowing for more constant distribution of the chemical agents within the organ [110,111,114]. In a study, it was reported that an average perfusion pressure of 8–12 mm Hg resulted in better preservation of the lobular structures in comparison to the native liver [5,115]. An oscillating pressure system was maintained to simulate the intra-abdominal pressure conditions for more efficient and uniform decellularization throughout the tissue [5,113,116].

8. Characterization of Decellularized Liver Samples

Decellularized liver tissues are preserved in 4% paraformaldehyde to prevent tissue degradation and preserve matrix architecture [110,111,117]. The sample slides were prepared for histology by dehydrating them using graded ethanol, followed by immersion in xylene and embedding in paraffin. In order to evaluate the cellular content and efficiency of decellularization, the samples were stained with hematoxylin, eosin, and 4′,6-diamidino-2-phenylindole (DAPI) [110,111,117]. The DNA content was evaluated with the help of a NanoDrop spectrophotometer based on the measurement of the normalized weight [110,111]. The ECM microstructure was evaluated with the help of scanning/transmission electron microscopy [104,109]. A colorimetric assay was performed to quantify the collagen in the ECM based on the detection of hydroxyproline found in the structural protein [111,118]. Another technique, namely immunohistochemistry, might also be used to indicate the presence of proteins, including collagen type I, collagen type III, collagen type IV, elastin, laminin, and fibronectin [3,5,107]. The GAG content in the ECM was quantified using a glycosaminoglycan assay based on the BlyscanTM dye-binding method [110,119]. The vascular integrity of the decellularized liver scaffold might be assessed by Digital Subtraction Angiography (DSA), with iodine used as the contrast agent delivered via the portal vein [104]. Biodegradation studies were also performed to evaluate the degradation rate of the prepared scaffolds upon incubation in collagenase for a period of about 48 h [120,121]. Figure 5 illustrates the overall fabrication of acellular liver scaffolds and the subsequent characterization procedures to evaluate the decellularization efficiency.

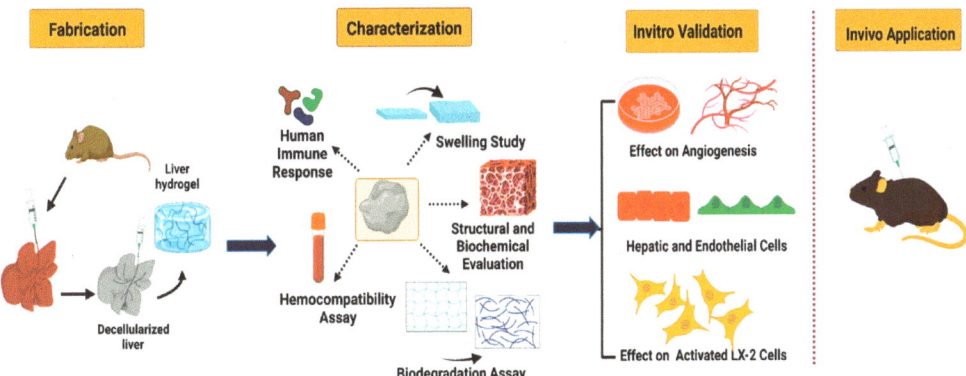

Figure 5. Schematic representation of the decellularization of whole organ liver and the successive characterization techniques [121].

9. Effects of Decellularization on ECM

Samples of decellularized liver appeared white and translucent, indicating the removal of cellular material [109,110]. The combinational use of the chemical agents resulted in the removal of a larger percentage of cellular and nuclear material. However, this also reduced the total ECM protein content that is essential for cell adhesion, growth, and mechanical integrity of the matrix [6,110,113]. Some studies revealed an average DNA removal efficiency of greater than 90% for both protocols [110,111]. Certain studies using the Triton X-100 procedure revealed substantially more DNA fragments than the ones using the SDS protocol [122].

Analytical procedures revealed that ECM proteins such as collagen and sGAGs were present in larger concentrations than in native liver tissue due to the elimination of cellular debris [113,120]. However, it was shown that the elastin content in the acellular liver was slightly lower than in fresh liver samples [107,120]. When examined using a scanning/transmission electron microscope, the 3D architecture and ultrastructure of the ECM were discovered to be intact, suggesting that the connective fibers retained the polygonal-like architecture and the ECM structural proteins, including collagen, fibronectin, and laminin were also conserved [104,107,109,116,123]. According to Hussein et al., 77% of collagen degradation occurred during the first three hours of placing the samples in collagenase. However, Baptista et al. reported 80% collagen degradation within the first six hours of placement and complete degradation in 48 h, indicative of the possible instability of the acellular samples upon enzymatic action [120,121].

Following decellularization using the suggested procedure, an intact vasculature was also observed, which is essential to maintain the delivery of growth factors, nutrients, and oxygen to the newly repopulated cells. [104,116,120]. However, certain studies have indicated possible ECM damage at higher SDS concentrations; therefore, lower proportions for longer durations were recommended [113]. Table 2 presents a comparative analysis of different techniques conducted under varying conditions and their impact on ECM.

Table 2. A comparison of various protocols implemented under various settings and their implications on liver ECM.

Protocol	Effects on ECM	References
1% Triton X-100	adequate clearance of cellular debris, a high DNA removal efficiency of about 96%, better collagen retention	[110,124]
0.1% SDS	high cell elimination efficacy complete removal of genetic material retained the structural proteins and integrity of the ECM	[105,124,125]
1% SDS	complete cell removal highly efficient in DNA removal with an efficiency of about 99% disrupted the microvasculature of ECM	[111,113,122]
1% Triton X-100 + 1% SDS	effective removal of cellular components and complete elimination of nuclear material preserved the vasculature and mechanical integrity of the ECM	[113,126]
4% Triton X-100/0.02% EGTA solution and 0.5% SDS aqueous solution	Decellularized whole liver organ as an ex vivo model with a unique native environment and vasculature for vascular embolization evaluation.	[127]
Free-thaw + Triton X-100/SDS + DNase/RNase	Sequentially perfusing the organ with SDS and Triton X-100, resulting in the generation of translucent acellular liver matrices within just 9 h. This approach offers a more streamlined and effective method for decellularization.	[128]
1% Triton X-100 + 0.05% EDTA + 30 µg/mL DNase	A unidirectional, one-way perfusion flow improved and accelerated the decellularization approach. Most significantly, decellularization preserved liver extracellular matrix integrity and cell adhesion and proliferation, enabling recellularization.	[129]
Enzymatic	Utilizes enzymes (e.g., trypsin, DNase) to digest cellular material while leaving the ECM intact.	[120]
Physical	Involves physical disruption of cells through mechanical agitation, shear, or pressure to remove cellular material.	[130]

10. Applications of Various Decellularized Liver Matrices and the Techniques Involved

Liver decellularized matrix is a promising biomaterial for fabricating 3D-bio printed, nanoparticle-incorporated, electrospun, and freeze–dried scaffolds. This is attributed to the microenvironment created by the matrix that closely resembles that of the native tissue, thereby promoting cellular functions such as proliferation and differentiation [131,132].

10.1. 3D Bioprinting of Decellularized Hepatic Extracellular Matrix

The use of 3D bioprinting involves layer-by-layer deposition of a material, permitting the fabrication of a highly controlled and desired 3D structure with improved resolution [132–134]. This method is extensively used because of its ability to mimic the complex, intricate structure of the liver ECM and its wide usage with a variety of biomaterials and cell types [135,136]. Additionally, the 3D structures offer biomechanical and biochemical cues stimulating numerous cellular processes since they preserve the native ECM and its structural integrity [137,138]. In this procedure, a bioink is developed, which is essentially a compound of suitable biomaterial and decellularized liver matrices (Figure 6) [134,135]. These materials are reinforced into the decellularized liver ECM for enhanced support, mechanical stability, printing resolution, rheological properties, and bioink ejection [139–141].

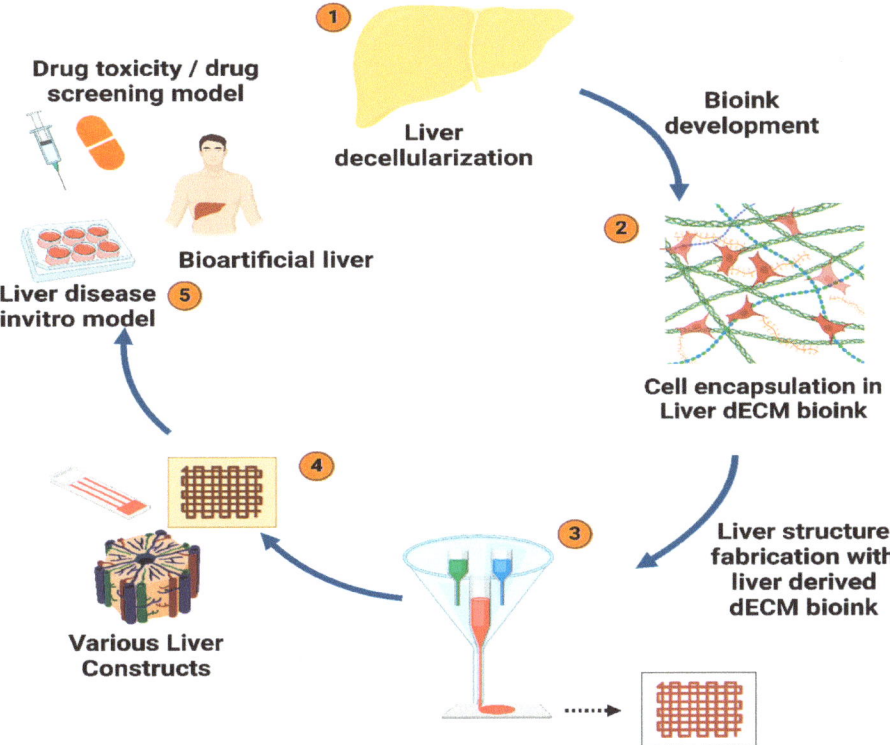

Figure 6. Illustrates the bioprinting approach using decellularized liver ECM bioink to create 3D liver constructs [135].

It is important to choose appropriate biomaterials that demonstrate biocompatibility, printability, sufficient mechanical strength, and resemblance to native liver morphology [139,141,142]. Naturally derived biomaterials such as collagen, gelatin, agarose, chitosan, hyaluronic acid, and others are most commonly used to prepare bioinks [135,142]. To prepare the bioink, the decellularized liver matrix is first lyophilized and powdered, then dissolved in acidic solutions of appropriate concentrations, such as 0.1 M acetic acid or 0.1 N hydrochloric acid, for around 4 days. Subsequently, the obtained solution is centrifuged at 3000–3500× g rpm for around 10 min to eliminate larger particles. The pH of the resultant solution can be modified to 7.4 by adding 10 M sodium hydroxide (NaOH) or phosphate-buffered saline (PBS) solution [135,138,140]. Similarly, bio-inks made of gelatin, collagen, and other materials, or their combinations, can be made by dissolving the corresponding components in appropriate solutions (for instance, collagen in 0.5 M acetic acid) and correcting the pH of the resulting solution with 10 M NaOH solution. Finally, the desired bioink may be prepared by combining the acquired mixture with the decellularized liver ECM bioink [135,143–145].

The prepared bioink loaded into a syringe is extruded out of the nozzle using pneumatic or mechanical forces and deposited over the print bed to create 3D structures [133,134]. Certain studies have utilized UV light for crosslinking to facilitate a more uniform and better printing resolution; however, this resulted in an alteration in cell behaviors upon extended usage [135,138,139].

10.2. Nanoparticles-Incorporated Decellularized Extracellular Matrices

Nanoparticles may be integrated into decellularized liver scaffolds for enhanced healing of damaged tissue, cellular growth, structural stability, antibacterial activities, and sustained release of growth factors [146–148]. Additionally, certain nanomaterials, such as polydiacetylene (PDA), may be reinforced into decellularized liver matrices to facilitate blood detoxification due to their antidotal behavior [149]. These nanoparticles are claimed to bind to matrices by ionic or covalent bonding, where the latter is dependent on the functional groups present on their surface [148].

Various studies have tested the functioning of silver nanoparticles conjugated in the matrices, and it is reported that they facilitated crosslinking due to their high affinity for collagen, thereby increasing the overall structural stability and resistance to biodegradation in vivo. Moreover, such conjugated scaffolds have demonstrated biocompatibility, anti-inflammatory activities, cytocompatibility, and less immunogenicity [147,148]. Figure 7 depicts the nanoparticles-incorporated extracellular matrix system and its overall benefits.

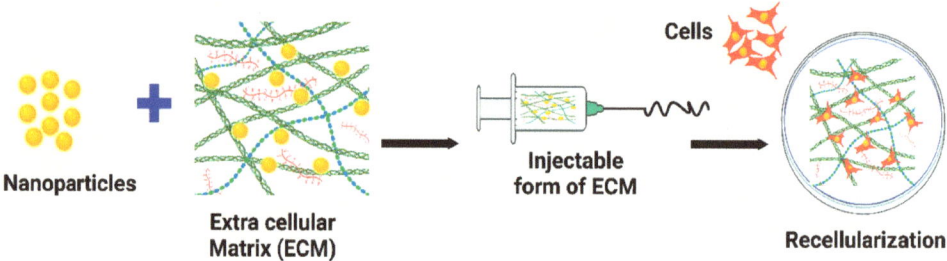

Figure 7. Schematic illustration of the extracellular cellular matrix-nanoparticles conjugated system and its numerous advantages, including improving structural stability and electrical conductivity, sustained release of growth factors, improving cellularity, adding antibacterial activities, and antitoxin functionalization [147].

10.3. Electrospinning

Electrospinning is a prevalent technique to produce micro- or nanofibers with precisely controlled diameters and a high surface-to-volume ratio, mimicking the structure of the extracellular matrix (ECM) in native tissues [150–152]. The fabrication of electrospun fibrous scaffolds using decellularized extracellular matrices blended with polymers reportedly produced design-driven constructs that are capable of retaining tissue-specific phenotypes, enhancing the proliferation and differentiation of seeded cells [153]. Figure 8 shows the general scheme of scaffold fabrication using decellularized ECM and electrospinning.

Decellularized porcine liver extracellular matrix (PLECM) and collagen type I were dissolved in 1,1,1,3,3,3-hexafluoro-2-propanol (HFIP) solvent and electrospun into porous 3D nanofibrous scaffolds. These scaffolds were then used to culture Primary Human Hepatocytes (PHH) alone or in combination with non-parenchymal cells such as 3T3-J2 murine embryonic fibroblasts and liver sinusoidal endothelial cells. Cells cultured on the fibrous scaffolds displayed superior urea synthesis, albumin secretion, and cytochrome-P450 1A2, 2A6, 2C9, and 3A4 enzyme activities compared with those cultured on conventionally adsorbed 2D ECM controls [154].

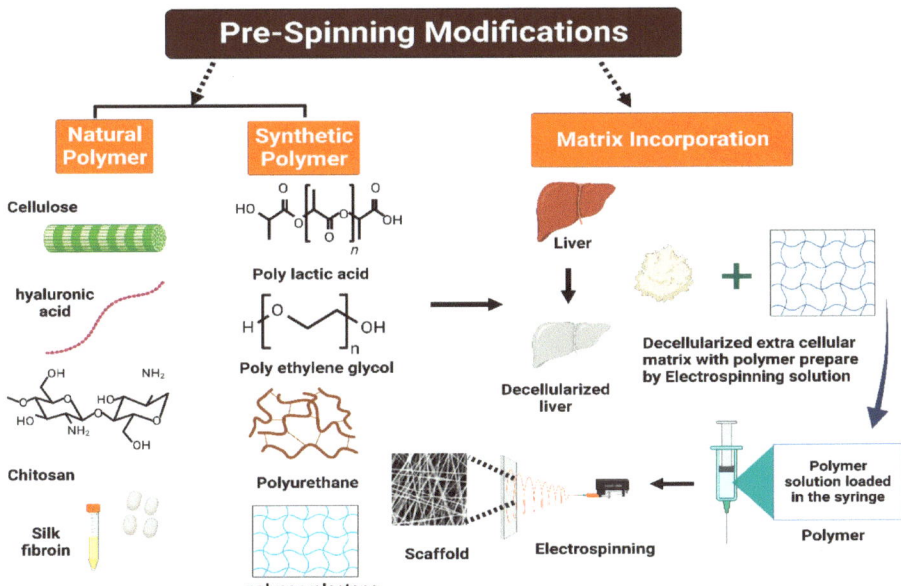

Figure 8. General scheme of scaffold fabrication using electrospinning and decellularized extracellular matrix–polymer blend solution [155].

Another study incorporated a decellularized human liver ECM directly into the fibers of an electrospun polylactic acid (PLA) matrix to create a bioactive protein–polymer scaffold to enhance the proliferation of THLE-3 hepatocytes [156]. A different method involved seeding a layer of bladder epithelium that produces ECM onto electrospun polycaprolactone (PCL) fibers to create hybrid polymer–ECM scaffolds. The initial layer was removed through detergent-based decellularization, and liver-representative cells (HepG2) were then grown on the scaffolds. The use of such scaffolds has proven to have a positive impact on the gene expression profile, albumin production, attachment, and survival of liver cells, which cannot be achieved by individual ECM components alone [153,157].

10.4. Lyophilization

Lyophilization or freeze–drying, a well-known method for fabricating scaffolds with controllable porosities, has been employed to enhance the shelf-life of decellularized heart valves in sheep [158]. A renal matrix scaffold was fabricated by extracting sheep kidney cells through decellularization followed by freeze-drying and chemical crosslinking in order to enhance the mechanical properties and pore structure [37,159,160].

In another study, researchers explored the possibility of developing a hemostatic and liver wound-healing nanocomposite material using a non-solubilized, powdered, decellularized liver extracellular matrix (L-ECM). The L-ECM was anchored to thrombin by lyophilization, and a TEMPO-oxidized cellulose nanofiber/chitosan/ECM-thrombin nanocomposite was developed. Figure 9 represents the procedure for the fabrication of the CN/CS/ECM-Th scaffold by means of the freeze–drying approach. The resultant biomaterial exhibited rapid pro-coagulation ability, highlighting its potential as a liver regeneration scaffold [161].

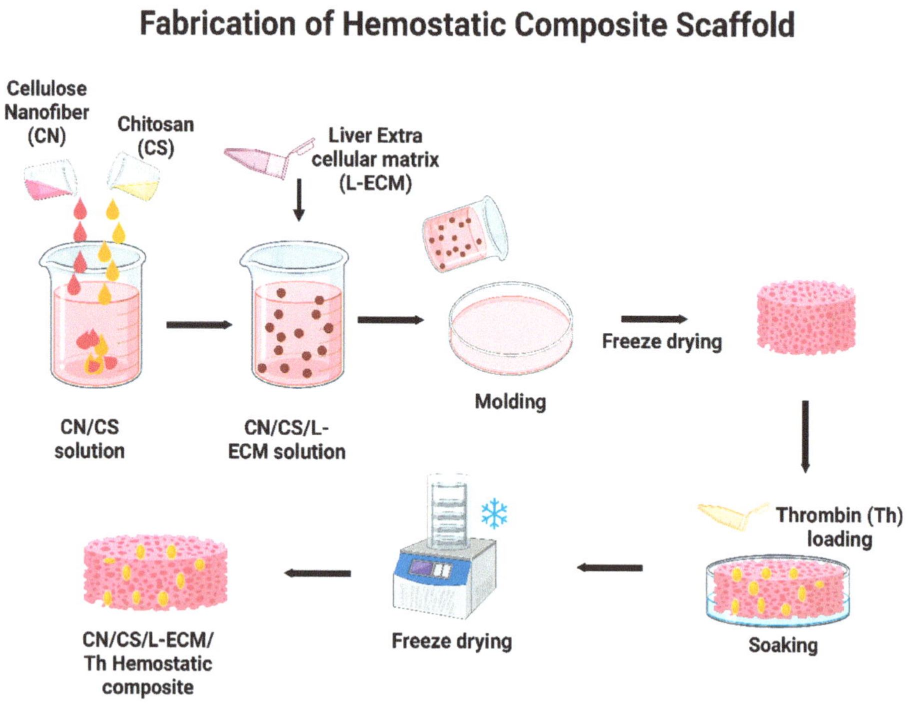

Figure 9. Schematic representation of the fabrication of CN/CS/ECM-Th Hemostatic composite using freeze drying [161].

11. Conclusions

The process of tissue decellularization, which belongs to the broad categories of tissue engineering and regenerative medicine, has garnered significant attention due to its ability to generate scaffolds that closely mimic the biological environment of the human body. This advancement retains the potential for enhancing the efficacy of tissue regeneration, restoration, and replacement. In recent years, the scarcity of available donor organs and the potential risks of immunogenic rejections post-transplantation have prompted researchers to explore alternative approaches for tissue repair and regeneration. One such approach acquiring significant attention is the utilization of decellularized tissues, which harness the patient's own cells for these purposes. This article aims to delve into the growing interest in decellularized tissues as a potential solution to address the aforementioned challenges in the field of transplantation and tissue engineering. The efficacy of tissue regeneration is dependent upon the successful elimination of cells and the triggering substances that induce an immunological response. In spite of the diverse range of methods available for cell isolation and scaffold preparation, the selection of an appropriate decellularization technique holds significant importance. The selection of an appropriate decellularization procedure is crucial and should be tailored to the specific tissue or organ under investigation, taking into account its unique extracellular matrix (ECM) structure and composition. The present study aims to evaluate the effectiveness of perfusion as a widely utilized process for achieving successful decellularization of the liver while preserving the organ's structural integrity. The present study aims to investigate the efficacy of a particular procedure in eliminating cellular and nuclear material. Multiple reports have indicated that this procedure exhibits promising results in achieving this objective. However, it is evident from various reports that although this procedure has been successful in eliminating the cellular and nuclear material to a large extent, care must be taken to ensure the chemical agents are introduced at appropriate concentrations to prevent any damage to the ECM microarchitecture. Therefore, it is imperative to conduct further investigations in order to substantiate the current knowledge and expedite the development of promising decellularization techniques, enabling preferable alternatives to conventional medical therapies.

Author Contributions: I.A.: Original draft preparation, data curation, validation, and writing. A.K.S.: Original draft preparation, data curation, validation, and writing. M.K.: validation, reviewing, and editing. S.G.: generated the figures, writing—review and editing. A.S.: Supervision, Project administration, reviewing, and editing. All authors have read and agreed to the published version of the manuscript.

Funding: This research work received no external funding.

Data Availability Statement: Data sharing is not applicable since no new data were generated.

Acknowledgments: We would like to express our gratitude to Biorender (licensed version) for providing us with the ability to generate scientific graphics.

Conflicts of Interest: The authors declare no conflict of interest.

References

1. Fu, R.-H.; Wang, Y.-C.; Liu, S.-P.; Shih, T.-R.; Lin, H.-L.; Chen, Y.-M.; Sung, J.-H.; Lu, C.-H.; Wei, J.-R.; Wang, Z.-W.; et al. Decellularization and Recellularization Technologies in Tissue Engineering. *Cell Transplant.* **2014**, *23*, 621–630. [CrossRef] [PubMed]
2. Gratzer, P.F. Decellularized Extracellular Matrix. In *Encyclopedia of Biomedical Engineering*; Elsevier: Amsterdam, The Netherlands, 2019; pp. 86–96; ISBN 978-0-12-805144-3.
3. Shimoda, H.; Yagi, H.; Higashi, H.; Tajima, K.; Kuroda, K.; Abe, Y.; Kitago, M.; Shinoda, M.; Kitagawa, Y. Decellularized Liver Scaffolds Promote Liver Regeneration after Partial Hepatectomy. *Sci. Rep.* **2019**, *9*, 12543. [CrossRef]
4. Chen, Y.; Geerts, S.; Jaramillo, M.; Uygun, B.E. Preparation of Decellularized Liver Scaffolds and Recellularized Liver Grafts. In *Decellularized Scaffolds and Organogenesis*; Turksen, K., Ed.; Methods in Molecular Biology; Springer: New York, NY, USA, 2017; Volume 1577, pp. 255–270; ISBN 978-1-4939-7655-3.
5. Dai, Q.; Jiang, W.; Huang, F.; Song, F.; Zhang, J.; Zhao, H. Recent Advances in Liver Engineering with Decellularized Scaffold. *Front. Bioeng. Biotechnol.* **2022**, *10*, 831477. [CrossRef] [PubMed]
6. Dias, M.L.; Paranhos, B.A.; Goldenberg, R.C.D.S. Liver Scaffolds Obtained by Decellularization: A Transplant Perspective in Liver Bioengineering. *J. Tissue Eng.* **2022**, *13*, 204173142211053. [CrossRef] [PubMed]
7. Moffat, D.; Ye, K.; Jin, S. Decellularization for the Retention of Tissue Niches. *J. Tissue Eng.* **2022**, *13*, 204173142211011. [CrossRef]
8. Abdel-Misih, S.R.Z.; Bloomston, M. Liver Anatomy. *Surg. Clin. North. Am.* **2010**, *90*, 643–653. [CrossRef]
9. Arias, I.M. (Ed.) *The Liver: Biology and Pathobiology*, 6th ed.; Wiley-Blackwell: Hoboken, NJ, USA, 2020; ISBN 978-1-119-43684-3.
10. Bram, Y.; Nguyen, D.-H.T.; Gupta, V.; Park, J.; Richardson, C.; Chandar, V.; Schwartz, R.E. Cell and Tissue Therapy for the Treatment of Chronic Liver Disease. *Annu. Rev. Biomed. Eng.* **2021**, *23*, 517–546. [CrossRef]
11. Ishibashi, H.; Nakamura, M.; Komori, A.; Migita, K.; Shimoda, S. Liver Architecture, Cell Function, and Disease. *Semin. Immunopathol.* **2009**, *31*, 399–409. [CrossRef]
12. Kaur, S.; Tripathi, D.M.; Venugopal, J.R.; Ramakrishna, S. Advances in Biomaterials for Hepatic Tissue Engineering. *Curr. Opin. Biomed. Eng.* **2020**, *13*, 190–196. [CrossRef]
13. Sembulingam, K.; Sembulingam, P. *Essentials of Medical Physiology*, 6th ed.; Jaypee Brothers Medical Publishers: New Delhi, India, 2013; ISBN 978-93-5025-936-8.
14. Akay, E.M.; Okumus, Z.; Yildirim, O.S.; Bokhari, M.A.; Akay, G. *Synthetic Organs for Transplant and Bio-Mimic Reactors for Process Intensification Using Nano-Structured Micro-Porous Materials*; WIT Press: Riga, Latvia, 2011; pp. 383–394.
15. Krishna, M. Microscopic Anatomy of the Liver. *Clin. Liver Dis.* **2013**, *2*, S4–S7. [CrossRef]
16. Hall, J.E.; Guyton, A.C. *Guyton and Hall Textbook of Medical Physiology*, 12th ed.; Saunders/Elsevier: Philadelphia, PA, USA, 2011; ISBN 978-1-4160-4574-8.
17. Khurana, I. *Medical Physiology for Undergraduate Students: Illustrated Synopsis of Dermatology and Sexually Transmitted Diseases*, 1st ed.; Elsevier: New Delhi, India, 2014; ISBN 978-81-312-3622-2.
18. Fausto, N.; Campbell, J.S.; Riehle, K.J. Liver Regeneration. *Hepatology* **2006**, *43*, S45–S53. [CrossRef] [PubMed]
19. Hosseini, V.; Maroufi, N.F.; Saghati, S.; Asadi, N.; Darabi, M.; Ahmad, S.N.S.; Hosseinkhani, H.; Rahbarghazi, R. Current Progress in Hepatic Tissue Regeneration by Tissue Engineering. *J. Transl. Med.* **2019**, *17*, 383. [CrossRef] [PubMed]
20. Mitra, V.; Metcalf, J. Metabolic Functions of the Liver. *Anaesth. Intensive Care Med.* **2012**, *13*, 54–55. [CrossRef]
21. Dawson, P.A. Bile Formation and the Enterohepatic Circulation. In *Physiology of the Gastrointestinal Tract*; Elsevier: Amsterdam, The Netherlands, 2018; pp. 931–956; ISBN 978-0-12-809954-4.

22. Kalra, A.; Yetiskul, E.; Wehrle, C.J.; Tuma, F. Physiology, Liver. In *StatPearls*; StatPearls Publishing: Treasure Island, FL, USA, 2023.
23. Stec, D.E.; John, K.; Trabbic, C.J.; Luniwal, A.; Hankins, M.W.; Baum, J.; Hinds, T.D. Bilirubin Binding to PPARα Inhibits Lipid Accumulation. *PLoS ONE* **2016**, *11*, e0153427. [CrossRef] [PubMed]
24. Wang, X.; Chowdhury, J.R.; Chowdhury, N.R. Bilirubin Metabolism: Applied Physiology. *Curr. Paediatr.* **2006**, *16*, 70–74. [CrossRef]
25. Mazza, G.; Al-Akkad, W.; Rombouts, K.; Pinzani, M. Liver Tissue Engineering: From Implantable Tissue to Whole Organ Engineering. *Hepatol. Commun.* **2018**, *2*, 131–141. [CrossRef]
26. Asrani, S.K.; Devarbhavi, H.; Eaton, J.; Kamath, P.S. Burden of Liver Diseases in the World. *J. Hepatol.* **2019**, *70*, 151–171. [CrossRef]
27. Burra, P.; Becchetti, C.; Germani, G. NAFLD and Liver Transplantation: Disease Burden, Current Management and Future Challenges. *JHEP Rep.* **2020**, *2*, 100192. [CrossRef]
28. Teng, M.L.; Ng, C.H.; Huang, D.Q.; Chan, K.E.; Tan, D.J.; Lim, W.H.; Yang, J.D.; Tan, E.; Muthiah, M.D. Global Incidence and Prevalence of Nonalcoholic Fatty Liver Disease. *Clin. Mol. Hepatol.* **2023**, *29*, S32–S42. [CrossRef]
29. Huang, D.Q.; Terrault, N.A.; Tacke, F.; Gluud, L.L.; Arrese, M.; Bugianesi, E.; Loomba, R. Global Epidemiology of Cirrhosis—Aetiology, Trends and Predictions. *Nat. Rev. Gastroenterol. Hepatol.* **2023**, *20*, 388–398. [CrossRef]
30. Sudo, R. Multiscale Tissue Engineering for Liver Reconstruction. *Organogenesis* **2014**, *10*, 216–224. [CrossRef] [PubMed]
31. Heydari, Z.; Najimi, M.; Mirzaei, H.; Shpichka, A.; Ruoss, M.; Farzaneh, Z.; Montazeri, L.; Piryaei, A.; Timashev, P.; Gramignoli, R.; et al. Tissue Engineering in Liver Regenerative Medicine: Insights into Novel Translational Technologies. *Cells* **2020**, *9*, 304. [CrossRef] [PubMed]
32. Uygun, B.E.; Soto-Gutierrez, A.; Yagi, H.; Izamis, M.-L.; Guzzardi, M.A.; Shulman, C.; Milwid, J.; Kobayashi, N.; Tilles, A.; Berthiaume, F.; et al. Organ Reengineering through Development of a Transplantable Recellularized Liver Graft Using Decellularized Liver Matrix. *Nat. Med.* **2010**, *16*, 814–820. [CrossRef] [PubMed]
33. Zhang, X.; Chen, X.; Hong, H.; Hu, R.; Liu, J.; Liu, C. Decellularized Extracellular Matrix Scaffolds: Recent Trends and Emerging Strategies in Tissue Engineering. *Bioact. Mater.* **2022**, *10*, 15–31. [CrossRef] [PubMed]
34. Prestwich, G.D.; Atzet, S. Engineered Natural Materials. In *Biomaterials Science*; Elsevier: Amsterdam, The Netherlands, 2013; pp. 195–209; ISBN 978-0-12-374626-9.
35. Chandra, P.K.; Atala, A.A. Use of Matrix and Seeding with Cells for Vasculature of Organs. In *Reference Module in Biomedical Sciences*; Elsevier: Amsterdam, The Netherlands, 2018; p. B9780128012383110785; ISBN 978-0-12-801238-3.
36. Wu, I.; Elisseeff, J. Biomaterials and Tissue Engineering for Soft Tissue Reconstruction. In *Natural and Synthetic Biomedical Polymers*; Elsevier: Amsterdam, The Netherlands, 2014; pp. 235–241; ISBN 978-0-12-396983-5.
37. Gundu, S.; Sahi, A.K.; Varshney, N.; Varghese, J.; Vishwakarma, N.K.; Mahto, S.K. Fabrication and in Vitro Characterization of Luffa-Based Composite Scaffolds Incorporated with Gelatin, Hydroxyapatite and Psyllium Husk for Bone Tissue Engineering. *J. Biomater. Sci. Polym. Ed.* **2022**, *33*, 2220–2248. [CrossRef] [PubMed]
38. Allu, I.; Kumar Sahi, A.; Kumari, P.; Sakhile, K.; Sionkowska, A.; Gundu, S. A Brief Review on Cerium Oxide (CeO_2NPs)-Based Scaffolds: Recent Advances in Wound Healing Applications. *Micromachines* **2023**, *14*, 865. [CrossRef]
39. Lin, P.; Chan, W.C.W.; Badylak, S.F.; Bhatia, S.N. Assessing Porcine Liver-Derived Biomatrix for Hepatic Tissue Engineering. *Tissue Eng.* **2004**, *10*, 1046–1053. [CrossRef]
40. Choudhury, D.; Yee, M.; Sheng, Z.L.J.; Amirul, A.; Naing, M.W. Decellularization Systems and Devices: State-of-the-Art. *Acta Biomater.* **2020**, *115*, 51–59. [CrossRef]
41. Martinez-Hernandez, A.; Amenta, P.S. The Hepatic Extracellular Matrix: I. Components and Distribution in Normal Liver. *Vichows Arch. A Pathol. Anat.* **1993**, *423*, 1–11. [CrossRef]
42. Laurila, P.; Leivo, I. Basement Membrane and Interstitial Matrix Components Form Separate Matrices in Heterokaryons of PYS-2 Cells and Fibroblasts. *J. Cell Sci.* **1993**, *104*, 59–68. [CrossRef]
43. Bedossa, P.; Paradis, V. Liver Extracellular Matrix in Health and Disease: Liver Extracellular Matrix. *J. Pathol.* **2003**, *200*, 504–515. [CrossRef] [PubMed]
44. Mak, K.M.; Mei, R. Basement Membrane Type IV Collagen and Laminin: An Overview of Their Biology and Value as Fibrosis Biomarkers of Liver Disease: Type IV Collagen and Laminin. *Anat. Rec.* **2017**, *300*, 1371–1390. [CrossRef] [PubMed]
45. Rescan, P.Y.; Loréal, O.; Hassell, J.R.; Yamada, Y.; Guillouzo, A.; Clément, B. Distribution and Origin of the Basement Membrane Component Perlecan in Rat Liver and Primary Hepatocyte Culture. *Am. J. Pathol.* **1993**, *142*, 199–208. [PubMed]
46. Iredale, J.P.; Thompson, A.; Henderson, N.C. Extracellular Matrix Degradation in Liver Fibrosis: Biochemistry and Regulation. *Biochim. Biophys. Acta Mol. Basis Dis.* **2013**, *1832*, 876–883. [CrossRef] [PubMed]
47. Rauterberg, J.; Voss, B.; Pott, G.; Gerlach, U. Connective Tissue Components of the Normal and Fibrotic Liver: I. Structure, Local Distribution and Metabolism of Connective Tissue Components in the Normal Liver and Changes in Chronic Liver Diseases. *Klin. Wochenschr.* **1981**, *59*, 767–779. [CrossRef]
48. Xu, B.; Broome, U.; Uzunel, M.; Nava, S.; Ge, X.; Kumagai-Braesch, M.; Hultenby, K.; Christensson, B.; Ericzon, B.-G.; Holgersson, J.; et al. Capillarization of Hepatic Sinusoid by Liver Endothelial Cell-Reactive Autoantibodies in Patients with Cirrhosis and Chronic Hepatitis. *Am. J. Pathol.* **2003**, *163*, 1275–1289. [CrossRef]
49. Klaas, M.; Kangur, T.; Viil, J.; Mäemets-Allas, K.; Minajeva, A.; Vadi, K.; Antsov, M.; Lapidus, N.; Järvekülg, M.; Jaks, V. The Alterations in the Extracellular Matrix Composition Guide the Repair of Damaged Liver Tissue. *Sci. Rep.* **2016**, *6*, 27398. [CrossRef]

50. Thiele, M.; Johansen, S.; Gudmann, N.S.; Madsen, B.; Kjærgaard, M.; Nielsen, M.J.; Leeming, D.J.; Jacobsen, S.; Bendtsen, F.; Møller, S.; et al. Progressive Alcohol-related Liver Fibrosis Is Characterised by Imbalanced Collagen Formation and Degradation. *Aliment. Pharmacol. Ther.* **2021**, *54*, 1070–1080. [CrossRef]
51. Hoshiba, T.; Chen, G.; Endo, C.; Maruyama, H.; Wakui, M.; Nemoto, E.; Kawazoe, N.; Tanaka, M. Decellularized Extracellular Matrix as an In Vitro Model to Study the Comprehensive Roles of the ECM in Stem Cell Differentiation. *Stem Cells Int.* **2016**, *2016*, 6397820. [CrossRef]
52. Hynes, R.O. The Extracellular Matrix: Not Just Pretty Fibrils. *Science* **2009**, *326*, 1216–1219. [CrossRef]
53. Lopresti, S.T.; Brown, B.N. Host Response to Naturally Derived Biomaterials. In *Host Response to Biomaterials*; Elsevier: Amsterdam, The Netherlands, 2015; pp. 53–79; ISBN 978-0-12-800196-7.
54. Tao, M.; Ao, T.; Mao, X.; Yan, X.; Javed, R.; Hou, W.; Wang, Y.; Sun, C.; Lin, S.; Yu, T.; et al. Sterilization and Disinfection Methods for Decellularized Matrix Materials: Review, Consideration and Proposal. *Bioact. Mater.* **2021**, *6*, 2927–2945. [CrossRef] [PubMed]
55. Rajab, T.K.; O'Malley, T.J.; Tchantchaleishvili, V. Decellularized Scaffolds for Tissue Engineering: Current Status and Future Perspective. *Artif. Organs* **2020**, *44*, 1031–1043. [CrossRef]
56. Mendibil, U.; Ruiz-Hernandez, R.; Retegi-Carrion, S.; Garcia-Urquia, N.; Olalde-Graells, B.; Abarrategi, A. Tissue-Specific Decellularization Methods: Rationale and Strategies to Achieve Regenerative Compounds. *Int. J. Mol. Sci.* **2020**, *21*, 5447. [CrossRef] [PubMed]
57. Liao, J.; Xu, B.; Zhang, R.; Fan, Y.; Xie, H.; Li, X. Applications of Decellularized Materials in Tissue Engineering: Advantages, Drawbacks and Current Improvements, and Future Perspectives. *J. Mater. Chem. B* **2020**, *8*, 10023–10049. [CrossRef] [PubMed]
58. Gilpin, A.; Yang, Y. Decellularization Strategies for Regenerative Medicine: From Processing Techniques to Applications. *BioMed Res. Int.* **2017**, *2017*, 9831534. [CrossRef]
59. Boccafoschi, F.; Ramella, M.; Fusaro, L.; Catoira, M.C.; Casella, F. Biological Grafts: Surgical Use and Vascular Tissue Engineering Options for Peripheral Vascular Implants. In *Encyclopedia of Biomedical Engineering*; Elsevier: Amsterdam, The Netherlands, 2019; pp. 310–321; ISBN 978-0-12-805144-3.
60. Wang, X.; Chan, V.; Corridon, P.R. Decellularized Blood Vessel Development: Current State-of-the-Art and Future Directions. *Front. Bioeng. Biotechnol.* **2022**, *10*, 951644. [CrossRef]
61. Rabbani, M.; Zakian, N.; Alimoradi, N. Contribution of Physical Methods in Decellularization of Animal Tissues. *J. Med. Signals Sens.* **2021**, *11*, 1–11. [CrossRef]
62. Lange, P.; Greco, K.; Partington, L.; Carvalho, C.; Oliani, S.; Birchall, M.A.; Sibbons, P.D.; Lowdell, M.W.; Ansari, T. Pilot Study of a Novel Vacuum-Assisted Method for Decellularization of Tracheae for Clinical Tissue Engineering Applications: Vacuum-Assisted Decellularization. *J. Tissue Eng. Regen. Med.* **2017**, *11*, 800–811. [CrossRef]
63. Alizadeh, M.; Rezakhani, L.; Soleimannejad, M.; Sharifi, E.; Anjomshoa, M.; Alizadeh, A. Evaluation of Vacuum Washing in the Removal of SDS from Decellularized Bovine Pericardium: Method and Device Description. *Heliyon* **2019**, *5*, e02253. [CrossRef]
64. Butler, C.R.; Hynds, R.E.; Crowley, C.; Gowers, K.H.C.; Partington, L.; Hamilton, N.J.; Carvalho, C.; Platé, M.; Samuel, E.R.; Burns, A.J.; et al. Vacuum-Assisted Decellularization: An Accelerated Protocol to Generate Tissue-Engineered Human Tracheal Scaffolds. *Biomaterials* **2017**, *124*, 95–105. [CrossRef]
65. Lei, C.; Mei, S.; Zhou, C.; Xia, C. Decellularized Tracheal Scaffolds in Tracheal Reconstruction: An Evaluation of Different Techniques. *J. Appl. Biomater. Funct. Mater.* **2021**, *19*, 228080002110649. [CrossRef] [PubMed]
66. Alizadeh, M.; Rezakhani, L.; Khodaei, M.; Soleimannejad, M.; Alizadeh, A. Evaluating the Effects of Vacuum on the Microstructure and Biocompatibility of Bovine Decellularized Pericardium. *J. Tissue Eng. Regen. Med.* **2021**, *15*, 116–128. [CrossRef] [PubMed]
67. Crapo, P.M.; Gilbert, T.W.; Badylak, S.F. An Overview of Tissue and Whole Organ Decellularization Processes. *Biomaterials* **2011**, *32*, 3233–3243. [CrossRef] [PubMed]
68. Neishabouri, A.; Soltani Khaboushan, A.; Daghigh, F.; Kajbafzadeh, A.-M.; Majidi Zolbin, M. Decellularization in Tissue Engineering and Regenerative Medicine: Evaluation, Modification, and Application Methods. *Front. Bioeng. Biotechnol.* **2022**, *10*, 805299. [CrossRef]
69. Das, P.; Singh, Y.P.; Mandal, B.B.; Nandi, S.K. Tissue-Derived Decellularized Extracellular Matrices toward Cartilage Repair and Regeneration. In *Methods in Cell Biology*; Elsevier: Amsterdam, The Netherlands, 2020; Volume 157, pp. 185–221; ISBN 978-0-12-820174-9.
70. Funamoto, S.; Nam, K.; Kimura, T.; Murakoshi, A.; Hashimoto, Y.; Niwaya, K.; Kitamura, S.; Fujisato, T.; Kishida, A. The Use of High-Hydrostatic Pressure Treatment to Decellularize Blood Vessels. *Biomaterials* **2010**, *31*, 3590–3595. [CrossRef]
71. Zemmyo, D.; Yamamoto, M.; Miyata, S. Efficient Decellularization by Application of Moderate High Hydrostatic Pressure with Supercooling Pretreatment. *Micromachines* **2021**, *12*, 1486. [CrossRef]
72. Nouri Barkestani, M.; Naserian, S.; Uzan, G.; Shamdani, S. Post-Decellularization Techniques Ameliorate Cartilage Decellularization Process for Tissue Engineering Applications. *J. Tissue Eng.* **2021**, *12*, 204173142098356. [CrossRef]
73. Smagowska, B.; Pawlaczyk-Łuszczyńska, M. Effects of Ultrasonic Noise on the Human Body—A Bibliographic Review. *Int. J. Occup. Saf. Ergon.* **2013**, *19*, 195–202. [CrossRef]
74. Rubio, F.; Blandford, E.D.; Bond, L.J. Survey of Advanced Nuclear Technologies for Potential Applications of Sonoprocessing. *Ultrasonics* **2016**, *71*, 211–222. [CrossRef]
75. Lin, C.-H.; Hsia, K.; Su, C.-K.; Chen, C.-C.; Yeh, C.-C.; Ma, H.; Lu, J.-H. Sonication-Assisted Method for Decellularization of Human Umbilical Artery for Small-Caliber Vascular Tissue Engineering. *Polymers* **2021**, *13*, 1699. [CrossRef]

76. Phillips, M.; Maor, E.; Rubinsky, B. Nonthermal Irreversible Electroporation for Tissue Decellularization. *J. Biomech. Eng.* **2010**, *132*, 091003. [CrossRef]
77. Kim, B.; Kim, J.; So, K.; Hwang, N.S. Supercritical Fluid-Based Decellularization Technologies for Regenerative Medicine Applications. *Macromol. Biosci.* **2021**, *21*, 2100160. [CrossRef]
78. Arora, R. Mechanism of Freeze-Thaw Injury and Recovery: A Cool Retrospective and Warming up to New Ideas. *Plant Sci.* **2018**, *270*, 301–313. [CrossRef] [PubMed]
79. Burk, J.; Erbe, I.; Berner, D.; Kacza, J.; Kasper, C.; Pfeiffer, B.; Winter, K.; Brehm, W. Freeze-Thaw Cycles Enhance Decellularization of Large Tendons. *Tissue Eng. Methods* **2014**, *20*, 276–284. [CrossRef] [PubMed]
80. Cao, E.; Chen, Y.; Cui, Z.; Foster, P.R. Effect of Freezing and Thawing Rates on Denaturation of Proteins in Aqueous Solutions. *Biotechnol. Bioeng.* **2003**, *82*, 684–690. [CrossRef] [PubMed]
81. Cheng, J.; Wang, C.; Gu, Y. Combination of Freeze-Thaw with Detergents: A Promising Approach to the Decellularization of Porcine Carotid Arteries. *Bio-Med. Mater. Eng.* **2019**, *30*, 191–205. [CrossRef]
82. Poornejad, N.; Frost, T.S.; Scott, D.R.; Elton, B.B.; Reynolds, P.R.; Roeder, B.L.; Cook, A.D. Freezing/Thawing without Cryoprotectant Damages Native but Not Decellularized Porcine Renal Tissue. *Organogenesis* **2015**, *11*, 30–45. [CrossRef]
83. Santoso, E.G.; Yoshida, K.; Hirota, Y.; Aizawa, M.; Yoshino, O.; Kishida, A.; Osuga, Y.; Saito, S.; Ushida, T.; Furukawa, K.S. Application of Detergents or High Hydrostatic Pressure as Decellularization Processes in Uterine Tissues and Their Subsequent Effects on In Vivo Uterine Regeneration in Murine Models. *PLoS ONE* **2014**, *9*, e103201. [CrossRef]
84. Azhim, A.; Syazwani, N.; Morimoto, Y.; Furukawa, K.; Ushida, T. The Use of Sonication Treatment to Decellularize Aortic Tissues for Preparation of Bioscaffolds. *J. Biomater. Appl.* **2014**, *29*, 130–141. [CrossRef]
85. Syazwani, N.; Azhim, A.; Morimoto, Y.; Furukawa, K.S.; Ushida, T. Decellularization of Aorta Tissue Using Sonication Treatment as Potential Scaffold for Vascular Tissue Engineering. *J. Med. Biol. Eng.* **2015**, *35*, 258–269. [CrossRef]
86. Yusof, F.; Sha'ban, M.; Azhim, A. Development of Decellularized Meniscus Using Closed Sonication Treatment System: Potential Scaffolds for Orthopedics Tissue Engineering Applications. *Int. J. Nanomed.* **2019**, *14*, 5491–5502. [CrossRef] [PubMed]
87. Ho, M.P. Tissue Engineering with Electroporation. In *Handbook of Electroporation*; Miklavcic, D., Ed.; Springer International Publishing: Cham, Switzerland, 2016; pp. 1–21; ISBN 978-3-319-26779-1.
88. Koo, M.-A.; Jeong, H.; Hong, S.H.; Seon, G.M.; Lee, M.H.; Park, J.-C. Preconditioning Process for Dermal Tissue Decellularization Using Electroporation with Sonication. *Regen. Biomater.* **2022**, *9*, rbab071. [CrossRef]
89. Gerli, M.F.M.; Guyette, J.P.; Evangelista-Leite, D.; Ghoshhajra, B.B.; Ott, H.C. Perfusion Decellularization of a Human Limb: A Novel Platform for Composite Tissue Engineering and Reconstructive Surgery. *PLoS ONE* **2018**, *13*, e0191497. [PubMed]
90. Guyette, J.P.; Gilpin, S.E.; Charest, J.M.; Tapias, L.F.; Ren, X.; Ott, H.C. Perfusion Decellularization of Whole Organs. *Nat. Protoc.* **2014**, *9*, 1451–1468. [CrossRef]
91. Haniel, J.; de Souza Brandão, A.P.M.; Cruz, R.D.C.; Vale, M.; Soares, B.M.; Huebner, R. **Development of Equipment for Decellularization Using the Perfusion Method.** *Acta Sci. Technol.* **2018**, *40*, 35349. [CrossRef]
92. Zhang, J.; Hu, Z.Q.; Turner, N.J.; Teng, S.F.; Cheng, W.Y.; Zhou, H.Y.; Zhang, L.; Hu, H.W.; Wang, Q.; Badylak, S.F. Perfusion-Decellularized Skeletal Muscle as a Three-Dimensional Scaffold with a Vascular Network Template. *Biomaterials* **2016**, *89*, 114–126. [CrossRef] [PubMed]
93. Casali, D.M.; Handleton, R.M.; Shazly, T.; Matthews, M.A. A Novel Supercritical CO 2 -Based Decellularization Method for Maintaining Scaffold Hydration and Mechanical Properties. *J. Supercrit. Fluids* **2018**, *131*, 72–81. [CrossRef]
94. Chou, P.-R.; Lin, Y.-N.; Wu, S.-H.; Lin, S.-D.; Srinivasan, P.; Hsieh, D.-J.; Huang, S.-H. Supercritical Carbon Dioxide-Decellularized Porcine Acellular Dermal Matrix Combined with Autologous Adipose-Derived Stem Cells: Its Role in Accelerated Diabetic Wound Healing. *Int. J. Med. Sci.* **2020**, *17*, 354–367. [CrossRef]
95. Duarte, M.M.; Silva, I.V.; Eisenhut, A.R.; Bionda, N.; Duarte, A.R.C.; Oliveira, A.L. Contributions of Supercritical Fluid Technology for Advancing Decellularization and Postprocessing of Viable Biological Materials. *Mater. Horiz.* **2022**, *9*, 864–891. [CrossRef]
96. Srinivasan, P.; Hsieh, D.-J. Supercritical Carbon Dioxide Facilitated Collagen Scaffold Production for Tissue Engineering. In *Collagen Biomaterials*; Mazumder, N., Chakrabarty, S., Eds.; IntechOpen: Rijeka, Croatia, 2022; ISBN 978-1-80355-411-2.
97. Jiang, Y.; Li, R.; Han, C.; Huang, L. Extracellular Matrix Grafts: From Preparation to Application (Review). *Int. J. Mol. Med.* **2020**, *47*, 463–474. [CrossRef]
98. Yang, W. Nucleases: Diversity of Structure, Function and Mechanism. *Quart. Rev. Biophys.* **2011**, *44*, 1–93. [CrossRef] [PubMed]
99. Nokhbatolfoghahaei, H.; Paknejad, Z.; Bohlouli, M.; Rezai Rad, M.; Aminishakib, P.; Derakhshan, S.; Mohammadi Amirabad, L.; Nadjmi, N.; Khojasteh, A. Fabrication of Decellularized Engineered Extracellular Matrix through Bioreactor-Based Environment for Bone Tissue Engineering. *ACS Omega* **2020**, *5*, 31943–31956. [CrossRef] [PubMed]
100. Kim, Y.S.; Majid, M.; Melchiorri, A.J.; Mikos, A.G. Applications of Decellularized Extracellular Matrix in Bone and Cartilage Tissue Engineering. *Bioeng. Transl. Med.* **2019**, *4*, 83–95. [CrossRef]
101. Narciso, M.; Ulldemolins, A.; Júnior, C.; Otero, J.; Navajas, D.; Farré, R.; Gavara, N.; Almendros, I. Novel Decellularization Method for Tissue Slices. *Front. Bioeng. Biotechnol.* **2022**, *10*, 832178. [CrossRef]
102. Akbari Zahmati, A.H.; Alipoor, R.; Rezaei Shahmirzadi, A.; Khori, V.; Abolhasani, M.M. Chemical Decellularization Methods and Its Effects on Extracellular Matrix. *Intern. Med. Med. Investig. J.* **2017**, *2*, 76. [CrossRef]

103. Dussoyer, M.; Michopoulou, A.; Rousselle, P. Decellularized Scaffolds for Skin Repair and Regeneration. *Appl. Sci.* **2020**, *10*, 3435. [CrossRef]
104. Alaby Pinheiro Faccioli, L.; Suhett Dias, G.; Hoff, V.; Lemos Dias, M.; Ferreira Pimentel, C.; Hochman-Mendez, C.; Braz Parente, D.; Labrunie, E.; Souza Mourão, P.A.; Rogério de Oliveira Salvalaggio, P.; et al. Optimizing the Decellularized Porcine Liver Scaffold Protocol. *Cells Tissues Organs* **2022**, *211*, 385–394. [CrossRef]
105. Croce, S.; Peloso, A.; Zoro, T.; Avanzini, M.A.; Cobianchi, L. A Hepatic Scaffold from Decellularized Liver Tissue: Food for Thought. *Biomolecules* **2019**, *9*, 813. [CrossRef]
106. Hillebrandt, K.H.; Everwien, H.; Haep, N.; Keshi, E.; Pratschke, J.; Sauer, I.M. Strategies Based on Organ Decellularization and Recellularization. *Transpl. Int.* **2019**, *32*, 571–585. [CrossRef]
107. Mazza, G.; Rombouts, K.; Rennie Hall, A.; Urbani, L.; Vinh Luong, T.; Al-Akkad, W.; Longato, L.; Brown, D.; Maghsoudlou, P.; Dhillon, A.P.; et al. Decellularized Human Liver as a Natural 3D-Scaffold for Liver Bioengineering and Transplantation. *Sci. Rep.* **2015**, *5*, 13079. [CrossRef]
108. Coronado, R.E.; Somaraki-Cormier, M.; Natesan, S.; Christy, R.J.; Ong, J.L.; Halff, G.A. Decellularization and Solubilization of Porcine Liver for Use as a Substrate for Porcine Hepatocyte Culture: Method Optimization and Comparison. *Cell Transpl.* **2017**, *26*, 1840–1854. [CrossRef] [PubMed]
109. Lang, R.; Stern, M.M.; Smith, L.; Liu, Y.; Bharadwaj, S.; Liu, G.; Baptista, P.M.; Bergman, C.R.; Soker, S.; Yoo, J.J.; et al. Three-Dimensional Culture of Hepatocytes on Porcine Liver Tissue-Derived Extracellular Matrix. *Biomaterials* **2011**, *32*, 7042–7052. [CrossRef] [PubMed]
110. Willemse, J.; Verstegen, M.M.A.; Vermeulen, A.; Schurink, I.J.; Roest, H.P.; Van Der Laan, L.J.W.; De Jonge, J. Fast, Robust and Effective Decellularization of Whole Human Livers Using Mild Detergents and Pressure Controlled Perfusion. *Mater. Sci. Eng. C* **2020**, *108*, 110200. [CrossRef] [PubMed]
111. Wu, Q.; Bao, J.; Zhou, Y.; Wang, Y.; Du, Z.; Shi, Y.; Li, L.; Bu, H. Optimizing Perfusion-Decellularization Methods of Porcine Livers for Clinical-Scale Whole-Organ Bioengineering. *BioMed Res. Int.* **2015**, *2015*, 785474. [CrossRef] [PubMed]
112. Demko, P.; Hillebrandt, K.H.; Napierala, H.; Haep, N.; Tang, P.; Gassner, J.M.G.V.; Kluge, M.; Everwien, H.; Polenz, D.; Reutzel-Selke, A.; et al. Perfusion-Based Recellularization of Rat Livers with Islets of Langerhans. *J. Med. Biol. Eng.* **2022**, *42*, 271–280. [CrossRef]
113. Fathi, I.; Eltawila, A. Whole-Liver Decellularization: Advances and Insights into Current Understanding. In *Xenotransplantation-New Insights*; Miyagawa, S., Ed.; InTech: Rijeka, Croatia, 2017; ISBN 978-953-51-3355-1.
114. Nicholls, D.L.; Rostami, S.; Karoubi, G.; Haykal, S. Perfusion Decellularization for Vascularized Composite Allotransplantation. *SAGE Open Med.* **2022**, *10*, 205031212211238. [CrossRef]
115. Shaheen, M.F.; Joo, D.J.; Ross, J.J.; Anderson, B.D.; Chen, H.S.; Huebert, R.C.; Li, Y.; Amiot, B.; Young, A.; Zlochiver, V.; et al. Sustained Perfusion of Revascularized Bioengineered Livers Heterotopically Transplanted into Immunosuppressed Pigs. *Nat. Biomed. Eng.* **2019**, *4*, 437–445. [CrossRef]
116. Toprakhisar, B.; Verfaillie, C.M.; Kumar, M. Advances in Recellularization of Decellularized Liver Grafts with Different Liver (Stem) Cells: Towards Clinical Applications. *Cells* **2023**, *12*, 301. [CrossRef]
117. Maghsoudlou, P.; Georgiades, F.; Smith, H.; Milan, A.; Shangaris, P.; Urbani, L.; Loukogeorgakis, S.P.; Lombardi, B.; Mazza, G.; Hagen, C.; et al. Optimization of Liver Decellularization Maintains Extracellular Matrix Micro-Architecture and Composition Predisposing to Effective Cell Seeding. *PLoS One* **2016**, *11*, e0155324. [CrossRef]
118. Cissell, D.D.; Link, J.M.; Hu, J.C.; Athanasiou, K.A. A Modified Hydroxyproline Assay Based on Hydrochloric Acid in Ehrlich's Solution Accurately Measures Tissue Collagen Content. *Tissue Eng. Methods* **2017**, *23*, 243–250. [CrossRef]
119. Brézillon, S.; Untereiner, V.; Mohamed, H.T.; Hodin, J.; Chatron-Colliet, A.; Maquart, F.-X.; Sockalingum, G.D. Probing Glycosaminoglycan Spectral Signatures in Live Cells and Their Conditioned Media by Raman Microspectroscopy. *Analyst* **2017**, *142*, 1333–1341. [CrossRef]
120. Baptista, P.M.; Siddiqui, M.M.; Lozier, G.; Rodriguez, S.R.; Atala, A.; Soker, S. The Use of Whole Organ Decellularization for the Generation of a Vascularized Liver Organoid. *Hepatology* **2011**, *53*, 604–617. [CrossRef] [PubMed]
121. Hussein, K.H.; Park, K.-M.; Yu, L.; Kwak, H.-H.; Woo, H.-M. Decellularized Hepatic Extracellular Matrix Hydrogel Attenuates Hepatic Stellate Cell Activation and Liver Fibrosis. *Mater. Sci. Eng. C* **2020**, *116*, 111160. [CrossRef] [PubMed]
122. Wang, Y.; Bao, J.; Wu, Q.; Zhou, Y.; Li, Y.; Wu, X.; Shi, Y.; Li, L.; Bu, H. Method for Perfusion Decellularization of Porcine Whole Liver and Kidney for Use as a Scaffold for Clinical-Scale Bioengineering Engrafts. *Xenotransplantation* **2015**, *22*, 48–61. [CrossRef]
123. Washabau, R.J.; Day, M.J. Liver. In *Canine and Feline Gastroenterology*; Elsevier: Amsterdam, The Netherlands, 2013; pp. 849–957; ISBN 978-1-4160-3661-6.
124. Shupe, T.; Williams, M.; Brown, A.; Willenberg, B.; Petersen, B.E. Method for the Decellularization of Intact Rat Liver. *Organogenesis* **2010**, *6*, 134–136. [CrossRef] [PubMed]
125. Debnath, T.; Mallarpu, C.S.; Chelluri, L.K. Development of Bioengineered Organ Using Biological Acellular Rat Liver Scaffold and Hepatocytes. *Organogenesis* **2020**, *16*, 61–72. [CrossRef] [PubMed]
126. De Kock, J.; Ceelen, L.; De Spiegelaere, W.; Casteleyn, C.; Claes, P.; Vanhaecke, T.; Rogiers, V. Simple and Quick Method for Whole-Liver Decellularization: A Novel In Vitro Three-Dimensional Bioengineering Tool? *Arch. Toxicol.* **2011**, *85*, 607–612. [CrossRef]

127. Gao, Y.; Li, Z.; Hong, Y.; Li, T.; Hu, X.; Sun, L.; Chen, Z.; Chen, Z.; Luo, Z.; Wang, X.; et al. Decellularized Liver as a Translucent Ex Vivo Model for Vascular Embolization Evaluation. *Biomaterials* **2020**, *240*, 119855. [CrossRef]
128. Lu, S.; Cuzzucoli, F.; Jiang, J.; Liang, L.-G.; Wang, Y.; Kong, M.; Zhao, X.; Cui, W.; Li, J.; Wang, S. Development of a Biomimetic Liver Tumor-on-a-Chip Model Based on Decellularized Liver Matrix for Toxicity Testing. *Lab. Chip* **2018**, *18*, 3379–3392. [CrossRef]
129. Caires-Júnior, L.C.; Goulart, E.; Telles-Silva, K.A.; Araujo, B.H.S.; Musso, C.M.; Kobayashi, G.; Oliveira, D.; Assoni, A.; Carvalho, V.M.; Ribeiro-Jr, A.F.; et al. Pre-Coating Decellularized Liver with HepG2-Conditioned Medium Improves Hepatic Recellularization. *Mater. Sci. Eng. C* **2021**, *121*, 111862. [CrossRef]
130. Soto-Gutierrez, A.; Navarro-Alvarez, N.; Yagi, H.; Nahmias, Y.; Yarmush, M.L.; Kobayashi, N. Engineering of an Hepatic Organoid to Develop Liver Assist Devices. *Cell Transpl.* **2010**, *19*, 815–822. [CrossRef] [PubMed]
131. Chen, W.; Xu, Y.; Li, Y.; Jia, L.; Mo, X.; Jiang, G.; Zhou, G. 3D Printing Electrospinning Fiber-Reinforced Decellularized Extracellular Matrix for Cartilage Regeneration. *Chem. Eng. J.* **2020**, *382*, 122986. [CrossRef]
132. Wang, H.; Yu, H.; Zhou, X.; Zhang, J.; Zhou, H.; Hao, H.; Ding, L.; Li, H.; Gu, Y.; Ma, J.; et al. An Overview of Extracellular Matrix-Based Bioinks for 3D Bioprinting. *Front. Bioeng. Biotechnol.* **2022**, *10*, 905438. [CrossRef]
133. Khati, V. *Decellularized Liver Extracellular Matrix as a 3D Scaffold for Bioengineering Applications*; KTH Royal Institute of Technology: Stockholm, Sweden, 2022.
134. Zhang, C.-Y.; Fu, C.-P.; Li, X.-Y.; Lu, X.-C.; Hu, L.-G.; Kankala, R.K.; Wang, S.-B.; Chen, A.-Z. Three-Dimensional Bioprinting of Decellularized Extracellular Matrix-Based Bioinks for Tissue Engineering. *Molecules* **2022**, *27*, 3442. [CrossRef] [PubMed]
135. Lee, H.; Han, W.; Kim, H.; Ha, D.-H.; Jang, J.; Kim, B.S.; Cho, D.-W. Development of Liver Decellularized Extracellular Matrix Bioink for Three-Dimensional Cell Printing-Based Liver Tissue Engineering. *Biomacromolecules* **2017**, *18*, 1229–1237. [CrossRef]
136. Zhe, M.; Wu, X.; Yu, P.; Xu, J.; Liu, M.; Yang, G.; Xiang, Z.; Xing, F.; Ritz, U. Recent Advances in Decellularized Extracellular Matrix-Based Bioinks for 3D Bioprinting in Tissue Engineering. *Materials* **2023**, *16*, 3197. [CrossRef]
137. Agmon, G.; Christman, K.L. Controlling Stem Cell Behavior with Decellularized Extracellular Matrix Scaffolds. *Curr. Opin. Solid. State Mater. Sci.* **2016**, *20*, 193–201. [CrossRef]
138. Mao, Q.; Wang, Y.; Li, Y.; Juengpanich, S.; Li, W.; Chen, M.; Yin, J.; Fu, J.; Cai, X. Fabrication of Liver Microtissue with Liver Decellularized Extracellular Matrix (dECM) Bioink by Digital Light Processing (DLP) Bioprinting. *Mater. Sci. Eng. C* **2020**, *109*, 110625. [CrossRef]
139. Khati, V.; Ramachandraiah, H.; Pati, F.; Svahn, H.A.; Gaudenzi, G.; Russom, A. 3D Bioprinting of Multi-Material Decellularized Liver Matrix Hydrogel at Physiological Temperatures. *Biosensors* **2022**, *12*, 521. [CrossRef]
140. Kim, M.K.; Jeong, W.; Kang, H.-W. Liver dECM–Gelatin Composite Bioink for Precise 3D Printing of Highly Functional Liver Tissues. *J. Funct. Biomater.* **2023**, *14*, 417. [CrossRef]
141. Mir, T.A.; Nakamura, M.; Sakai, S.; Iwanaga, S.; Wani, S.I.; Alzhrani, A.; Arai, K.; Mir, B.A.; Kazmi, S.; Assiri, A.M.; et al. Mammalian-Specific Decellularized Matrices Derived Bioink for Bioengineering of Liver Tissue Analogues: A Review. *Int. J. Bioprint.* **2023**, *9*, 714. [CrossRef] [PubMed]
142. Dzobo, K.; Motaung, K.S.C.M.; Adesida, A. Recent Trends in Decellularized Extracellular Matrix Bioinks for 3D Printing: An Updated Review. *Int. J. Mol. Sci.* **2019**, *20*, 4628. [CrossRef] [PubMed]
143. Semba, J.A.; Mieloch, A.A.; Tomaszewska, E.; Cywoniuk, P.; Rybka, J.D. Formulation and Evaluation of a Bioink Composed of Alginate, Gelatin, and Nanocellulose for Meniscal Tissue Engineering. *Int. J. Bioprint.* **2022**, *9*, 621. [CrossRef] [PubMed]
144. Luo, W.; Song, Z.; Wang, Z.; Wang, Z.; Li, Z.; Wang, C.; Liu, H.; Liu, Q.; Wang, J. Printability Optimization of Gelatin-Alginate Bioinks by Cellulose Nanofiber Modification for Potential Meniscus Bioprinting. *J. Nanomater.* **2020**, *2020*, 3863428. [CrossRef]
145. Stepanovska, J.; Supova, M.; Hanzalek, K.; Broz, A.; Matejka, R. Collagen Bioinks for Bioprinting: A Systematic Review of Hydrogel Properties, Bioprinting Parameters, Protocols, and Bioprinted Structure Characteristics. *Biomedicines* **2021**, *9*, 1137. [CrossRef]
146. Ahmed, E.; Saleh, T.; Yu, L.; Song, S.; Park, K.; Kwak, H.; Woo, H. Decellularized Extracellular Matrix-rich Hydrogel–Silver Nanoparticle Mixture as a Potential Treatment for Acute Liver Failure Model. *J. Biomed. Mater. Res.* **2020**, *108*, 2351–2367. [CrossRef]
147. Saleh, T.; Ahmed, E.; Yu, L.; Hussein, K.; Park, K.-M.; Lee, Y.-S.; Kang, B.-J.; Choi, K.-Y.; Choi, S.; Kang, K.-S.; et al. Silver Nanoparticles Improve Structural Stability and Biocompatibility of Decellularized Porcine Liver. *Artif. Cells Nanomed. Biotechnol.* **2018**, *46*, 273–284. [CrossRef]
148. Saleh, T.M.; Ahmed, E.A.; Yu, L.; Kwak, H.-H.; Hussein, K.H.; Park, K.-M.; Kang, B.-J.; Choi, K.-Y.; Kang, K.-S.; Woo, H.-M. Incorporation of Nanoparticles into Transplantable Decellularized Matrices: Applications and Challenges. *Int. J. Artif. Organs* **2018**, *41*, 421–430. [CrossRef]
149. Xu, F.; Kang, T.; Deng, J.; Liu, J.; Chen, X.; Wang, Y.; Ouyang, L.; Du, T.; Tang, H.; Xu, X.; et al. Functional Nanoparticles Activate a Decellularized Liver Scaffold for Blood Detoxification. *Small* **2020**, *16*, 2001267. [CrossRef]
150. Sahi, A.K.; Varshney, N.; Poddar, S.; Mahto, S.K. Comparative Behaviour of Electrospun Nanofibers Fabricated from Acid and Alkaline Hydrolysed Gelatin: Towards Corneal Tissue Engineering. *J. Polym. Res.* **2020**, *27*, 344. [CrossRef]
151. Sahi, A.K.; Varshney, N.; Poddar, S.; Gundu, S.; Mahto, S.K. Fabrication and Characterization of Silk Fibroin-Based Nanofibrous Scaffolds Supplemented with Gelatin for Corneal Tissue Engineering. *Cells Tissues Organs* **2021**, *210*, 173–194. [CrossRef] [PubMed]

152. Kumar Sahi, A.; Gundu, S.; Kumari, P.; Klepka, T.; Sionkowska, A. Silk-Based Biomaterials for Designing Bioinspired Microarchitecture for Various Biomedical Applications. *Biomimetics* **2023**, *8*, 55. [CrossRef] [PubMed]
153. Santschi, M.; Vernengo, A.; Eglin, D.; D'Este, M.; Wuertz-Kozak, K. Decellularized Matrix as a Building Block in Bioprinting and Electrospinning. *Curr. Opin. Biomed. Eng.* **2019**, *10*, 116–122. [CrossRef]
154. Liu, J.S.; Madruga, L.Y.C.; Yuan, Y.; Kipper, M.J.; Khetani, S.R. Decellularized Liver Nanofibers Enhance and Stabilize the Long-Term Functions of Primary Human Hepatocytes In Vitro. *Adv. Healthc. Mater.* **2023**, *12*, 2202302. [CrossRef] [PubMed]
155. Vasudevan, A.; Tripathi, D.M.; Sundarrajan, S.; Venugopal, J.R.; Ramakrishna, S.; Kaur, S. Evolution of Electrospinning in Liver Tissue Engineering. *Biomimetics* **2022**, *7*, 149. [CrossRef]
156. Grant, R.; Hallett, J.; Forbes, S.; Hay, D.; Callanan, A. Blended Electrospinning with Human Liver Extracellular Matrix for Engineering New Hepatic Microenvironments. *Sci. Rep.* **2019**, *9*, 6293. [CrossRef]
157. Grant, R.; Hay, D.C.; Callanan, A. A Drug-Induced Hybrid Electrospun Poly-Capro-Lactone: Cell-Derived Extracellular Matrix Scaffold for Liver Tissue Engineering. *Tissue Eng.* **2017**, *23*, 650–662. [CrossRef]
158. Goecke, T.; Theodoridis, K.; Tudorache, I.; Ciubotaru, A.; Cebotari, S.; Ramm, R.; Höffler, K.; Sarikouch, S.; Vásquez Rivera, A.; Haverich, A.; et al. In Vivo Performance of Freeze-Dried Decellularized Pulmonary Heart Valve Allo- and Xenografts Orthotopically Implanted into Juvenile Sheep. *Acta Biomater.* **2018**, *68*, 41–52. [CrossRef]
159. Zheng, L.; Zheng, S.; Chen, Z.; Li, X.; Liu, C.; Bai, J.; Jiang, D.; Nie, Y.; Zhang, J.; Liu, T.; et al. Preparation and Properties of Decellularized Sheep Kidney Derived Matrix Scaffolds. *J. Phys. Conf. Ser.* **2022**, *2160*, 012014. [CrossRef]
160. Gundu, S.; Varshney, N.; Sahi, A.K.; Mahto, S.K. Recent Developments of Biomaterial Scaffolds and Regenerative Approaches for Craniomaxillofacial Bone Tissue Engineering. *J. Polym. Res.* **2022**, *29*, 73. [CrossRef]
161. Ibne Mahbub, M.S.; Bae, S.H.; Gwon, J.-G.; Lee, B.-T. Decellularized Liver Extracellular Matrix and Thrombin Loaded Biodegradable TOCN/Chitosan Nanocomposite for Hemostasis and Wound Healing in Rat Liver Hemorrhage Model. *Int. J. Biol. Macromol.* **2023**, *225*, 1529–1542. [CrossRef] [PubMed]

Disclaimer/Publisher's Note: The statements, opinions and data contained in all publications are solely those of the individual author(s) and contributor(s) and not of MDPI and/or the editor(s). MDPI and/or the editor(s) disclaim responsibility for any injury to people or property resulting from any ideas, methods, instructions or products referred to in the content.

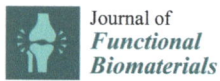 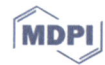

Article

Development and Functionalization of a Novel Chitosan-Based Nanosystem for Enhanced Drug Delivery

Carmen Grierosu [1,2], Gabriela Calin [1,*], Daniela Damir [3,*], Constantin Marcu [4,5], Radu Cernei [6,*], Georgeta Zegan [6], Daniela Anistoroaei [6], Mihaela Moscu [6], Elena Mihaela Carausu [6], Letitia Doina Duceac [1,4,7], Marius Gabriel Dabija [6,7], Geta Mitrea [4,8], Cristian Gutu [4,9], Elena Roxana Bogdan Goroftei [4,10] and Lucian Eva [1,7]

1. Faculty of Dental Medicine, "Apollonia" University of Iasi, 11 Pacurari Str., 700511 Iasi, Romania; grierosucarmen@yahoo.com (C.G.); letimedr@yahoo.com (L.D.D.); lucianeva74@yahoo.com (L.E.)
2. Orthopaedic Trauma Surgery Clinic, Clinical Rehabilitation Hospital, 14 Pantelimon Halipa Str., 700661 Iasi, Romania
3. Faculty of Medicine, "Grigore T. Popa" University of Medicine and Pharmacy Iasi, 16 Universitatii Str., 700115 Iasi, Romania
4. Faculty of Medicine and Pharmacy, University Dunarea de Jos, 47 Domneasca Str., 800008 Galati, Romania; marcu_saar@yahoo.de (C.M.); getamitrea@yahoo.com (G.M.); dr_cgutu@yahoo.com (C.G.); elenamed84@yahoo.com (E.R.B.G.)
5. Saarbrucken-Caritas Klinkum St. Theresia University Hospital, 66113 Saarbrücken, Germany
6. Faculty of Dental Medicine, "Grigore T. Popa" University of Medicine and Pharmacy Iasi, 16 Universitatii Str., 700115 Iasi, Romania; georgetazegan@yahoo.com (G.Z.); anistoroaei_daniela@yahoo.com (D.A.); mihaela_moscu@ymail.com (M.M.); mihaelacarausu@yahoo.com (E.M.C.); mariusdabija.md@gmail.com (M.G.D.)
7. "Prof. Dr. Nicolae Oblu" Neurosurgery Hospital Iasi, 2 Ateneului Str., 700309 Iasi, Romania
8. "St. Ap. Andrei" Emergency Clinical Hospital, 177 Brailei Str., 800578 Galati, Romania
9. "Dr. Aristide Serfioti" Emergency Military Hospital, 199 Traian Str., 800150 Galati, Romania
10. "Sf Ioan" Emergency Clinical Hospital, 2 Gheorghe Asachi Str., 800494 Galati, Romania
* Correspondence: m_gabriela2004@yahoo.com (G.C.); danadamir@yahoo.com (D.D.); cerneiradu@yahoo.com (R.C.)

Abstract: Nowadays, infection diseases are one of the most significant threats to humans all around the world. An encouraging strategy for solving this issue and fighting resistant microorganisms is to develop drug carriers for a prolonged release of the antibiotic to the target site. The purpose of this work was to obtain metronidazole-encapsulated chitosan nanoparticles using an ion gelation route and to evaluate their properties. Due to the advantages of the ionic gelation method, the synthesized polymeric nanoparticles can be applied in various fields, especially pharmaceutical and medical. Loading capacity and encapsulation efficiency varFied depending on the amount of antibiotic in each formulation. Physicochemical characterization using scanning electron microscopy revealed a narrow particle size distribution where 90% of chitosan particles were 163.7 nm in size and chitosan-loaded metronidazole nanoparticles were 201.3 nm in size, with a zeta potential value of 36.5 mV. IR spectra revealed characteristic peaks of the drug and polymer nanoparticles. Cell viability assessment revealed that samples have no significant impact on tested cells. Release analysis showed that metronidazole was released from the chitosan matrix for 24 h in a prolonged course, implying that antibiotic-encapsulated polymer nanostructures are a promising drug delivery system to prevent or to treat various diseases. It is desirable to obtain new formulations based on drugs encapsulated in nanoparticles through different preparation methods, with reduced cytotoxic potential, in order to improve the therapeutic effect through sustained and prolonged release mechanisms of the drug correlated with the reduction of adverse effects.

Keywords: polymer composite; bioactivity; biodegradability; metronidazole; biomedical application

1. Introduction

For many years, nanotechnology significantly contributed to biomedicine regarding prevention, diagnosis and treatment of various diseases [1–3]. Nanomaterials used as drug transporters are very important due to their small size and morphology [4,5]. These properties are relevant for active molecules loading and sustained release to the specific site of action [6–9]. A considerable issue is to design drug delivery systems in order to enhance the pharmaceutical impact of a drug and to limit its side effects [10,11].

Metronidazole (MET) is a broad-spectrum antibiotic used to combat anaerobic bacteria and some parasites. It is a nitro-imidazole (Figure 1) derived from the reduction of the nitro group on the molecule by the bacteria and thus determines the emergence of toxic metabolites. These compounds use their bactericidal action with molecular DNA destruction, stopping the DNA repair process. Metronidazole is a drug that penetrates bacteria through the mechanism of passive diffusion, and is activated in the cytoplasm where it is transformed into free nitrogen radical. Having cytotoxic activity, it inhibits synthesis and damages DNA, stopping the multiplication of bacteria. Furthermore, the DNA breakage caused by the metronidazole metabolites leads to bacterial cell damage. This drug treats surgical infections, duodenal ulcer caused by Helicobacter Pylori contamination, intestinal amoebiasis, etc. Nowadays, metronidazole is used as an antimicrobial agent for the cure of periodontal disease, including topical application after scaling and subgingival treatment. The pharmacokinetic profile of metronidazole shows that the active substance reaches a concentration of 10 mg/mL in plasma one hour after the administration of a dose of 500 mg.

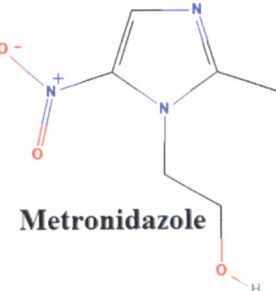

Figure 1. Chemical structure of metronidazole molecule.

Administration of MET can cause certain side effects such as nausea, mouth dryness, epigastric pain and others. A major disadvantage regarding conventional therapy refers to the accumulation of high drug concentrations in the liver and kidneys. Among the side effects caused by the administration of systemic antibiotics, gastrointestinal intolerances, hypersensitivity reactions and the establishment of bacterial resistance can be noted. There are studies that reveal that if the active substance does not reach the desired concentration at the site of action, systems for the prolonged release of drugs can be developed, reaching the desired concentration at the site of action and reducing adverse effects.

In order to combat adverse effects of metronidazole it is necessary to reformulate the antibiotic by developing a different drug delivery nanosystem which yields better targeted transport of the active molecule. Nowadays, researchers are focused on reducing antibiotic side effects as well as delivering the active molecule to the target site, enhancing drug efficiency [12–16]. MET is also currently used for the treatment of periodontal disease, especially as a topical administrative drug inhibiting anaerobic microorganisms [17,18].

Although many types of nanoparticles were studied as drug delivery systems, ample researches were developed on polymeric nanostructures for various active molecule transports. Polymeric nanosized architectures own excellent stability, reproducibility and biodegradability properties, making them suitable for the application in several pharmaceutical formulations [16].

Chitosan is a natural polymer obtained with the deacetylation of chitin. It is a biocompatible cationic polysaccharide metabolized with specific human enzymes, mainly lysozyme, which attributes chitosan to be a possibly efficient drug carrier [19–21]. Chemical structure of chitosan (Figure 2) contains copolymer units of N-acetyl-glucosamine and glucosamine. Structurally, the chitosan molecule presents functional groups that allow electrochemical interactions at the molecular and cellular level. Chitosan nanoparticles possess antimicrobial properties; therefore, they can be loaded with several bioactive molecules to obtain different formulations used in the medical field [22–25]. Due to chitosan's low solubility, some proposals for tailoring its structure were advanced in order to obtain various chitosan derivatives, and improved solubility was achieved by using free hydroxyl and amino groups based on the self-assembly feature.

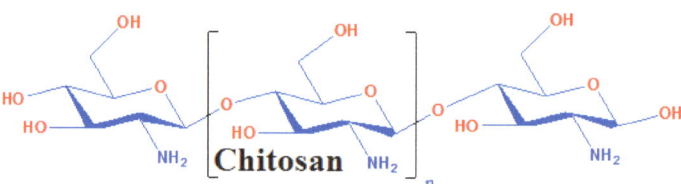

Figure 2. Structural representation of chitosan.

The significant properties of chitosan determined researchers to use it in various bio-medical formulations.

Studies on the synthesis of nanoparticles with the ionic gelation method have attracted the attention of researchers in recent years. This is because various compounds can be loaded into the polymer structure, thus constituting the drug delivery system and being able to be used later in various medical fields. Therefore, this biopolymer has been involved in several trials, namely drug delivery, with applications in many medical areas, such as dental medicine, tissue engineering, epidemiology, pulmonology, neurosurgery, neonatology, cardiology, emergency, regenerative medicine (including hard tissue and soft tissue due to its ability to protect unstable biomolecules), biodegradation, biocompatibility, mucosal tissue adhering, nontoxicity and antimicrobial activity. The use of such systems requires small amounts of the active substance as the absorption of the medicine is carried out in a sustained and controlled manner, thus reducing the side effects of antibiotics [26–31]. Although many drug-loaded chitosan nanoparticles were studied as carriers, this work proposes obtaining a novel formulation based on metronidazole-encapsulated chitosan nanoparticles and evaluating the cytotoxicity of these nanostructures according to physicochemical features and the drug release profile. Nowadays, biomedical application and development of polymer composites [32], which includes significant features such as bioactivity, low toxicity, molecules transport and biodegradability, is of major interest. Our study involved the preparation of a nanosystem based on chitosan nanoparticles loaded with metronidazole, which was structurally and morphologically characterized and evaluated for its cytotoxic effect. Formulation designs based on drug-loaded polymeric nanoparticles could provide improved therapeutic alternatives for currently administered drugs. Furthermore, this study proposed that the new drug delivery systems increase the therapeutic effect through biodegradation processes of the polymer matrix, deliver the active molecule to the target site and, implicitly, reduce side effects on the body.

2. Materials and Methods

2.1. Materials

Metronidazole active substance was offered by a research institute for free (Sigma–Aldrich, analytical standard, ≤100%, stable at room temperature). Chitosan (75–85% deacetylated) and sodium tri-polyphosphate was acquired from Sigma–Aldrich, Darmstadt, Germany. The other reagents used to obtain antibiotic-loaded chitosan nanoparticles were of analytical grade of purity.

2.2. Preparation Methods

Nanoparticles' Preparation

Chitosan nanoparticles (Chi) were obtained with ionic gelation method [31] using tri-polyphosphate (TPP) as cross-linking agent due to their counter ions which establish inter- and intra-molecular connections. This is a route to obtain nanoparticles based on the electrostatic interaction between compounds with opposite charges, with chitosan (cation) and TPP (anion) being the most frequently used. By adding TPP, drop by drop, to a solution containing chitosan, the polyanion binds to an amino group, which causes the polymer to suffer a gel ionization operation; then, nanoparticles were forms with centrifugation. The preparation of polymeric nanoparticles depends on the concentration of the polymer, its molecular weight, the chitosan/tri-polyphosphate ratio, the concentration of the bioactive principle, pH, the time and speed of stirring and centrifugation. This technique implies dissolution of chitosan polysaccharide in an aqueous acid solution (1% v/v glacial acetic acid) resulting in positively charged chitosan. Then, this solution is added to a TPP solution (0.1% w/v in ultrapure water) under stirring conditions and forms a positive–negative complex.

For preparation of antibiotic-loaded polymer nanoparticles, metronidazole (in different concentrations) was added to chitosan solution, and adjustment of the pH of each product at 5.0 was performed by using solutions of 0.1 N HCl and 1 N NaOH. The as prepared nanocomposites were centrifuged at 9000 rpm for 1 h at room temperature. After this step, the supernatant was kept at 2–6 °C until further assessment. Finally, the antibiotic-loaded chitosan nanoparticles were lyophilized for 48 h and analyzed to achieve the aims of this study. The ionic gelation method requires cheap and easy-to-use materials and equipment, and having the advantage of the electrostatic interaction mechanism, instead of chemical synthesis, leads to the avoidance of possible toxicity of the reagents; however, its disadvantage is that nanoparticles are not produced on a large scale with a uniform size distribution. This technique is widely used because it has proven to be useful for obtaining various formulations of polymeric nanoparticles loaded with drugs. Each formulation code is presented in Table 1, which comprises the concentration of the drug, polymer and crosslinking agent.

Table 1. The proportion of chitosan, TPP and metronidazole used in different formulations.

Code of Each Formulation	Chitosan (mg)	Crosslinking Agent, TPP (mg)	Metronidazole (mg)
Chi_1	100	50	-
Chi_2	150	50	-
Chi_3	200	50	-
ChiMet_2.1	150	50	100
ChiMet_2.2	150	50	150
ChiMet_2.3	150	50	200

After preparing the nanostructures, their characterization included particle size distribution (PSD), zeta potential, morphology (scanning electron microscope, SEM), encapsulation efficiency (EE), loading capacity (LC), Fourier transform infrared spectroscopy (FTIR) and spectrometry (UV-Vis). The characteristics of nanocomposites using these advanced techniques depended on the synthesis conditions.

2.3. Characterization Equipment

Characterization of the obtained samples was based on antibiotic-loaded polymer nanoparticles.

2.3.1. Evaluation of Loading Capacity and Encapsulation Efficiency

Loading capacity and encapsulation efficiency of each composite was established using a Cary 60 UV-Vis spectrometer at 319.5 nm to measure the absorption of each supernatant after centrifugation. Loading capacity and encapsulation efficiency are expressed by the following formula:

$$\text{Loading capacity (\%)} = \frac{W_t - W_f}{W_n} \times 100 \quad (1)$$

$$\text{Encapsulation efficiency (\%)} = \frac{W_t - W_f}{W_t} \times 100 \quad (2)$$

where

- W_t is the total content of metronidazole encapsulated initially into the polymer matrix;
- W_f represents the amount of drugs in the supernatant;
- W_n represents the weight of dried nanoparticles after lyophilization process.

Loading capacity is an indicator that reveals the amount of drugs that can be loaded into a quantity of nanocomposite; encapsulation efficiency is an index that shows the yield of the process of obtaining nanostructures.

Nanoparticles' Size Assessment

Particles' size distribution was established with DLS (dynamic light scattering) using a Zetasizer Nano ZS (Malvern, Germany), which evaluates the particle size, electrophoretic mobility and zeta potential.

2.3.2. Nanoparticles' Morphology

Morphological features of metronidazole-loaded chitosan nanoparticles were analyzed using scanning electron microscope (Thermo Fisher Scientific, Waltham, MA, USA) equipped with an energy dispersive spectrometer (EDS, EDAX Octane Elite, Thermo Fisher Scientific, Waltham, MA, USA), which allows high-resolution morphological investigations of these types of nanocomposites. Nanostructured samples were dried at room temperature by spreading the suspensions on a glass plate; then, they were coated with gold under vacuum before examination.

FTIR (Fourier transform infrared spectroscopy) characterization implied scanning of KBr tablets (in the spectral range of 4000 to 400 cm^{-1}) that were obtained by compressing a mixture containing small amounts of KBr and antibiotic-loaded polymer nanoparticles.

Release profiles were established at 37 °C in a horizontal shaker containing 50 mg/200 mL of drug-loaded chitosan nanoarchitectures by applying a few horizontal strikes. Dissolution media comprised phosphate-buffered saline solution pH 7.5, phosphate-buffered solution pH 7.0 and 0.1 N HCl solution pH 1.5. Metronidazole release operation was performed for 24 h and, at fixed intervals, 10 mL of sample was withdrawn and substituted with dissolution media then analyzed with UV-Vis spectrophotometer, at specific wavelengths to each dissolution media.

2.3.3. Cell Viability Assay

HeLa cells were used for testing cytotoxic effect of metronidazole-encapsulated chitosan nanoparticles. After 24 h of incubation, in presence of the tested compounds, cell viability was evaluated with MTT assay. HeLa cell line was maintained in DMEM (Dulbecco's Modified Eagle Medium, Biochrom AG, Berlin, Germany), and supplemented with 10% FSB (fetal bovine serum), 100 IU/mL penicillin and 100 µg/mL streptomycin at 37 °C in a humidified atmosphere of 5% CO_2 in air. Evaluation of viability was based on MTT assay. HeLa cells were seeded in 96-well plates (density of 5×10^3 cells/well), allowed to attach and grow overnight. Treatment with the polymeric nanoparticles anticipated the replacement of growth medium with new complete medium containing the NPs in doses ranging from 100 µg/mL to 0.01 µg/mL. After 24 h of treatment, the cells were washed and covered with 100 μL of fresh DMEM 10% FBS. An amount of 10 μL of MTT (5 mg/mL) was added into medium, and cells were incubated for another 3 h. DMSO (dimethyl sulfoxide, Merck, Darmstadt, Germany) was used to dissolve the formazan that was formed, and the absorbance was recorded at 570 nm.

3. Results

The loading capacity and encapsulation efficiency (Table 2) reveals that a higher antibiotic concentration determined a reduction in the loading capacity and an increase in the encapsulation efficiency.

Table 2. Loading capacity and encapsulation efficiency of the noncompounds.

Sample Code	Metronidazole/Chitosan Conc.	Loading Capacity, %	Encapsulation Efficiency, %
ChiMet_2.1	100/150	70	26
ChiMet_2.2	150/150	67	30
ChiMet_2.3	200/150	62	35

The results of particle size and zeta potential evaluation showed that the concentration of the antibiotic did not intercede with the size and the positive zeta potential of the metronidazole-loaded chitosan nanoparticles.

Figure 3A shows the representative nanoparticles size distribution of chitosan nanoparticles and drug-loaded polymer nanoparticles for the ChiMet_2.2 formulation. The results revealed that ninety percent of chitosan nanoparticles had a size of 163.7 nm and metronidazole-loaded chitosan nanoparticles had a size of 201.3 nm. Thus, this confirmed that a small increase occurs when the drug molecules are encapsulated into the polymer structure. The zeta potential (Figure 3B) is based on the electrophoretic scattering of light for molecules, particles and surfaces in the size range of 0.3 nm–10 μm. The electrokinetic potential (zeta) represents the difference between the electric charges on the surface of the solid nanoparticles in the dispersing medium and the charges of the diffused electric layer. It also reveals the degree of repulsion of particles with the same charge. In the case of the new prepared formulations, a higher zeta potential indicated the stability of the dispersions that do not allow the aggregation of polymer nanoparticles loaded with antibiotics.

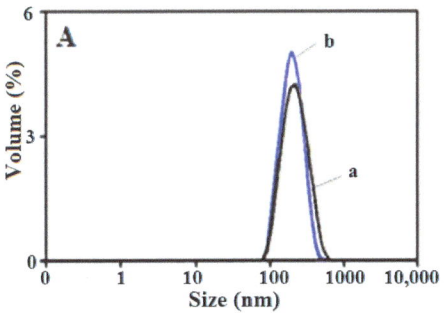 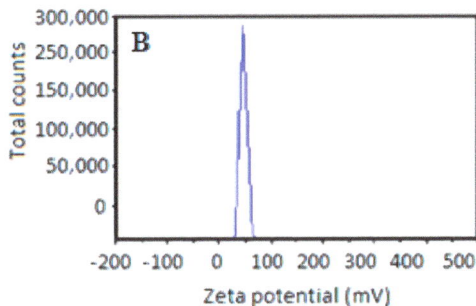

Figure 3. Nanoparticles' size distribution representation: (A) chitosan particles (a) and metronidazole-loaded chitosan nanoparticles (b) and (B) zeta potential of chitosan-loaded metronidazole nanoparticles.

SEM micrographs, Figure 4A,B of the ChiMet_2.2 sample, show varied and dense nanoparticles, which are spherical in shape and have a porous chitosan matrix texture.

By comparing the morphology of antibiotic-loaded polymeric nanoparticles and non-loaded nanoparticles, it was observed that loading the drug into the chitosan structure did not significantly change the textural properties of the nanoparticles.

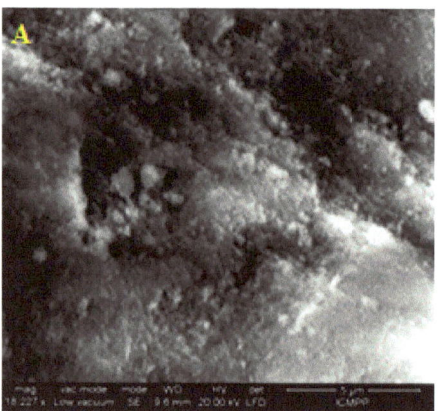 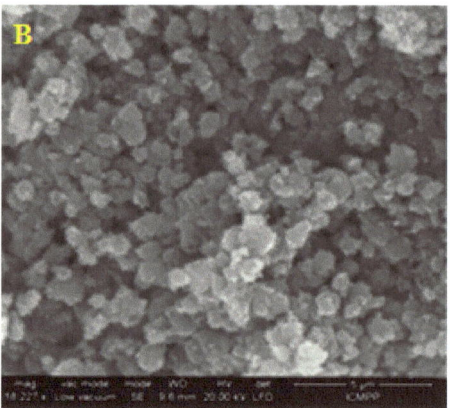

Figure 4. (**A**) SEM micrograph of chitosan. (**B**) SEM image of metronidazole-loaded chitosan nanoparticles.

3.1. FTIR Characterization

Figure 5 displays the IR spectrum of the drug, polymer and metronidazole-encapsulated chitosan nanoparticles (ChiMet_2.2 sample). Pure metronidazole revealed characteristic peaks at 270 cm^{-1} attributed to the C-O stretching vibration, a N-O stretching at 1370 cm^{-1}, a C-N stretching vibration at 1540 cm^{-1} and a O-H bond at 3230 cm^{-1}. The IR spectrum of chitosan showed characteristic peaks at 3450 cm^{-1} assigned to the –OH and NH$_2$ stretching vibration, and peaks at 1650 cm^{-1} attributed to the amide group.

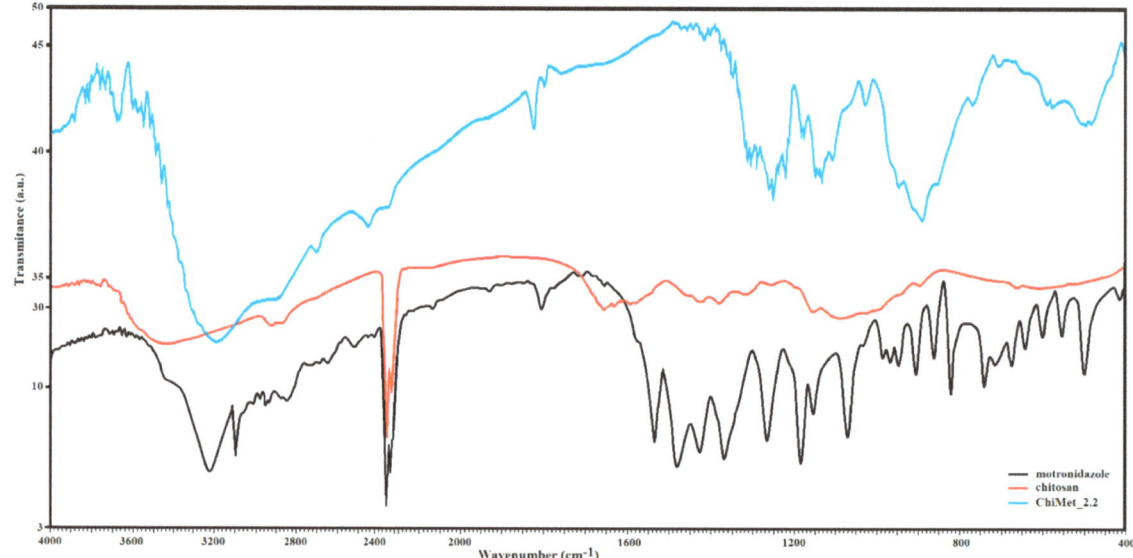

Figure 5. IR spectrum of pure metronidazole. IR spectrum of pure chitosan and IR spectrum of ChiMet_2.2 (metronidazole-loaded chitosan nanoparticles).

IR spectrum of ChiMet_2.2 sample presented peaks at 1670 cm^{-1} corresponding to the amide group in chitosan, and peaks at 1490 cm^{-1} attributed to the –NO$_3$ group in the metronidazole molecule and peaks at 1420 cm^{-1} assigned to the intermolecular hydrogen stretching vibration.

From the analysis of the IR spectra, it can be assumed that the efficiency of the incorporated active principle depends on the technique of loading the drug into the polymer structure.

3.2. Drug Release Profile

The in vitro release profiles of the antibiotic from the polymeric nanoparticles in different dissolution media (Figure 6A,B): phosphate-buffered saline (pH 7.5), phosphate buffer (pH 7.0) and 0.1 N HCl (pH 1.5). Up to one hour, there was an initial rapid release of about 30% of metronidazole, probably caused by the dissolution of the metronidazole crystals located on the surface of the chitosan nanoparticles. In the next 24 h, a prolonged release followed, possibly due to the diffusion of the antibiotic through the polymer matrix.

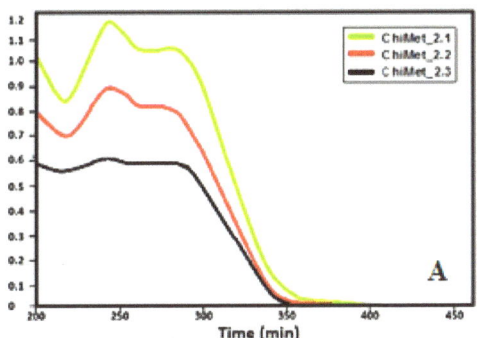
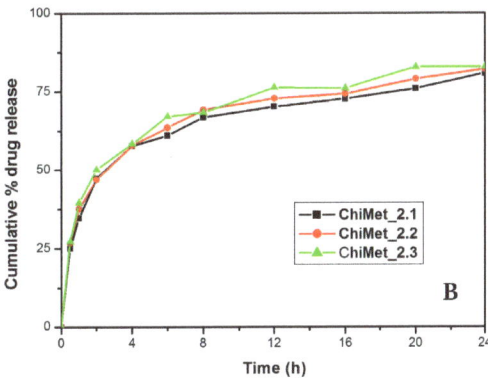

Figure 6. (**A**) UV–VIS spectrum of ChiMet_2.1, ChiMet_2.2, ChiMet_2.3. and (**B**) drug release profile of metronidazole-loaded chitosan nanoparticles.

The release of metronidazole from the polymeric nanostructures shows that these drug carriers allow sustained and prolonged release of the drug at the target site, increasing the bioavailability of the drug and minimizing its adverse effects.

The release profile of metronidazole with different concentrations in the formulation showed that the release rate of the drug tended to increase as the amount of the drug in the sample increased, which lead to differences in the diffusion mechanism.

3.3. Cell Viability Assay

Cellular viability (%) (Figure 7) was calculated according to the following formula: % cell viability = [absorbance]sample/[absorbance]control × 100. Investigating the action of different concentrations of the ChiMet_2.2 sample on the viability of HeLa cell cultures revealed a moderate cytotoxic impact of these compounds, with cell viability reductions between 36.8% and 23.3%.

No significant differences were recorded between the different concentrations used in terms of the cytotoxic impact. However, even if the value of the cytotoxic impact is around 30%, from the point of view of the antitumor response, it has no therapeutic significance.

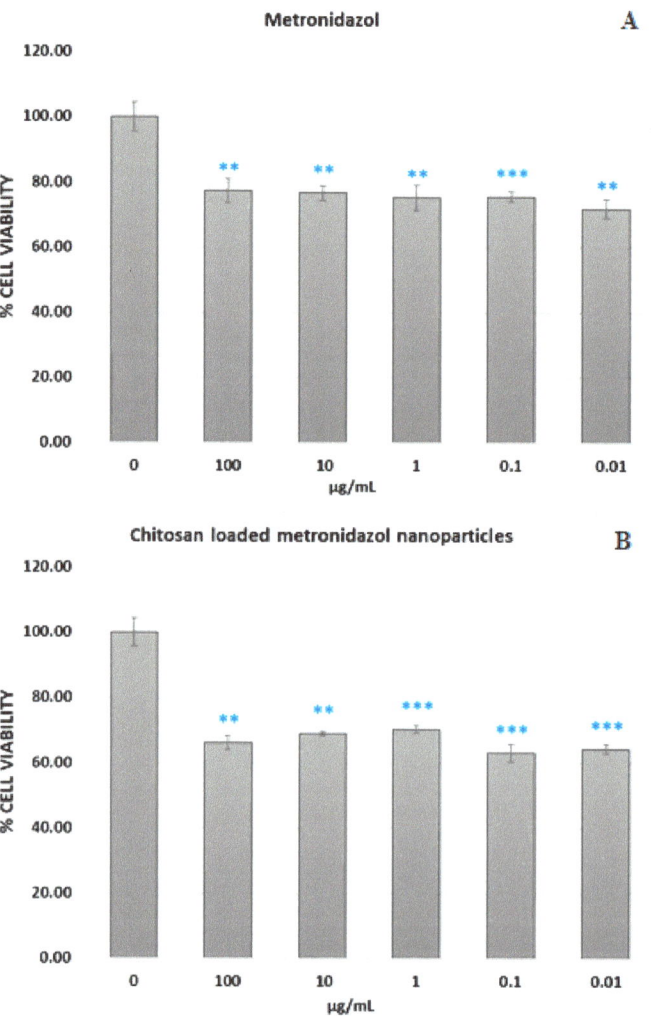

Figure 7. Viability of HeLa cells determined with MTT assay at 24 h after the treatment with chitosan-loaded metronidazol nanoparticles (**B**) or metronidazol NPs (**A**). Statistical significance was evaluated with paired *t* test, with significance thresholds of <0.05. ** = <0.01; *** = <0.001.

4. Discussion

The continuous development and improvement of drug delivery nanosystems is of major importance for the technologies used in the pharmaceutical field. Thus, obtaining nanostructures that act as a matrix for different active principles is significant due to the stability and control of drug release. Recently, the use of drug delivery systems in nanomedicine enhanced prevention, diagnosis and treatment of some threatening diseases by targeting the affected site while minimizing adverse effects. By using the ionic gelation method, bioactive molecules can be encapsulated in the polymer matrix to improve their effectiveness. Changing the amount of the drug in nanocomposites determined a loading capacity in the range of 70–62% and an entrapment efficiency in the range of 26–35%. The encapsulation capacity variation occurs due to the fact that chitosan nanoparticles precipitate faster, inhibiting the incorporation of the drug, which is followed by an increase in the diffusion of the drug when its amount in the formulation increases. Particle size distribution and zeta potential indicated no considerable modification when the antibiotic molecule was encapsulated into the polymer structure. The method used for the preparation of chitosan nanoparticles loaded with metronidazole led to a narrow size distribution of the nanocomposites. The complexity of the formation mechanism of the new nanostructures is probably due to the presence of phenomena, such as nucleation, growth, self-assembly and aggregation, that take place at the same time, thus determining the characteristics of the newly prepared formulations. If the predominant phenomenon is nucleation, a larger number of nanoparticles with smaller sizes are obtained; if it is molecular growth, self-assembly or aggregation predominates, and larger nanoparticles are formed. The conditions predetermined with the preparation method of the new compounds determine the predominant phenomenon, with them being the factors that influence the morphology and size distribution of the obtained nanoarchitectures. It was observed that an increase in the amount of the drug in the formulation implies a slight increase in the size of chitosan nanoparticles loaded with metronidazole from 163.7 nm to 201.3 nm, thus suggesting that the incorporation of the active molecule in the polymer matrix does not significantly change the size of the nanostructure. Morphology analysis performed with scanning electron microscopy indicated a porous surface of pure chitosan nanoparticles and spherical-shaped particles of the tested metronidazole-immobilized chitosan nanoparticles. A difference in the degree of agglomeration in nanocomposites compared to chitosan nanoparticles can also be observed. The IR spectra were recorded at the wavenumber range of 4000–400 cm^{-1} to evaluate chemical interactions between metronidazole and polymer molecules. FTIR spectral investigations, performed to analyze the alteration of chemical structure, revealed no significant physicochemical interaction between metronidazole and chitosan, concluding that these compounds are compatible with each other. The small changes in the absorption spectra of the new formulation of chitosan nanoparticles loaded with metronidazole possibly occurred due to the antibiotic molecule that changes the functional groups in the polymer. The dissolution assay indicated that the antibiotic was immobilized in the polymer structure due to the crosslinked gelation technique. The release profile suggests that the active substance was released in a controlled, prolonged manner from the polymer matrix with a non-Fickian behavior, indicating a transport of the active principle via diffusion, which is associated with polymer relaxation. Changing the metronidazole concentration did not significantly change the release profile of the drug from the tested samples and reached 80% for a 24 h period. The swelling and relaxation of the polymer could have a significant role in the release mechanism of the embedded substance. This could be due to the rapid dissolution of the drug on the surface of the chitosan nanoparticles that created pores, and its release from the polymeric nanostructure would have occurred through those pores. Towards the end of the delivery time, a decrease in the release speed could be observed due to the increase in the diffusion path of the drug. MTT testing is a quantitative method used on a large scale to determine, in vitro, the cytotoxic effects of some products (biomaterials, drugs, hybrid compounds) on cell lines. The cytotoxicity test was used to evaluate the possibility of the new formulation based on chitosan nanoparticles loaded with metronidazole having a therapeutic action without toxic effects on the cells. These findings presume promising applications of drug carriers in pharmacological and medical areas. Nowadays, there is a particular interest in obtaining polymeric nanoparticles through the ionic gelation method, which can be later loaded with new active ingredients and used both to prevent and to treat serious infections caused by various pathogens. This research aimed to highlight the possibility of expanding the field of applications of drug carriers based on polymeric nanoparticles loaded with different active principles to prevent and treat dangerous infections but also to reduce the side effects of drugs. An important aspect to consider refers to the chemical structure of the active molecule; therefore, the chemical affinity between the polymer and the drug can reveal surface interactions. Considering this factor in the design of new formulations could lead to the functionalization of the surface of polymeric nanoparticles to improve their performance as controlled drug release systems. This work aimed to obtain a new formulation of polymeric nanoparticles loaded with an antibiotic in which the structural and morphological characteristics were evaluated according to the conditions and methods of preparation and thus obtaining nanoparticulate systems with prolonged release of the drug without significant cytotoxicity. Further research should focus on testing chitosan nanoparticles loaded with metronidazole in different medical fields, and is expected to obtain a special performance of the transport and release of the drug at the target site. The prepared nanoparticles were characterized for their use in the delivery of active principles in biological systems, focusing on new formulations that reduce the adverse effects of drugs.

5. Conclusions

This study presents the synthesis and characterization of metronidazole-loaded chitosan nanoparticles as carriers for the antibiotic target site. The ionic gelation technique was used to prepare polymer nanoparticles. Chitosan is a natural polymer obtained with the deacetylation of chitin in an alkaline environment which is then metabolized by a human enzyme such as lysozyme. It is a cheap and easy to obtain, biocompatible, biodegradable and non-toxic compound that acts as a matrix for the inclusion of active principles. They also have a prolonged release at the site of action, which is followed by the dissolution of the host. Structural and morphological properties of as prepared delivery systems were performed using FTIR, SEM techniques and UV-VIS spectroscopy in order to investigate the release behavior. FTIR and SEM analyses indicate that the loading of the polymer matrix with an active principle does not significantly change its structural and textural characteristics. Moreover, the prolonged and controlled release of the molecule helps modern medicine in the diagnosis, prevention and treatment of many diseases. The results of the particle size distribution indicated a slight increase from 163.7 nm, in the case of uncharged polymer nanoparticles, to 210.3 nm, in the case of chitosan nanoparticles loaded with metronidazole. The cytotoxicity profile revealed that the cytotoxic impact was insignificant. Based on the obtained results, drug carriers can be successfully used for enhancing the encapsulation and biodistribution of metronidazole at the target site. Chitosan possesses low toxicity, indicating that it can be used in the biomedical field as a drug delivery nanosystem, thus promising various formulations which enhance drug therapy and limit side effects. Incorporating the antibiotic into the structure of chitosan nanoparticles can offer multiple advantages in the creation of transport systems and the localization of the active substance. The characteristics of nanocarriers such as the shape, size, release profile and cytotoxicity are significant in the design of drug delivery systems. Moreover, a promising strategy to combat antibiotic-resistant microorganisms and to reduce nosocomial infections is to use drug-loaded nanocarriers.

Author Contributions: All authors contributed equally to this work. Conceptualization, C.G. (Carmen Grierosu) and D.D.; project administration, C.M.; data curation, R.C.; formal analysis, G.Z., M.G.D. and L.D.D.; investigation, D.A., M.M. and E.M.C.; resources, G.M. and C.G. (Cristian Gutu); visualization, E.R.B.G.; validation, L.E.; investigation and writing—review and editing, G.C. and D.D.; methodology, G.C. and G.M. All authors have read and agreed to the published version of the manuscript.

Funding: This research received no external funding.

Conflicts of Interest: The authors declare no conflict of interest.

References

1. Vasquez Marcano, R.; Tominaga, T.T.; Khalil, N.M.; Pedroso, L.S.; Mainardes, R.M. Chitosan functionalized poly (epsilon-caprolactone) nanoparticles for amphotericin B delivery. *Carbohydr. Polym.* **2018**, *202*, 345–354. [CrossRef]
2. Hsiao, M.H.; Mu, Q.; Stephen, Z.R.; Fang, C.; Zhang, M. Hexanoyl-Chitosan-PEG Copolymer Coated Iron Oxide Nanoparticles for Hydrophobic Drug Delivery. *ACS Macro Lett.* **2015**, *4*, 403–407. [CrossRef]

3. Bhavsar, C.; Momin, M.; Gharat, S.; Omri, A. Functionalized and graft copolymers of chitosan and its pharmaceutical applications. *Expert Opin. Drug Deliv.* **2017**, *14*, 1189–1204. [CrossRef]
4. Wang, Z.; Luo, T.; Cao, A.; Sun, J.; Jia, L.; Sheng, R. Morphology-Variable Aggregates Prepared from Cholesterol-Containing Amphiphilic Glycopolymers: Their Protein Recognition/Adsorption and Drug Delivery Applications. *Nanomaterials* **2018**, *8*, 136. [CrossRef]
5. Ferji, K.; Venturini, P.; Cleymand, F.; Chassenieux, C.; Six, J.-L. In situ glyco-nanostructure formulation via photo-polymerization induced self-assembly. *Polym. Chem.* **2018**, *9*, 2868–2872. [CrossRef]
6. Sohail, M.F.; Hussain, S.Z.; Saeed, H.; Javed, I.; Sarwar, H.S.; Nadhman, A.; Huma, Z.E.; Rehman, M.; Jahan, S.; Hussain, I.; et al. Polymeric nanocapsules embedded with ultra-small silver nanoclusters for synergistic pharmacology and improved oral delivery of Docetaxel. *Sci. Rep.* **2018**, *8*, 13304–13314. [CrossRef]
7. Park, J.H.; Saravanakumar, G.; Kim, K.; Kwon, I.C. Targeted delivery of low molecular drugs using chitosan and its derivatives. *Adv. Drug Deliv. Rev.* **2010**, *62*, 28–41. [CrossRef]
8. Hoop, M.; Mushtaq, F.; Hurter, C.; Chen, X.Z.; Nelson, B.J.; Pane, S. A smart multifunctional drug delivery nanoplatform for targeting cancer cells. *Nanoscale* **2016**, *8*, 12723–12728. [CrossRef]
9. Li, J.; Cai, C.; Li, J.; Li, J.; Li, J.; Sun, T.; Wang, L.; Wu, H.; Yu, G. Chitosan-Based Nanomaterials for Drug Delivery. *Molecules* **2018**, *23*, 2661. [CrossRef]
10. Qi, L.; Xu, Z.; Jiang, X.; Hu, C.; Zou, X. Preparation and antibacterial activity of chitosan nanoparticles. *Carbohydr. Res.* **2004**, *339*, 2693–2700. [CrossRef]
11. Devi, K.T.; Venkateswarlu, B.S. Formulation and Characterization of Metronidazole Loaded Polymeric Nanoparticles. *Int. J. Pharm. Biol. Sci.-IJPBSTM* **2019**, *9*, 422–433.
12. Choughury, P.K.; Murthy, P.N.; Tripathy, N.K.; Panigraphy, R.; Behera, S. Investigation of drug polymer compatibility: Formulation and characterization of metronidazole microspheres for colonic delivery. *Pharm. Sci.* **2012**, *3*, 1–20.
13. Emara, L.; Abdo, A.; El-Ashmawy, A.; Mursi, N. Preparation and evaluation of metronidazole sustained release floating tablets. *Int. J. Pharm. Pharm. Sci.* **2014**, *6*, 198–204.
14. Rima, K.; Dima, M.; Cherine, S.; Paolo, Y. Encapsulation of metronidazole in polycaprolactone microspheres. *J. Drug Deliv. Ther.* **2019**, *9*, 190–194.
15. Omar, S.; Aldosari, B.; Refai, H.; Gohary, O.A. Colon-specific drug delivery for mebeverine hydrochloride. *J. Drug Target.* **2007**, *15*, 691–700. [CrossRef]
16. Englert, C.; Brendel, J.C.; Majdanski, T.C.; Yildirim, T.; Schubert, S.; Gottschaldt, M.; Windhab, N.; Schubert, U.S. Pharmapolymers in the 21st century: Synthetic polymers in drug delivery applications. *Prog. Polym. Sci.* **2018**, *87*, 107–164. [CrossRef]
17. Toskic-Radojicic, M. Effects of topical application of Metronidazole-containing mucoadhesive lipogel in periodontal pockets. *Vojn. Pregl.* **2005**, *62*, 565–568. [CrossRef]
18. Adha, N.; Ervina, I.; Agusnar, H. The effectiveness of metronidazole gel based chitosan inhibits the growth of bacteria Aggregatibacter actinomycetemcomitans, Porphyromonas gingivalis, Fusobacterium nucleatum (In vitro). *Int. J. Appl. Dent. Sci.* **2017**, *3*, 30–37.
19. Rinaudo, M. Chitin and chitosan: Properties and applications. *Prog. Polym. Sci.* **2006**, *31*, 603–632. [CrossRef]
20. Chaubey, P.; Patel, R.R.; Mishra, B. Development and optimization of curcumin-loaded mannosylated chitosan nanoparticles using response surface methodology in the treatment of visceral leishmaniasis. *Expert Opin. Drug Deliv.* **2014**, *11*, 1163–1181. [CrossRef]
21. Khan, G.; Yadav, S.K.; Patel, R.R.; Nath, G.; Bansal, M.; Mishra, B. Development and Evaluation of Biodegradable Chitosan Films of Metronidazole and Levofloxacin for the Management of Periodontitis. *AAPS PharmSciTech* **2016**, *17*, 1312–1325. [CrossRef]
22. Prabaharan, M. Review paper: Chitosan derivatives as promising materials for controlled drug delivery. *J. Biomater. Appl.* **2008**, *23*, 5–36. [CrossRef] [PubMed]
23. Kean, T.; Thanou, M. Biodegradation, biodistribution and toxicity of chitosan. *Adv. Drug Deliv. Rev.* **2010**, *62*, 3–11. [CrossRef] [PubMed]
24. Woraphatphadung, T.; Sajomsang, W.; Rojanarata, T.; Ngawhirunpat, T.; Tonglairoum, P.; Opanasopit, P. Development of Chitosan-Based pH-Sensitive Polymeric Micelles Containing Curcumin for Colon-Targeted Drug Delivery. *AAPS PharmSciTech* **2018**, *19*, 991–1000. [CrossRef] [PubMed]
25. Wang, Y.; Li, B.; Xu, F.; Han, Z.; Wei, D.; Jia, D.; Zhou, Y. Tough Magnetic Chitosan Hydrogel Nanocomposites for Remotely Stimulated Drug Release. *Biomacromolecules* **2018**, *19*, 3351–3360. [CrossRef]
26. Liu, D.; Li, J.; Pan, H.; He, F.; Liu, Z.; Wu, Q.; Bai, C.; Yu, S.; Yang, X. Potential advantages of a novel chitosan-N-acetylcysteine surface modified nanostructured lipid carrier on the performance of ophthalmic delivery of curcumin. *Sci. Rep.* **2016**, *6*, 28796–28809. [CrossRef]
27. Zhao, X.; Zhou, L.; Li, Q.; Zou, Q.; Du, C. Biomimetic mineralization of carboxymethyl chitosan nanofibers with improved osteogenic activity in vitro and in vivo. *Carbohydr. Polym.* **2018**, *195*, 225–234. [CrossRef]
28. Ho, D.K.; Frisch, S.; Biehl, A.; Terriac, E.; De Rossi, C.; Schwarzkopf, K.; Lautenschlager, F.; Loretz, B.; Murgia, X.; Lehr, C.M. Farnesylated Glycol Chitosan as a Platform for Drug Delivery: Synthesis, Characterization, and Investigation of Mucus-Particle Interactions. *Biomacromolecules* **2018**, *19*, 3489–3501. [CrossRef]

29. Ali, A.; Ahmed, S. A review on chitosan and its nanocomposites in drug delivery. *Int. J. Biol. Macromol.* **2018**, *109*, 273–286. [CrossRef]
30. Martinez-Martinez, M.; Rodriguez-Berna, G.; Gonzalez-Alvarez, I.; Hernandez, M.J.; Corma, A.; Bermejo, M.; Merino, V.; Gonzalez-Alvarez, M. Ionic Hydrogel Based on Chitosan Cross-Linked with 6-Phosphogluconic Trisodium Salt as a Drug Delivery System. *Biomacromolecules* **2018**, *19*, 1294–1304. [CrossRef]
31. Patil, J.S. Ionotropic Gelation and Polyelectrolyte Complexation: The Novel Techniques to Design Hydrogels Particulate Sustained, Modulated Drug Delivery System: A Review. *Dig. J. Nanomater. Biostruct.* **2010**, *5*, 241–248.
32. Bayan, M.F.; Marji, S.M.; Salem, M.S.; Begum, M.Y.; Chidambaram, K.; Chandrasekaran, B. Development of Polymeric-Based Formulation as Potential Smart Colonic Drug Delivery System. *Polymers* **2022**, *14*, 3697. [CrossRef] [PubMed]

Disclaimer/Publisher's Note: The statements, opinions and data contained in all publications are solely those of the individual author(s) and contributor(s) and not of MDPI and/or the editor(s). MDPI and/or the editor(s) disclaim responsibility for any injury to people or property resulting from any ideas, methods, instructions or products referred to in the content.

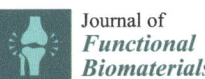

Communication

Montmorillonite-Sodium Alginate Oral Colon-Targeting Microcapsule Design for WGX-50 Encapsulation and Controlled Release in Gastro-Intestinal Tract

Yibei Jiang [1], Zhou Wang [1], Ke Cao [2], Lu Xia [3], Dongqing Wei [4,*] and Yi Zhang [1,*]

- [1] Department of Inorganic Materials, School of Minerals Processing and Bioengineering, Central South University, Changsha 410083, China; 215611016@csu.edu.cn (Y.J.); zhouwang@csu.edu.cn (Z.W.)
- [2] Department of Oncology, The Third Xiangya Hospital of Central South University, Changsha 410078, China; csucaoke@163.com
- [3] Center for Medical Genetics & Hunan Key Laboratory of Medical Genetics, School of Life Sciences, Central South University, Changsha 410078, China; xialu@sklmg.edu.cn
- [4] State Key Laboratory of Microbial Metabolism, School of Life Sciences and Biotechnology, Shanghai Jiao Tong University, Shanghai 200240, China
- * Correspondence: dqwei@sjtu.edu.cn (D.W.); yee_z10@csu.edu.cn (Y.Z.)

Abstract: The montmorillonite-sodium alginate (MMT-SA) colon-targeting microcapsules have been designed as a WGX-50 encapsulation and controlled release vehicle used in oral administration. The MMT-SA microcapsule was formed from a cross-linking reaction, and the stable micropore in the microcapsule changed with a different MMT-SA mixed mass ratio. The MMT-SA microcapsule has a reinforced micropore structure and an enhanced swell–dissolution in SIF and SCF with alkaline environment, which is attributed to the incorporated MMT. The MMT-SA microcapsule exhibited a high WGX-50 encapsulation rate up to 98.81 ± 0.31% and an obvious WGX-50 controlled release in the simulated digestive fluid in vitro. The WGX-50 loaded with MMT-SA microcapsule showed a weak minimizing drug loss in SGF (Simulated Gastric Fluid) with an acidic environment, while it showed a strong maximizing drug release in SIF (Simulated Intestinal Fluid) and SCF (Simulated Colonic Fluid) with an alkaline environment. These features make the MMT-SA microcapsule a nominated vehicle for colon disease treatment used in oral administration.

Keywords: montmorillonite; sodium alginate; microcapsule; controlled drug release; oral administration

1. Introduction

Drugs for oral administration with controlled release used in the digestive tract result in long-term stable release in large doses and have a high mass fraction therapeutic effect in target-specific sites [1]. There are some unique characteristics that should be taken into account, such as drug transport across the biologic barriers, drug release in the digestive tract microenvironment, and the drug molecule's absorption, distribution, metabolism, and excretion in the digestive tract, etc. [2–4]. WGX-50 is an amide compound extracted from Zanthoxylum Bungeanum Maxim, exhibiting a beneficial therapeutic effect on colon disease management through modulating the innate immune response. WGX-50 exhibits swift oral absorption, posing challenges in achieving uniform systemic distribution and targeted delivery to the colonic site, thereby limiting its therapeutic efficacy. Furthermore, the acidic milieu of the stomach may induce structural modifications in WGX-50. WGX-50 in oral administration should avoid an uncontrollable release in an inconvenient location [5–8]. Therefore, a WGX-50 encapsulation and controlled release vehicle used in oral administration should be designed for minimizing drug loss within the gastric tract microenvironment and accelerating drug absorption in the intestinal tract, and further facilitating therapeutic effects in the target-specific site [9–13].

Sodium alginate (SA) hydrogel microcapsules formed from an SA solution in various cross-linking reactions are water-swollen biomaterial with a three-dimensional network structure that exhibit remarkable features, such as a tunable microporous structure, non-toxicity, biodegradable and biocompatible, etc., which could be used as a drug encapsulation and controlled release vehicle used in oral administration [14–17]. Several studies on functionalized hydrogel microcapsules with enhanced mechanical structures for sustained and controlled drug release have been conducted, but undesired leakage makes them inefficient, i.e., encapsulating the drug molecule in a reinforced micropore structured microcapsule [18–20]. Montmorillonite (MMT) is a US Food and Drug Administration-approved active and inactive ingredient for diverse biomedical applications owing to its characteristics such as its two-dimensional structure in micronano scale and dual-charged distribution in structure while having a net negative charge in aqueous suspension, its high swelling behavior and inherent stiffness, non-toxicity and biocompatibility, etc. [21]. Hence, our foremost consideration revolves around the controlled release of the pharmaceutical agent and ensuring the safety and stability of the carrier. The hydrogel microcapsule functionalized with MMT-SA as a reinforced vehicle against chemical issues from the digestive tract microenvironment and even accelerating the drug molecule's absorption, distribution, metabolism, and excretion in the intestinal tract is an essential choice for drug encapsulation and controlled release vehicle used in oral administration [22,23].

The novelty of this work is that an oral colon-specific drug delivery system (MMT-SA microcapsules) has been designed taking into account the digestive tract microenvironment, which could benefit from targeted controlled release, efficient delivery, and even a reduction in initial losses for WGX-50. The microcapsule formation mechanism and the main influence factors at different stages are discussed in detail. The ratio of MMT to SA was adjusted to obtain microcapsules with optimal particle size, pore distribution, and thermal stability. The cytotoxicity of the microcapsules towards human cell lines associated with colon diseases has been evaluated. Additionally, the storage and release of WGX-50 in simulated digestive fluid in vitro provide an enhanced verification model in certain colon disease treatments.

2. Materials and Methods

2.1. Materials

Medical Montmorillonite (MMT, 98%, Product No.: SD1004) was obtained from Sand Technology Co., Ltd. (Ezhou City, China) Sodium alginate (SA, AR, 90%, CAS No.: 9005-38-3) was obtained from Maclin Biochemical Technology Co., Ltd. (Shanghai, China). Calcium chloride (AR, 96%, CAS No.: 1004-52-4) was purchased from Sinopharm Chemical Reagent Co., Ltd. (Shanghai, China). WGX-50 (MW: 311.384, CAS No.: 29946-61-0) was obtained from Sigma-Aldrich (Shanghai, China).

2.2. Preparation of MMT-SA Microcapsule

From the working solutions, MMT and SA were mixed with different mass ratios in 10 mL aqueous solution and stirred at room temperature. The mixing was carried out with a mixing time of 60 min and a mixing rate of 500 rpm, to ensure thorough mixing. Later, the mixed suspension was added to a 0.4 M $CaCl_2$ solution, and the 30 min cross-linking was there to ensure the completed reaction, i.e., the cross-linking reaction time is 30 min. Then, the microspheres were collected through filtration and washed with deionized water three times. Liquid nitrogen freeze-drying was used to ensure microsphere transformed into a microcapsule. The mixed mass ratios for the MMT-SA microcapsule to obtain different phases are presented in Supplementary Material Table S1.

2.3. Characterization

SEM images were evaluated using a Mira3 LMU SEM (Tescan, Brno, The Czech Republic) with a vacuum set to below 5×10^{-3} Pa, accelerating voltage was 20 kV, and spot size was 5.5–6.5 nm. Platinum was used as the gold-spraying material and the gold-spraying time was set to 120 s to increase the conductivity of the samples. The differential thermal analysis was analyzed using the STA449C (NETZSCH Machinery and Instruments, Selb, Germany), which ranged from 30 to 600 °C under constant argon purging with 10 °C/min rate of rise. The zeta potential values were measured using a Malvern Zetasizer Nano S90 (Malvern Instruments, Malvern, UK). The gel precursor, dissolved in buffer solutions with varying pH levels, was placed in a quartz cuvette. The values of zeta potential were obtained from three measurements. The diffuse reflectance spectrum was measured using a Fourier transform infrared spectrometer (Shimadzu FTIR 8120 spectrometer, SHIMADZU, Kyoto, Japan) in the range from 400 to 4000 cm^{-1}.

2.4. Cell Culture and Cytotoxicity Evaluation

Human intestinal epithelial cells 6 (HIEC-6) and human colonic epithelial cells (NCM460) were obtained from Abiowell Biotechnology Co., Ltd. (Changsha, China). HIEC-6 and NCM460 cells were cultured in RPMI 1640 medium containing 10% FBS and 1% Pen/Strep at 37 °C with 5% CO_2 atmosphere.

The culture medium was removed and replenished with RPMI 1640 culturing medium containing MMT-SA mixture ranging from 1 μg/mL to 300 μg/mL, and then incubated for 24 h at 37 °C. The viable cell counts were measured using Cell Counting Kit-8 (CCK-8) according to the manufacturer's instructions (Beijing Lablead Biotech, CK001-3000T, Beijing, China). The absorbance at 450 nm was measured using BIOTEK ELX800 Universal Microplate Reader (Thermo Fisher Scientific, Waltham, MA, USA).

2.5. Drug Encapsulation Measurement

WGX-50 with amounts ranging from 25 mg to 200 mg was dissolved in the aforementioned 10 mL MMT-SA initial mixed solution, and then stirred at room temperature for 60 min. The resulting mixture was added into 40 mL 0.4 M $CaCl_2$ solution in 30 min. The MMT-SA microcapsule containing WGX-50 (WGX-50/MMT-SA) was filtered and washed three times with deionized water to remove the residual WGX-50 on the microcapsule surface. The absorbance of the residual WGX-50 at 277.5 nm was measured using a UV-Vis spectrophotometer (UV2600, Thermo Fisher Scientific, Waltham, MA, USA).

The encapsulation rate (EE, %) and the drug loading rate (DL, %) were calculated using the following Equations (1) and (2) [24]:

$$EE(\%) = \left(W_{Fed} - W_{Non-encapsulated}\right)/W_{Fed} \times 100\% \tag{1}$$

$$DL(\%) = \left(W_{Fed} - W_{Non-encapsulated}\right)/W_{Total} \times 100\% \tag{2}$$

where W_{Fed} is the initial WGX-50 amount in total, $W_{Non-encapsulated}$ is residual WGX-50 amount in filtrate, and W_{Total} is the microcapsule amount containing WGX-50.

2.6. Drug Release In Vitro

In vitro WGX-50 release experiments were carried out in an alkaline environment (pH 6.8 in PBS solution, Simulated Intestinal Fluid, SIF; pH 7.4 in PBS solution, Simulated Colonic Fluid, SCF) and in an acidic environment (pH 1.2 in PBS solution, Simulated Gastric Fluid, SGF). To simulate the sequential pH changes that occur during the in vivo process, an in vitro release study mimicking the gastrointestinal tract was conducted for 30 h. Here, 30 mg WGX-50/MMT-SA microcapsules were sequentially immersed in 200 mL of SCF, SIF, and SGF for 2 h, 3 h, and 24 h at 37 °C 100 rpm. Then, 5 mL suspension was centrifuged at 3000 rpm in selected time intervals, the supernatants were measured using UV-Vis (λ = 277.5 nm) spectrophotometer, and the sediments were redispersed in 5 mL PBS solution to replenish the total volume. All the experiments were performed at least in triplicate.

3. Results and Discussion
3.1. Fabrication of the MMT-SA Microcapsule

Schematic illustration, digital photographs, and the representative SEM images for MMT-SA microcapsules are shown in Figure 1. The MMT was mixed with the SA solution, and the resulting mixed solution is a turbid colloidal suspension with viscosity and opacity, indicating that the MMTs were well scattered within the SA solution without obvious aggregation. Moreover, the mixed turbid colloidal suspension was flexible and stretchable, allowing it to be shaped into letters. This property is beneficial for fabricating hydrogel microspheres with a stable microstructure. Later, the mixed solution was added with the calcium chloride solution to form hydrogel microspheres, and the initial hydrogel microsphere exhibited opacity and hydrophobicity. Subsequently, the microcapsule was formed from freeze-dried hydrogel microspheres, and the irregular micropores in the microcapsule were created through the sublimation of ice crystals. Those microcapsules exhibited near-spherical shape in appearance and distinct ripple-like cell walls with a clear skeleton structure in their internal structure. Additionally, the oven-dried microcapsules have a smoother surface but lacked micropores compared to the freeze-dried microcapsules (Figure S1).

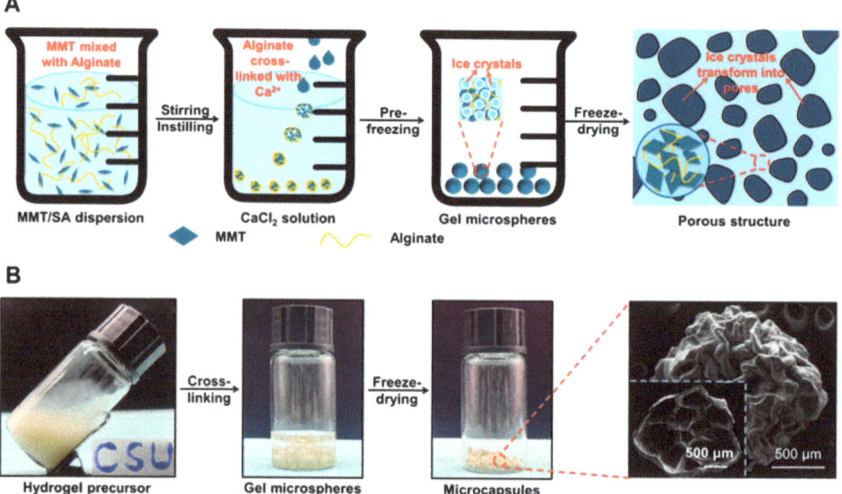

Figure 1. (**A**) Schematic illustration, (**B**) digital photographs and the representative SEM images for MMT-SA microcapsules.

3.2. Different Phases of the MMT-SA Microcapsule

The schematic illustration and the corresponding digital photographs and SEM images for MMT-SA microcapsule with different phases are shown in Figure 2. Figure 2A illustrates MMT and SA with different mixed mass ratios, resulting in various states, ranging from a mixed turbid colloidal suspension to a stable spherical microcapsule. The stable spherical microcapsules exhibited a smooth shell in wet state and uniform micropores in freeze-dried microspheres, which is beneficial to enhance drug encapsulation and controlled release in target-specific sites [25]. Additionally, the MMT agglomerates in the stable walls are presented in Figure S1. FTIR was used to record the characteristic peaks in the MMT-SA microcapsule in Figure S2. Peaks at 3485 cm^{-1}, 2925 cm^{-1}, 1612 cm^{-1}, 1417 cm^{-1}, and 821 cm^{-1} were attributed to SA [26]. Peaks at 3629 cm^{-1}, 3417 cm^{-1}, 1639 cm^{-1}, 1432 cm^{-1}, and 1030 cm^{-1} were attributed to MMT [27]. Peak at 1030 cm^{-1} shifting to 1040 cm^{-1} indicated a cross-linking reaction between MMT and SA. The TG–DSC curves of MMT (Figure S3A) exhibited endothermic peaks at 98 °C and 369 °C, indicating the loss of physically absorbed water molecules and the elimination of the water lattice in the compound. The thermal degradation of the MMT-SA composite ranged from 13.82% to 16.45% at temperatures between 121 °C and 137 °C, with an observed endothermic peak at 136 °C attributed to the removal of adsorbed surface water moisture in the composite (Figure S3B–E). The exothermic peak observed at temperatures ranging from 231 °C to 287 °C corresponds to the breakdown of alginate chains in the hybrid composite, as evidenced by its absence in the DSC curve of unblended MMT [28,29]. Another thermal decomposition was observed between 752 °C and 757 °C due to volatilization of residual SA carbons (Figure S3C–E) [30].

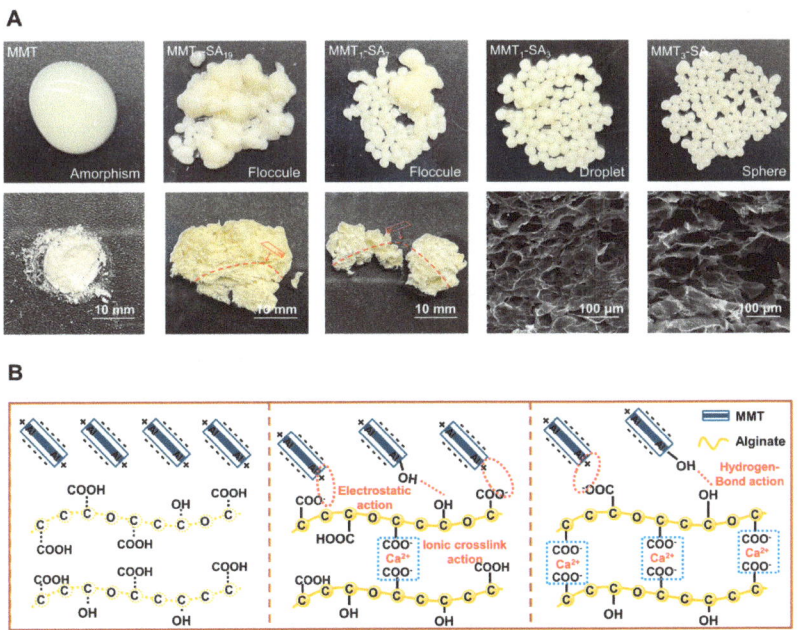

Figure 2. (**A**) The digital photographs, SEM images, and (**B**) the corresponding schematic illustration for MMT-SA microcapsule with different mixed mass ratios.

The MMT-SA microcapsule was fabricated using a cross-linking technique, as shown in Figure 2B. The layered MMT consists of one Al-octahedral sheet sandwiched between two opposing Si-tetrahedral sheets. The hydroxyl groups in silanol (Si–OH) and/or aluminol (Al–OH) groups existed in the internal, the external, and the edge surface areas. MMT's total negative charge originates from constant charge from the isomorphic substitution-induced charge compensating cations, variable charge from the active groups on the surface, and an opposite charge from various exchangeable cations [31]. SA consists of (1, 4)-linked β-D-mannuronic acid and α-L-guluronic acid units. There are abundant carboxyl groups along its backbone, which could be used to connect to other compounds. SA's total negative charge originates from protonated carboxyl groups in acidic conditions [32]. SA interacted with MMT to form complexes through anion–cation interaction and electrostatic attraction and absorption, which was almost simultaneous with the cross-linking reaction. It should be noted that multiple factors in SA absorbed on the MMT surface were not discussed in this manuscript, such as functional groups in SA, exchangeable cations in MMT, and charge value in all components, etc. Moreover, SA did not undergo intercalation into MMT.

Insufficient SA amount resulted in an inadequate cross-linking reaction, leading to the formation of an unstably structured microsphere that disintegrated with a slight disturbance or deformation with a changing environment. With an increased SA amount, the abundant COO⁻ from SA reacts with the Ca^{2+} from the $CaCl_2$ solution to form a cross-linked Ca-alginate. The cross-linking reaction is not controlled due to the $CaCl_2$ solution being water-soluble. The stable structured microsphere with a three-dimensional network structure has an obvious advantage in minimizing drug leakage within the digestive tract microenvironment [33].

3.3. Different Mixed Mass Ratios for the MMT-SA Microcapsule

Digital photographs, the cross-sectional SEM images, and the corresponding size distribution of the MMT-SA microcapsules with different mixed mass ratios are shown in Figure 3. The stable spherical microcapsule exhibited a smooth shell and was non-transparent white in a wet state and shrunken and wrinkled in appearance in a freeze-dried state, while exhibiting uniform micropores as a freeze-dried microsphere. As the MMT amount increases, the stable spherical microcapsule exhibits a darker appearance in the wet state, a larger size in the freeze-dried state from 1.4 mm to 2.1 mm, and a more intact and serried microcellular structure of the freeze-dried microsphere. The MMT-SA microcapsule with mass ratio of 300:75 was selected as the optimized drug-encapsulation and controlled-release vehicle used in oral administration, which resulted from overall considerations og MMT's toxic effects mentioned in the literature and the good microcellular structure in this condition [34].

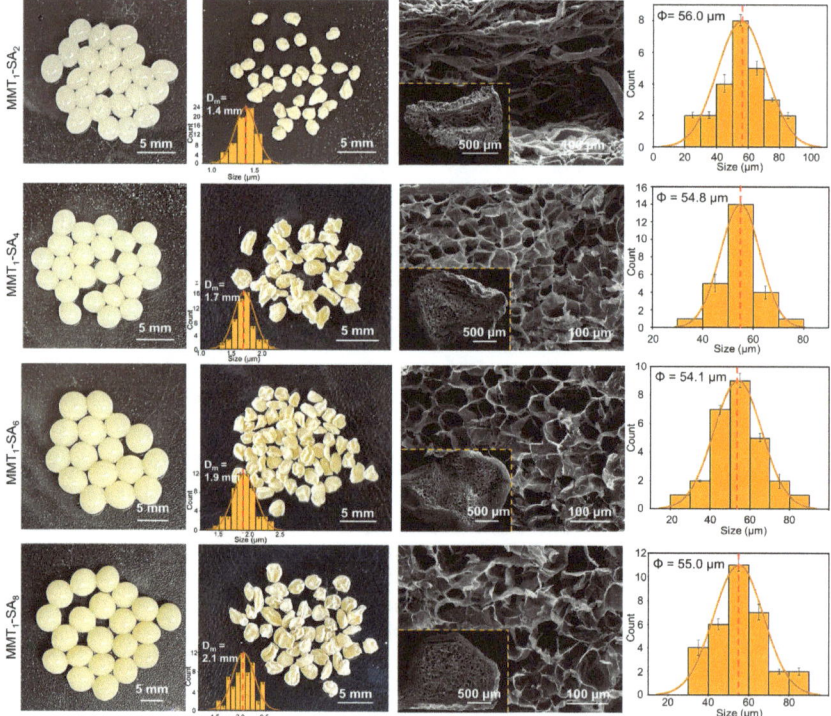

Figure 3. Digital photographs, the cross-sectional SEM images, and the corresponding size distribution for MMT-SA microcapsule with different mixed mass ratios.

Additionally, the MMT-SA microcapsule showed a negative charge as shown in Figure S4 and indicated that it could be adsorbed on the inflamed tissue in the intestinal tract through electrostatic interaction [35]. Due to certain biological differences between humans and other animals, the use of human-derived cells can better mimic biological processes in the human body and, thus, more accurately assess the safety and efficacy of drugs. The MMT-SA microcapsule was non-toxic towards the intestinal drug absorption-associated cells (human intestinal epithelial cells, HIEC-6 cells and human colonic epithelial cells, NCM460 cells) as shown in Figure S5, according to the ISO-10993 Standard [36,37].

3.4. Drug Encapsulation and Release In Vitro for the WGX-50 Coated with MMT-SA Microcapsule

The WGX-50 encapsulation and release in vitro for the WGX-50/MMT-SA microcapsule is shown in Figure 4. The WGX-50 encapsulation rate and loading rate is shown in Figure 4A, and the WGX-50 concentration calibration curve is shown in the lower-right corner. The WGX-50 encapsulation rate reached more than 90% when the WGX-50 amount was under 50 mg and followed a slow growth in WGX-50 encapsulation rate with an increasing WGX-50 amount. Hence, the optimal initial WGX-50 amount was 50 mg according to the cost-effectiveness research, and the WGX-50 encapsulation rate in the MMT-SA microcapsule was 99.60%.

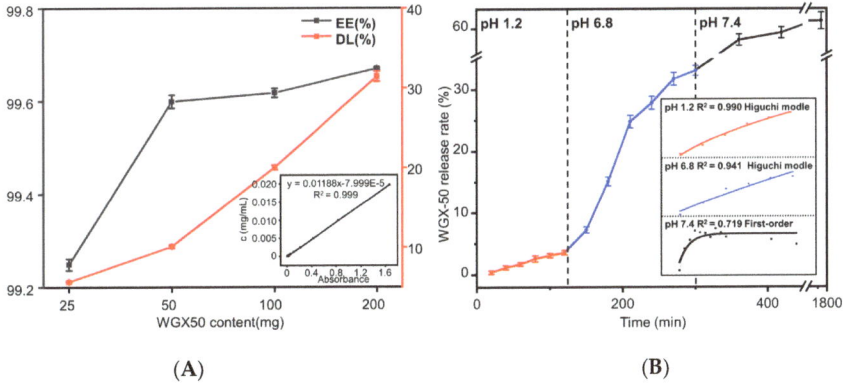

Figure 4. The WGX-50 encapsulation, where x is the absorbance (**A**) and release (**B**) in vitro for the WGX-50/MMT-SA microcapsule.

FTIR was used to record the characteristic peaks of the WGX-50/MMT-SA microcapsule in Figure S6. Peaks at 1657 cm^{-1}, 1534 cm^{-1}, 1513 cm^{-1}, 1330 cm^{-1}, 1280 cm^{-1}, and 1260 cm^{-1} were attributed to WGX-50. Peaks at 1657 cm^{-1}, 1534 cm^{-1}, and 1513 cm^{-1} in the WGX-50/MMT-SA microcapsule indicated that WGX-50 was encapsulated in MMT-SA microcapsule with surface adsorption rather than chemical bonding, which was beneficial for drug encapsulation and controlled release. To investigate the phase transition characteristics of the WGX-50/MMT-SA microcapsule, TG-DSC analyses were conducted, as shown in Figure S7. The mass loss of WGX-50 occurred within the temperature range of 280–440 °C, indicating the complete degradation of the compound. The endothermic peaks observed at 130 °C and 404 °C correspond to the melting point and decomposition of the crystalline WGX-50, respectively. However, in the DSC traces of WGX-50/MMT-SA, the sharp peak associated with crystalline WGX-50 was no longer present. This suggests that the WGX-50 lost its crystal structure during the encapsulation process within the MMT-SA composite, transforming into an amorphous state within the microcapsules [38].

WGX-50 release behavior from the WGX-50/MMT-SA microcapsule in simulated digestive fluid in vitro is shown in Figure 4B. The WGX-50/MMT-SA microcapsule showed a controlled fast release (32.42% and 61.66%) in alkaline environment (Simulated Intestinal Fluid, SIF; Simulated Colonic Fluid, SCF), followed by a snail-like slow release (3.46%) in an acidic environment (Simulated Gastric Fluid, SGF). WGX-50 release behavior from the WGX-50/MMT-SA microcapsule in SGF and SIF seems to fit the Higuchi model, and the release mechanism is Fick diffusion, indicating that WGX-50 adsorbed on the shell surface in small amounts while stored within the microcapsule in large amounts. The WGX-50 adsorbed on the shell surface could affect monitoring the adverse reactions but do not affect the therapeutic effects. The WGX-50 release behavior from WGX-50/MMT-SA microcapsule in SCF seems to fit with the First-order model, and the WGX-50 release rate correlates with initial WGX-50 concentration [39]. Additionally, the release component n, the rate constant k, and the correlation coefficient R^2 for the WGX-50/MMT-SA microcapsule in simulated digestive fluid in vitro are listed in Table S3.

3.5. Drug Release Mechanism and the Swell–Dissolution Model for the WGX50 Coated with MMT-SA Microcapsule

The WGX-50 release mechanism and the swell–dissolution model for the WGX-50/MMT-SA microcapsule are discussed in Figure 5. In SGF with an acidic environment, the microcapsule structure was compact with a low swelling rate. This is attributed to the –COOH of alginate being partially protonated and forming hydrogen bonds. The formation of hydrogen bonds leads to increased intermolecular interactions, resulting in a denser molecular network, making it more difficult for water molecules to enter the interior of the microcapsule, thus reducing the swelling rate of the microcapsule.

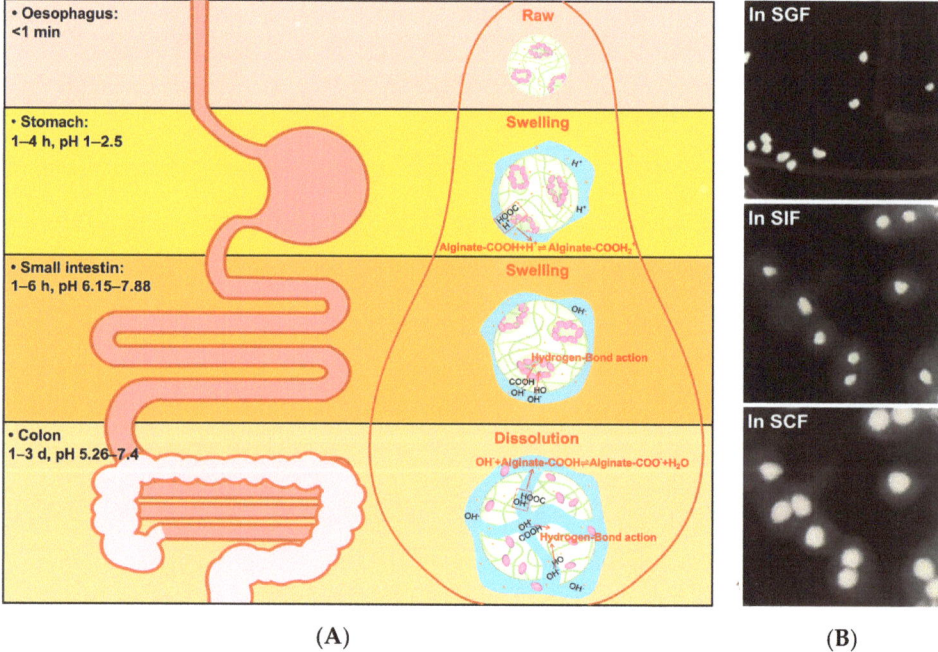

Figure 5. The WGX-50 release mechanism (**A**) and the swell–dissolution model (**B**) for WGX-50/MMT-SA microcapsule.

The total WGX50 slow release consists of surface desorption from WGX-50 adsorbed on the microcapsule surface and microporous diffusion from WGX-50 stored within the microcapsule. In SIF and SCF with an alkaline environment, the microcapsule structure was loose with a high swelling rate. This phenomenon can be attributed to the increased levels of OH^- interacting with the –COOH and –OH within the microcapsules to form hydrogen bonds, thereby weakening the intermolecular interactions and reducing the degree of coiling and entanglement of the calcium alginate molecular chains, resulting in a looser microcapsule structure and increased swelling [40]. Additionally, MMT could accelerate the water molecules' absorption, resulting in further swelling and dissolution of the MMT-

SA microcapsule. The total WGX-50 burst release was attributed to the alkali corrosion and microcapsule dissolution. Hence, the structural construction of the microcapsule is beneficial for drug encapsulation and controlled release at a target-specific site.

4. Conclusions

In this study, we successfully prepared MMT-SA microcapsules with different ratios as a delivery system for WGX-50, aiming to enhance the drug's bioavailability. The addition of MMT as a filler enabled the formation of spherical microcapsules with a dense and uniform internal pore structure. The successful encapsulation of WGX-50 within the microcapsules was confirmed through FTIR analysis. The WGX-50 loaded with MMT-SA microcapsules exhibited minimal drug loss in the acidic environment of SGF, while demonstrating significant drug release in the alkaline environments of SIF and SCF. MMT-SA microcapsules are considered to be an ideal drug-encapsulation and controlled-release vehicle for oral treatment of colon diseases due to their good biosafety for human gastrointestinal cells (HIEC-6 cells and NCM460 cells) as well as the improved microporous structure with enhanced swell–dissolution properties in SIF and SCF (alkaline environment). And then, the in-depth discussion on the absorption, distribution, metabolism, and excretion of the drug molecule in the digestive tract, etc., is a starting point for the following work.

Supplementary Materials: The following supporting information can be downloaded at: https://www.mdpi.com/article/10.3390/jfb15010003/s1. Figure S1. Freeze-dried microcapsules (A-B) and oven-dried microcapsules (C-D). Figure S2. FTIR of SA, MMT, MMT_1-SA_3, MMT_3-SA_5 and MMT_1-SA_2 microcapsule. Figure S3. TG-DSC curves for (A) MMT, (B)MMT_1-SA_{19}, (C) MMT_1-SA_7 (D) MMT_1-SA_3 and (E) MMT_3-SA_5. Figure S4. Zeta potentials of MMT1-SA4, MMT1-SA6, MMT1-SA8 in different pH. Figure S5. Cytotoxicity evaluation of MMT-SA to (A) HIEC-6 cells and (B) NCM-460 cells. Figure S6. FTIR of WGX-50, MMT-SA and WGX-50/MMT-SA microcapsule. Figure S7. TG (A) and DSC (B) of MMT, MMT-SA, WGX-50 and WGX-50/MMT-SA microcapsule. Table S1. The mixed mass ratios and labels of MMT-SA microcapsule. Table S2. In vitro release data of WGX-50. Table S3. Fitting results of WGX-50 release kinetics parameters using different models at pH 1.2, 6.8 and 7.4.

Author Contributions: Y.J.: Data curation, formal analysis, investigation, methodology, writing—original draft. Z.W.: Data curation, investigation, methodology. L.X.: Supervision, funding acquisition, resources. D.W.: Conceptualization, supervision, funding acquisition. K.C.: Conceptualization, supervision, writing—review and editing. Y.Z.: Conceptualization, supervision, writing—review and editing. All authors have read and agreed to the published version of the manuscript.

Funding: This research was funded by the National Natural Science Foundation of China (82101246), the Science and Technology Major Project of Hunan Province in China (2021SK1010), the Science and Technology Innovation Program of Hunan Province in China (2022RC1069), and the APC was funded by the Central South University Innovation-Driven Research Program (2023CXQD041).

Data Availability Statement: The data presented in this study are available on request from the corresponding author.

Conflicts of Interest: The authors declare no conflict of interest.

References

1. Peng, S.; Xu, W.; Liu, H. Drug controlled releasing system based on polypyrrole modified multi-responsive hydrogel constructed from methacrylic acid and N-isopropylacrylamide. *Colloid Surf. A Physicochem. Eng. Asp.* **2023**, *669*, 131514. [CrossRef]
2. Zhao, H.; Ye, H.; Zhou, J.; Tang, G.; Hou, Z.; Bai, H. Montmorillonite-enveloped zeolitic imidazolate framework as a nourishing oral nano-platform for gastrointestinal drug delivery. *ACS Appl. Mater. Interfaces* **2020**, *12*, 49431–49441. [CrossRef] [PubMed]
3. Chu, J.; Traverso, G. Foundations of gastrointestinal-based drug delivery and future developments. *Nat. Rev. Gastroenterol. Hepatol.* **2022**, *19*, 219–238. [CrossRef] [PubMed]
4. Zarenezhad, E.; Marzi, M.; Abdulabbas, H.T.; Jasim, S.A.; Kouhpayeh, S.A.; Barbaresi, S.; Ahmadi, S.; Ghasemian, A. Bilosomes as nanocarriers for the drug and vaccine delivery against gastrointestinal infections: Opportunities and challenges. *J. Funct. Biomater.* **2023**, *14*, 453. [CrossRef]
5. Arévalo-Pérez, R.; Maderuelo, C.; Lanao, J. Recent advances in colon drug delivery systems. *J. Control. Release* **2020**, *327*, 703–724. [CrossRef] [PubMed]

6. Azehaf, H.; Benzine, Y.; Tagzirt, M.; Skiba, M.; Karrout, Y. Microbiota-sensitive drug delivery systems based on natural polysaccharides for colon targeting. *Drug Discov. Today* **2023**, *28*, 103606. [CrossRef] [PubMed]
7. Zheng, J.; Fan, R.; Wu, H.; Yao, H.; Yan, Y.; Liu, J.; Ran, L.; Sun, Z.; Yi, L.; Dang, L.; et al. Directed self-assembly of herbal small molecules into sustained release hydrogels for treating neural inflammation. *Nat. Commun.* **2019**, *10*, 1604. [CrossRef] [PubMed]
8. Tang, M.; Wang, Z.; Zhou, Y.; Xu, W.; Li, S.; Wang, L.; Wei, D.; Qiao, Z. A novel drug candidate for Alzheimer's disease treatment: Gx-50 derived from zanthoxylum bungeanum. *J. Alzheimers Dis.* **2013**, *34*, 203–213. [CrossRef]
9. Jaberifard, F.; Arsalani, N.; Ghorbani, M.; Mostafavi, H. Incorporating halloysite nanotube/carvedilol nanohybrids into gelatin microsphere as a novel oral pH-sensitive drug delivery system. *Colloid Surf. A Physicochem. Eng. Asp.* **2022**, *637*, 128122. [CrossRef]
10. Sun, J.; Xu, Z.; Hou, Y.; Yao, W.; Fan, X.; Zheng, H.; Piao, J.; Li, F.; Wei, Y. Hierarchically structured microcapsules for oral delivery of emodin and tanshinone IIA to treat renal fibrosis. *Int. J. Pharm.* **2022**, *616*, 121490. [CrossRef]
11. Wang, X.; Gao, S.; Yun, S.; Zhang, M.; Peng, L.; Li, Y.; Zhou, Y. Microencapsulating alginate-based polymers for probiotics delivery systems and their application. *Pharmaceuticals* **2022**, *15*, 644. [CrossRef] [PubMed]
12. Yu, C.; Naeem, A.; Liu, Y.; Guan, Y. Ellagic acid inclusion complex-loaded hydrogels as an efficient controlled release system: Design, fabrication and in vitro evaluation. *J. Funct. Biomater.* **2023**, *14*, 278. [CrossRef]
13. Kaushik, A.C.; Kumar, A.; Deng, Z.; Khan, A.; Junaid, M.; Ali, A.; Bharadwaj, S.; Wei, D. Evaluation and validation of synergistic effects of amyloid-beta inhibitor–gold nanoparticles complex on Alzheimer's disease using deep neural network approach. *J. Mater. Res.* **2019**, *34*, 1845–1853. [CrossRef]
14. Prakash, J.; Kumar, T.; Venkataprasanna, K.; Niranjan, R.; Kaushik, M.; Samal, D.; Venkatasubbu, G. PVA/alginate/hydroxyapatite films for controlled release of amoxicillin for the treatment of periodontal defects. *Appl. Surf. Sci.* **2019**, *495*, 143543. [CrossRef]
15. Yang, I.; Chen, Y.; Li, J.; Liang, Y.J.; Lin, T.; Jakfar, S.; Thacker, M.; Wu, S.; Lin, F. The development of laminin-alginate microspheres encapsulated with Ginsenoside Rg1 and ADSCs for breast reconstruction after lumpectomy. *Bioact. Mater.* **2021**, *6*, 1699–1710. [CrossRef] [PubMed]
16. Wang, J.; Deng, H.; Sun, Y.; Yang, C. Montmorillonite and alginate co-stabilized biocompatible pickering emulsions with multiple-stimulus tunable rheology. *J. Colloid Interface Sci.* **2020**, *562*, 529–539. [CrossRef]
17. Dattilo, M.; Patitucci, F.; Prete, S.; Parisi, O.I.; Puoci, F. Polysaccharide-based hydrogels and their application as drug delivery systems in cancer treatment: A review. *J. Funct. Biomater.* **2023**, *14*, 55. [CrossRef]
18. Yadav, H.; Agrawal, R.; Panday, A.; Patel, J.; Maiti, S. Polysaccharide-silicate composite hydrogels: Review on synthesis and drug delivery credentials. *J. Drug Deliv. Sci. Technol.* **2022**, *74*, 103573. [CrossRef]
19. Yuan, Y.; Xu, X.; Gong, J.; Mu, R.; Li, Y.; Wu, C.; Pang, J. Fabrication of chitosan-coated konjac glucomannan/sodium alginate/graphene oxide microspheres with enhanced colon-targeted delivery. *Int. J. Biol. Macromol.* **2019**, *131*, 209–217. [CrossRef]
20. Li, W.; Chen, J.; Zhao, S.; Huang, T.; Ying, H.; Trujillo, C.; Molinaro, G.; Zhou, Z.; Jiang, T.; Liu, W.; et al. High drug-loaded microspheres enabled by controlled in-droplet precipitation promote functional recovery after spinal cord injury. *Nat. Commun.* **2022**, *13*, 1262. [CrossRef]
21. Nielsen, R.B.; Kahnt, A.; Dillen, L.; Wuyts, K.; Snoeys, J.; Nielsen, U.G.; Holm, R.; Nielsen, C.U. Montmorillonite-surfactant hybrid particles for modulating intestinal P-glycoprotein-mediated transport. *Int. J. Pharm.* **2019**, *571*, 118696. [CrossRef] [PubMed]
22. Gaharwar, A.; Cross, L.; Peak, C.; Gold, K.; Carrow, J.; Brokesh, A.; Singh, K. 2D nanoclay for biomedical applications: Regenerative medicine, therapeutic delivery, and additive manufacturing. *Adv. Mater.* **2019**, *31*, 1900332. [CrossRef] [PubMed]
23. Khatoona, N.; Chu, M.; Zhou, C. Nanoclay-based drug delivery systems and their therapeutic potentials. *J. Mat. Chem.* **2020**, *8*, 7335–7351. [CrossRef] [PubMed]
24. Ayazi, H.; Akhavan, O.; Raoufi, M.; Varshochian, R.; Motlagh, N.; Atyabi, F. Graphene aerogel nanoparticles for in-situ loading/pH sensitive releasing anticancer drugs. *Colloid Surf. B Biointerfaces* **2020**, *186*, 110712. [CrossRef] [PubMed]
25. Wang, T.; Yi, W.; Zhang, Y.; Wu, H.; Fan, H.; Zhao, J.; Wang, S. Sodium alginate hydrogel containing platelet-rich plasma for wound healing. *Colloid Surf. B Biointerfaces* **2023**, *222*, 113096. [CrossRef] [PubMed]
26. Dong, X.; Li, Y.; Huang, G.; Xiao, J.; Guo, L.; Liu, L. Preparation and characterization of soybean Protein isolate/chitosan/sodium alginate ternary complex coacervate phase. *LWT Food Sci. Technol.* **2021**, *150*, 112081. [CrossRef]
27. Wang, W.; Ni, J.; Chen, L.; Ai, Z.; Zhao, Y.; Song, S. Synthesis of carboxymethyl cellulose-chitosan-montmorillonite nanosheets composite hydrogel for dye effluent remediation. *Int. J. Biol. Macromol.* **2020**, *165*, 1–10. [CrossRef] [PubMed]
28. You, Y.; Qu, K.; Huang, Z.; Ma, R.; Shi, C.; Li, X.; Liu, D.; Dong, M.; Guo, Z. Sodium alginate templated hydroxyapatite/calcium silicate composite adsorbents for efficient dye removal from polluted water. *Int. J. Biol. Macromol.* **2019**, *141*, 1035–1043. [CrossRef]
29. Da Silva Fernandes, R.; de Moura, M.R.; Glenn, G.M.; Aouada, F.A. Thermal, microstructural, and spectroscopic analysis of Ca^{2+} alginate/clay nanocomposite hydrogel beads. *J. Mol. Liq.* **2018**, *265*, 327–336. [CrossRef]
30. Ahamed, A.F.; Manimohan, M.; Kalaivasan, N. Fabrication of Biologically Active Fish Bone Derived Hydroxyapatite and Montmorillonite Blended Sodium Alginate Composite for In-Vitro Drug Delivery Studies. *J. Inorg. Organomet. Polym. Mater.* **2022**, *32*, 3902–3922. [CrossRef]
31. Zhong, L.; Hu, S.; Yang, X.; Yang, M.; Zhang, T.; Chen, L.; Zhao, Y.; Song, S. Difference in the preparation of two-dimensional nanosheets of montmorillonite from different regions: Role of the layer charge density. *Colloid Surf. A Physicochem. Eng. Asp.* **2021**, *617*, 126364. [CrossRef]
32. Guo, H.; Qin, Q.; Chang, J.-S.; Lee, D.-J. Modified alginate materials for wastewater treatment: Application prospects. *Bioresour. Technol.* **2023**, *387*, 129639. [CrossRef] [PubMed]

33. Xu, P.; Song, J.; Dai, Z.; Xu, Y.; Li, D.; Wu, C. Effect of Ca^{2+} cross-linking on the properties and structure of lutein-loaded sodium alginate hydrogels. *Int. J. Biol. Macromol.* **2021**, *193*, 53–63. [CrossRef] [PubMed]
34. Sharifzadeh, G.; Hezaveh, H.; Muhamad, I.; Hashim, S.; Khairuddin, N. Montmorillonite-based polyacrylamide hydrogel rings for controlled vaginal drug delivery. *Biomater. Adv.* **2020**, *110*, 110609. [CrossRef] [PubMed]
35. Zhao, S.; Li, Y.; Liu, Q.; Li, S.; Cheng, Y.; Cheng, C.; Sun, Z.; Du, Y.; Butch, C.; Wei, H. An orally administered CeO_2@Montmorillonite nanozyme targets inflammation for inflammatory bowel disease therapy. *Adv. Funct. Mater.* **2020**, *30*, 2004692. [CrossRef]
36. García-Guzmán, P.; Medina-Torres, L.; Calderas, F.; Bernad-Bernad, M.J.; Gracia-Mora, J.; Marcos, X.; Correa-Basurto, J.; Núñez-Ramírez, D.M.; Manero, O. Rheological mucoadhesion and cytotoxicity of montmorillonite clay mineral/hybrid microparticles biocomposite. *Appl. Clay Sci.* **2019**, *180*, 105202. [CrossRef]
37. *ISO 10993-5: 2009(en)*; Biological Evaluation of Medical Devices—Part 5: Tests for In Vitro Cytotoxicity. ISO: Geneva, Switzerland, 2009.
38. Christoforidou, T.; Giasafaki, D.; Andriotis, E.G.; Bouropoulos, N.; Theodoroula, N.F.; Vizirianakis, I.S.; Steriotis, T.; Charalambopoulou, G.; Fatouros, D.G. Oral Drug Delivery Systems Based on Ordered Mesoporous Silica Nanoparticles for Modulating the Release of Aprepitant. *Int. J. Mol. Sci.* **2021**, *22*, 1896. [CrossRef] [PubMed]
39. Li, X.; Zhang, C.; Wu, S.; Chen, X.; Mai, J.; Chang, M.W. Precision Printing of Customized Cylindrical Capsules with Multifunctional Layers for Oral Drug Delivery. *ACS Appl. Mater. Interfaces* **2019**, *11*, 39179–39191. [CrossRef]
40. Jing, H.; Huang, X.; Du, X.; Mo, L.; Ma, C.; Wang, H. Facile synthesis of pH-responsive sodium alginate/carboxymethyl chitosan hydrogel beads promoted by hydrogen bond. *Carbohydr. Polym.* **2022**, *278*, 118993. [CrossRef]

Disclaimer/Publisher's Note: The statements, opinions and data contained in all publications are solely those of the individual author(s) and contributor(s) and not of MDPI and/or the editor(s). MDPI and/or the editor(s) disclaim responsibility for any injury to people or property resulting from any ideas, methods, instructions or products referred to in the content.

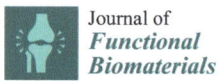
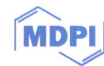

Article

Surface Properties of a Biocompatible Thermoplastic Polyurethane and Its Anti-Adhesive Effect against *E. coli* and *S. aureus*

Elisa Restivo [1,2], Emanuela Peluso [1,2], Nora Bloise [1,2,3,*], Giovanni Lo Bello [4], Giovanna Bruni [5], Marialaura Giannaccari [1,2], Roberto Raiteri [4], Lorenzo Fassina [6,*] and Livia Visai [1,2,3]

[1] Department of Molecular Medicine, Centre for Health Technologies (CHT), Consorzio Interuniversitario Nazionale per la Scienza e la Tecnologia dei Materiali (INSTM), Research Unit (UdR) Pavia, University of Pavia, 27100 Pavia, Italy; elisa.restivo01@universitadipavia.it (E.R.); emanuela.peluso01@universitadipavia.it (E.P.); marialaura.giannaccari01@universitadipavia.it (M.G.); livia.visai@unipv.it (L.V.)

[2] Interuniversity Center for the Promotion of the 3Rs Principles in Teaching and Research (Centro 3R), University of Pavia Unit, 27100 Pavia, Italy

[3] Medicina Clinica-Specialistica, UOR5 Laboratorio di Nanotecnologie, ICS Maugeri, IRCCS, 27100 Pavia, Italy

[4] Department of Informatics, Bioengineering, Robotics and System Engineering—DIBRIS, University of Genoa, 16145 Genoa, Italy; giovanni.lobello@edu.unige.it (G.L.B.); roberto.raiteri@unige.it (R.R.)

[5] Department of Chemistry, Physical Chemistry Section, University of Pavia, 27100 Pavia, Italy; giovanna.bruni@unipv.it

[6] Department of Electrical, Computer and Biomedical Engineering, Centre for Health Technologies (CHT), University of Pavia, 27100 Pavia, Italy

* Correspondence: nora.bloise@unipv.it (N.B.); lorenzo.fassina@unipv.it (L.F.); Tel.: +39-0382-987723 (N.B.); +39-0382-985266 (L.F.)

Abstract: Thermoplastic polyurethane (TPU) is a polymer used in a variety of fields, including medical applications. Here, we aimed to verify if the brush and bar coater deposition techniques did not alter TPU properties. The topography of the TPU-modified surfaces was studied via AFM demonstrating no significant differences between brush and bar coater-modified surfaces, compared to the un-modified TPU (TPU Film). The effect of the surfaces on planktonic bacteria, evaluated by MTT assay, demonstrated their anti-adhesive effect on *E. coli*, while the bar coater significantly reduced staphylococcal planktonic adhesion and both bacterial biofilms compared to other samples. Interestingly, Pearson's R coefficient analysis showed that R_a roughness and Haralick's correlation feature were trend predictors for planktonic bacterial cells adhesion. The surface adhesion property was evaluated against NIH-3T3 murine fibroblasts by MTT and against human fibrinogen and human platelet-rich plasma by ELISA and LDH assay, respectively. An indirect cytotoxicity experiment against NIH-3T3 confirmed the biocompatibility of the TPUs. Overall, the results indicated that the deposition techniques did not alter the antibacterial and anti-adhesive surface properties of modified TPU compared to un-modified TPU, nor its bio- and hemocompatibility, confirming the suitability of TPU brush and bar coater films in the biomedical and pharmaceutical fields.

Keywords: thermoplastic polyurethane (TPU); brush; bar coater; topography; atomic force microscopy (AFM); Haralick texture analysis; bacteria; cell adhesion; hemocompatibility

1. Introduction

Microbial colonization and biofilm formation on medical devices is a major public health concern [1]. Scientists are searching for effective strategies to prevent device-associated infections because the implantable devices such as prostheses, mechanical heart valves, stents, or urinary catheters, although they may improve patients' lives, they could be colonized by planktonic bacteria aggregating in biofilms and causing infectious diseases [2,3], which can become chronic and difficult to treat with antibiotics [4,5].

Today, the antimicrobial resistance is responsible for circa 700,000 deaths per year [6], a number that is expected to rise to 10 million by 2050, according to the World Health Organization (WHO) [7].

In the field of biomaterial science, researchers are designing devices that, thanks to their properties (e.g., surface texture), modifications (e.g., physical, chemical) [8], or presence of antimicrobial agents, could be able to hinder the bacterial adhesion [6]. Prior to the functionalization of a biomaterial with antimicrobial agents, it is very important to demonstrate its biocompatibility [9–12] and to characterize its surface properties since they can influence the cell behavior [13,14] and differentiation [15]. Properties such as topography, roughness, pore size [13], which determine the biomaterial surface texture, can affect the protein adsorption and consequently the cell adhesion [12,13,16], so that studying them is fundamental.

Various methods, such as atomic force microscopy (AFM), transmission electron microscopy (TEM), field emission scanning electron microscopy (FESEM), X-ray diffraction [17,18], and Fourier transform infrared (FTIR) spectroscopy [19], are known to study the surface characteristics. However, an interesting and innovative method, based on the analysis of an image of the material surface, is the measure of the Haralick's features [20]: a gray-level co-occurrence matrix (GLCM) is extracted from the image and reveals the distribution of co-occurring pixel grayscale values [21]. For instance, the GLCM and its Haralick features (e.g., contrast, variance, and correlation) are used in medicine to analyze tumor heterogeneity [22], in magnetic resonance imaging (MRI) or X-ray images, as well as to predict the prokaryotic and eukaryotic cell behavior onto a biomaterial.

A very versatile biomaterial used in medical applications such as catheters, wound dressings, coatings, and drug delivery systems is represented by polyurethane (PU) [23–26], in particular by thermoplastic PU (TPU). This polymer is composed of soft and hard segments, polyols and isocyanates, respectively [24,26], whose proportions determine a different degree of flexibility, toughness, and softness [23] and confer good mechanical properties. In addition, TPUs have been shown to be durable, biocompatible, biostable [27], and hemocompatible [28–30], making them suitable for biomedical applications.

TPUs could be also functionalized with antibacterial molecules, including antibiotics and/or nanoparticles [31], which can be released after bacterial contact or by physicochemical surface modifications [8] to either prevent or reduce the bacterial adhesion, for example, in the medical or food industry [32], where the antimicrobial property is required [33].

In our previous works [34,35], compression-molded TPU films were prepared and characterized for different mechanical (e.g., tensile and adhesive properties) and thermal characteristics. Different agents such as titanium dioxide, chitosan and silver nanoparticles were added in the TPU mother solutions, which were used to coat the surface of TPU films, in order to provide antibacterial activities with the aim to use these materials as medical devices (e.g., probes, catheters, dynamic stents). In the cited work [35], we studied the antibacterial effect of modified polyurethane films, whose modification consisted in depositing the antibacterial coatings with brush and bar coater applicators to homogenously distribute the solution and have an equal release of antibacterial agents from the surfaces. Bare TPU solutions (non-containing antibacterial agents) were deposited with a brush and bar coater on TPU films as well to be used as control [35].

In the present work, we used the bare TPU films modified on the surface by the brush and bar coater to provide a further characterization of surface topography through AFM in order to verify whether the surface modification would not have altered the biocompatible properties of TPU Brush and Bar Coater films compared to the un-modified sample, that is, the TPU Film. We evaluated the anti-adhesive effect of the surfaces against the planktonic and biofilm cultures of Gram-negative *Escherichia coli* and the Gram-positive *Staphylococcus aureus* bacteria. Interestingly, we performed a Pearson's R coefficient analysis, which showed that both R_a roughness and Haralick's correlation feature were trend predictors for the adhesion of planktonic bacteria. Moreover, in this work, we provided a preliminary study of the hemocompatibility (via human fibrinogen adsorption and human platelets adhesion) and further biocompatibility characterization, not performed in the previous works, of the TPU-modified surfaces.

2. Materials and Methods

2.1. Material Preparation and Characterization

The thermoplastic polyurethane films studied in the present work were fabricated and characterized as previously described [34,35]. Briefly, TPU films were prepared by compression molding as substrate (named TPU Film) while TPU Brush and Bar Coater were obtained by depositing mother solutions of TPU using a brush and a bar coater method, respectively, which allowed a homogeneous distribution of the polymer solutions. The materials' characterizations like NMR spectroscopy, X-ray diffraction, thermogravimetric analysis, differential scanning calorimetry as well as the wettability, have been described in our previous works. In particular, the characterization analyses of TPU samples including the main tensile properties (elastic modulus ($E = 26.2 \pm 1.4$ MPa), maximum stress ($\sigma_{max} = 36.4 \pm 1.6$ MPa), elongation at break ($\varepsilon_{break} = 1075 \pm 44\%$), and wettability ($\theta = \sim 90°$) were published in the previous work [34], while the adhesion test results (maximum force ~ -0.3 N for compression and ~ 0.3 N for tension) of the bare TPU mother solution were published in [35]. For further characterization, refer to the cited works.

2.2. Scanning Electron Microscopy (SEM)

TPU film, brush, and bar coater were observed using a Zeiss EVO-MA10 scanning electron microscope (Zeiss, Oberkochen, Germany) with an accelerating voltage of 20 kV, at 10k× and 40k× magnification.

2.3. Atomic Force Microscopy (AFM)

AFM topography images were obtained using a Nanowizard 4XP AFM (Bruker Nano GmbH, Berlin, Germany) coupled to an upright optical microscope (Axio Zoom.V16, Carl Zeiss, Iena, Germany). All measurements were conducted at room temperature (RT) in water solution (NaCl 0.9%). Topography was measured in contact mode, using a commercial AFM rectangular cantilever characterized by a conical tip with a hard diamond-like coating in order to prevent wearing over different scans (model HQ:CSC17/Hard/AI BS, μ-Masch, Tallinn, Estonia). The tip radius is less than 20 nm with a full cone angle of 40° and a nominal tip height of 15 μm. The cantilever spring constant was determined by means of the Sader method [36] and resulted to be K = 0.18 N/m. For each sample, topography images (512×512 pixel) were collected on at least ten different, randomly selected, 100×100 μm^2 areas using a force setpoint of 30 nN.

AFM images were processed using the instrument software (JPKSPM Data Processing) in order to remove tilt and calculate three surface roughness parameters: R_a (Arithmetic Average Roughness), R_q (Root Mean Square Roughness), and R_t (Maximum Peak-to-Valley Roughness).

2.4. Bacterial Cell Adhesion and Biofilm Formation

2.4.1. Bacterial Strains and Culture Conditions

The used microbial strains were *Escherichia coli* ATCC (American Type Culture Collection, Manassas, VA, USA) 25922 (*E. coli*) and *Staphylococcus aureus* ATCC 25923 (*S. aureus*). *E. coli* bacteria were grown in Luria Bertani (LB) broth (ForMedium, Norfolk, UK), overnight, under aerobic conditions at 37 °C using a shaker incubator (VDRL Stirrer 711/CT, Asal S.r.l., Milan, Italy) and *S. aureus* in Tryptic Soy Broth (TSB) (ForMedium). The number of bacterial cells/mL of both cultures was determined by comparing the optical density (OD_{600}) of the sample with a standard curve relating the OD to the cell number [37].

2.4.2. MTT Assay

Bacteria (10^5/sample) were inoculated for 6 h at 37 °C on sterile TPU samples and in tissue culture plates (TCP) used as control. Planktonic bacteria contained in the supernatant, after the desired incubation time, were removed and the samples were gently washed with PBS 1×. They were transferred in clean wells where the viability of adherent bacteria was evaluated through 3-(4,5-dimethylthiazol-2-yl)-2,5-diphenyltetrazolium bromide (MTT) colorimetric assay (Sigma-Aldrich, St. Louis, MO, USA) as described in our previous work [35]. The experiment was performed in triplicate and repeated twice.

2.4.3. Biofilm Formation

Overnight cultures of bacteria were diluted to 10^7/sample in LB containing 0.5% glucose for *E. coli* and 0.25% for *S. aureus* [38] and incubated for 24 h at 37 °C on TPU film, brush, and bar coater samples contained in 96-well culture plates (Euroclone S.p.a., Pero, Italy). After the incubation time, the surfaces were washed and transferred, and the biofilm viability assay was performed as previously described. The experiment was performed in triplicate and repeated twice.

2.5. Texture Analysis of SEM Images

The texture of a gray-level image can be calculated through Haralick features; therefore, it is possible to correlate these data with the observed biological parameters, namely the number of bacteria in planktonic culture. For each SEM image of the materials without bacteria, we have selected at least two regions of interest (ROIs) to measure the gray-level co-occurrence matrix (GLCM) [39]. Then, for each GLCM, we have calculated one Haralick's feature: the "correlation" [20]. The correlation computes the amount of similarity inside the GLCM and is a measure of the image's pixel homogeneity.

2.6. Platelets' Adhesion

Human platelet-rich plasma (hPRP) was obtained from Fondazione IRCCS Policlinico San Matteo, Pavia (Italy). hPRP was isolated according to "Decreto Ministero della Salute 2 November 2015 n.69, Disposizioni relative ai requisiti di qualità e sicurezza del sangue e degli emocomponenti" and "Accordo Stato-Regioni n.225/CSR 13 December 2018, Schema-tipo di convenzione per la cessione del sangue e dei suoi prodotti per uso di laboratorio e per la produzione di dispositivi medico-diagnostici in vitro". The quantification of platelets' adhesion to TPU samples was determined through lactate dehydrogenase (LDH) assay (Sigma-Aldrich). Human platelets were diluted in 10 mM EDTA (VWR Chemicals, Milan, Italy) at a concentration of 2×10^8 platelets/mL and seeded on sterile samples (film, brush, bar coater) for 1 h at 37 °C [29]. After the incubation time, the supernatant was removed, the samples washed three times with sterile PBS 1× and transferred into clean Eppendorfs. Lysis of adherent platelets was performed with 300 µL of 1% Triton X-100 on ice [29], for 30 min. The Eppendorfs were centrifuged at 15,000 rpm, for 30 min, at 4 °C and the supernatant was used to quantify LDH release according to the manufacturer's instructions. A titration curve with known concentration of platelets/mL was used to plot the obtained absorbance.

2.7. Enzyme-Linked Immunosorbent Assay (ELISA)

Human fibrinogen (10 µg/mL) was immobilized on the three TPU types, overnight at 4 °C, on agitation. The wells were washed three times with PBST (PBS 1× + 0.05% Tween 20) and then blocked with BSA (bovine serum albumin) 3% in PBST at RT. After that, anti-fibrinogen-HRP conjugated antibody (1:10,000) (Rockland Immunochemicals Inc., Pottstown, PA, USA) was incubated for 1 h at RT, on agitation. The wells were washed, and the reaction was developed through OPD tablets (Sigma-Aldrich). The absorbance was read at 450 nm with a reference wavelength of 620 nm [12]. The obtained absorbance was related to a calibration curve containing known amounts of fibrinogen and expressed as [µg/mL]/cm^2.

2.8. Fibroblasts' Viability

NIH-3T3 murine fibroblast cell line (ATCC CRL-1658) was obtained from the American Type Culture Collection (ATCC, Manassas, VA, USA) and cultured as described in [40]. They were seeded either in wells or onto TPU samples to evaluate the biocompatibility of TPU materials.

2.8.1. Indirect Experiment

DMEM medium was incubated overnight at 37 °C + 5% CO_2 on TPU Film, Brush, and Bar Coater to evaluate the sample's cytotoxicity. At the end of the incubation time, the solution was 2-fold serial diluted and incubated with NIH-3T3 cells (2×10^4/well) for 24 h at 37 °C + 5% CO_2. After incubation, the cells were washed with PBS 1× and incubated with MTT (Sigma-Aldrich) for 3 h at 37 °C + 5% CO_2 [41]. The reaction was read at 595 nm with the reference wavelength of 655 nm. Titration curve interpolation was used to express the number of cells in each sample. The results were normalized to the number of cells grown in a tissue culture plate (TCP), which was used as a control.

2.8.2. Direct Experiment

NIH-3T3 cells (6×10^4) were seeded on TPU film, brush, and bar coater for 24 h at 37 °C + 5% CO_2. Viability of cells was evaluated through MTT as previously described.

2.9. SEM of Cells and Platelets

Bacteria (planktonic cultures and biofilms), platelets, and fibroblasts were incubated on the three surfaces as previously described. After the desired incubation time, the samples were gently washed with PBS 1× and fixed with glutaraldehyde 2.5% (Sigma-Aldrich) and treated as described in [12]. Images of bacterial planktonic adhesion were acquired at 6k× and 15k× magnifications, with biofilms acquired at 6k× and 30k×, platelets at 3k× and 10k×, and fibroblasts at 3k×.

2.10. Statistical Analysis

Statistics regarding biological data was carried out by considering the mean of the results (in triplicate) obtained from two separate experiments. The analysis was performed using GraphPad Prism 9 (GraphPad Inc., Boston, MA, USA). The analysis was performed using Student's unpaired, two-sided *t*-test (significance level of 0.05) in comparison to the TCP control. In addition, one-way analysis of variance (ANOVA), followed by Bonferroni's multiple comparisons test, was performed [12].

3. Results

3.1. Evaluation of Morphological and Topographical Properties of TPUs

Scanning electron microscopy (SEM) and atomic force microscopy (AFM) were used to visualize the surface (Figure 1A) and the topography (Figure 1B) of the TPU Film (a,d–g), Brush (b,h–m), and Bar Coater (c,n–q). Figure 1B reports representative images of the topography of each of the three samples under investigation: Film (d–g), Brush (h–m), and Bar Coater (n–q). Images were obtained by scanning a 100×100 µm² area in different regions over the surface. No sample-distinctive structural features could be observed. Yet it can be observed that the bar coater-modified surface (n–q) looked flatter than the others. The roughness of the surface was calculated through AFM (C).

Figure 1C shows the distributions of the three surface roughness parameters that have been measured from each topography image; it can be observed that the lowest roughness values were obtained for the TPU Bar Coater, providing an indication of a smoother surface among the three samples.

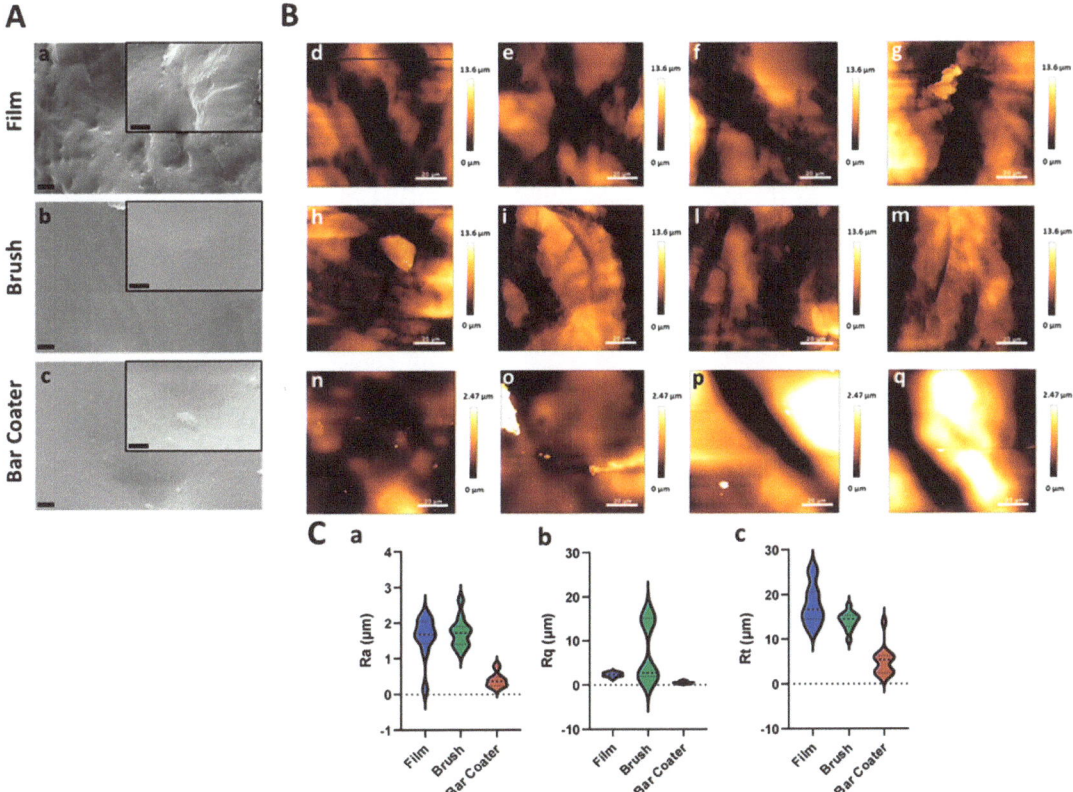

Figure 1. Thermoplastic polyurethane surface. Microscopic images (**A**) of thermoplastic polyurethane (TPU) Film (**a**), Brush (**b**), and Bar Coater (**c**). SEM images were acquired at 10k× magnification (scale bar 2 µm), and insets at 40k× (scale bar 1 µm). Morphological analysis (**B**) in four different areas of TPU Film (**d–g**), Brush (**h,i,l,m**), and Bar Coater (**n,o,p,q**). Roughness values (**C**) calculated for the three samples on $n = 10$ images (topography 100×100 µm^2). Average Roughness R_a (**a**), RMS Roughness R_q (**b**), Peak-to-Valley Roughness R_t (**c**) for Film (blue), Brush (green), and Bar Coater (red).

3.2. Evaluation of Planktonic Bacterial Adhesion on TPUs

The ability of planktonic bacteria to adhere on the TPU Film, Brush, and Bar Coater was evaluated through an MTT viability assay (Figure 2A). Figure 2 shows the *E. coli* viability (A,a) and distribution (B,a–c) on the three samples after 6 h of adhesion time, whereas in panels (A,b) and (B,d–f) *S. aureus* data are reported.

Figure 2A shows that only 1% of Gram-negative *E. coli* (a) was viable after 6 h of adhesion on TPU with respect to the TCP control, represented by bacteria which adhered on the well surface. The non-adhesive properties of TPU against *E. coli* are independent from the type of deposition method. Panel (b) shows, on the contrary, the opposite behavior of Gram-positive *S. aureus* on TPUs: *S. aureus* was viable on Film (~50%), Brush (~70%), and Bar Coater (~25%). A comparative summary table (Table 1) is reported as follow. The data are supported by SEM images (Figure 2B).

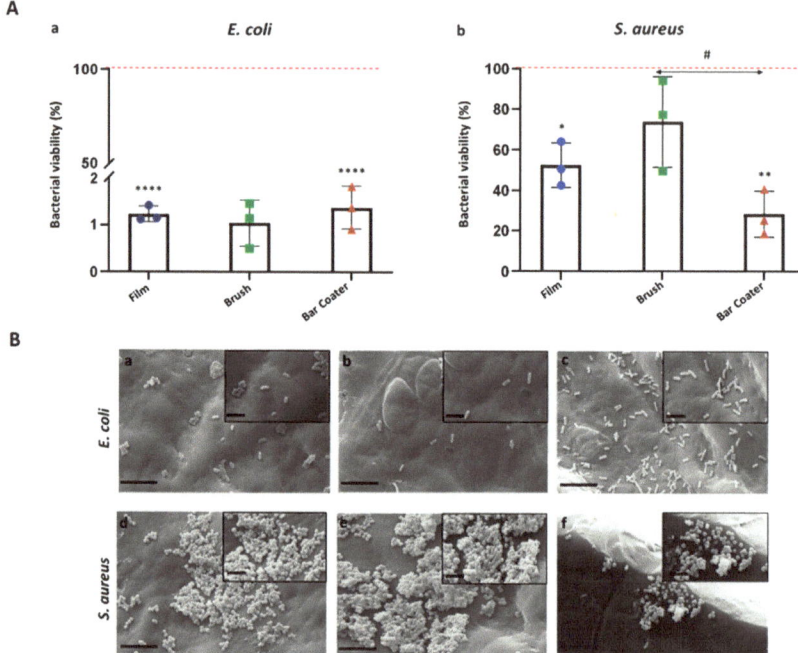

Figure 2. Bacterial adhesion on TPUs. *E. coli* (**A**, **a**; **B**, **a–c**) and *S. aureus* (**A**, **b**; **B**, **d–f**) were incubated for 6 h at 37 °C on Film, Brush, and Bar Coater. After removal of supernatant, the viability of adherent bacteria has been determined through MTT (**A**). Cell viability (%) was represented with respect to the TCP control, consisting of bacteria grown in medium and set as 100% (red line). Data are represented as the mean values of the replicates (n = 3) ± the standard deviation (SD), represented by the error bars. Statistical analysis (*, #) indicates the analysis vs. TCP: $p < 0.0001$ (****), $p < 0.01$ (**), $p < 0.05$ (*). One-way analysis of variance (ANOVA), followed by Bonferroni's test between samples (#) within bacterium ($p < 0.05$), was performed. Data not significant ($p > 0.05$) for *E. coli*. SEM images (**B**) of *E. coli* (**a–c**) and *S. aureus* (**d–f**) bacterial adhesion on Film (**a,d**), Brush (**b,e**) and Bar Coater (**c,f**) were acquired at 6k× magnification (scale bar 8 μm), and insets at 15k× (scale bar 2 μm).

Table 1. Summary of the adhesion onto TPU surfaces.

TPU Surface	Adhesion						
	Planktonic Behavior Predicted by Haralick Analysis		Biofilm		PLTs	hFg	NIH-3T3
	E. coli	*S. aureus*	*E. coli*	*S. aureus*			
Film	~1%	~50%	80%	50%	<0.5%	~15%	<2.5%
Brush	~1%	~70%	70%	70%	<0.5%	~15%	<2.5%
Bar Coater	~1%	~25%	60%	20%	<0.5%	~20%	<2.5%

3.3. TEXTURE Analysis of the SEM Images for the Prediction of the Bacteria Number in Planktonic Cultures

The Haralick's texture analysis was performed on the TPU Film, Brush, and Bar Coater. SEM images, at 40k× magnification, were used to extract the Haralick correlation feature and to analyze the link between this feature and the bacterial adhesion (Figure 3). Moreover, we have correlated the R_a roughness to the bacterial adhesion (Figure 4).

In order to link the Haralick correlation feature of the material surface to the number of bacteria in planktonic culture onto that surface, we have performed a Pearson analysis: the Pearson R coefficient is the most common method to study a linear relationship; it is a number between -1 and 1 that measures the strength and the direction of the relationship between two variables, in our work, the Haralick correlation feature and the number of bacteria in planktonic culture.

In Figure 3, we can see that the Haralick correlation is a trend predictor for the number of bacteria (in fact, $|R| > 0.9$ for both bacteria). In particular, for *E. coli*, the number of bacteria increases with an increasing Haralick's correlation; on the other hand, for *S. aureus*, the number of bacteria decreases with an increasing Haralick's correlation. In addition, major differences were found for the brush-modified surface, whereas minor differences were found for the bar coater-modifiedsurface.

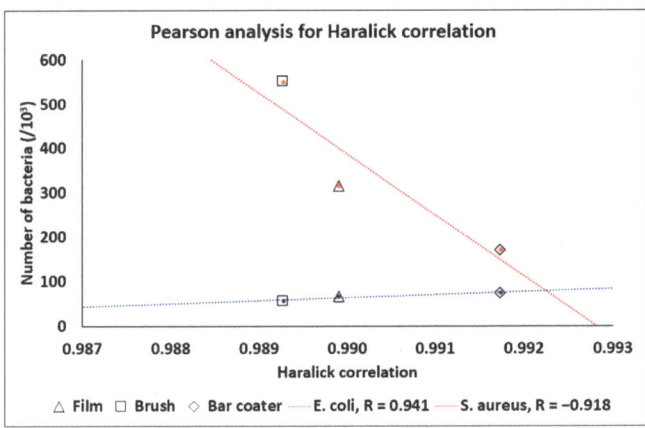

Figure 3. Pearson analysis for Haralick correlation.

Figure 4 reports the rugosity R_a, which is a trend predictor for the number of bacteria (in fact, $|R| > 0.85$ for both bacteria). In particular, for *E. coli*, the number of bacteria decreases with an increasing rugosity R_a; on the other hand, for *S. aureus*, the number of bacteria increases with an increasing rugosity R_a. In addition, major differences were found for the Brush surface, whereas minor differences were observed for the Bar Coater surface.

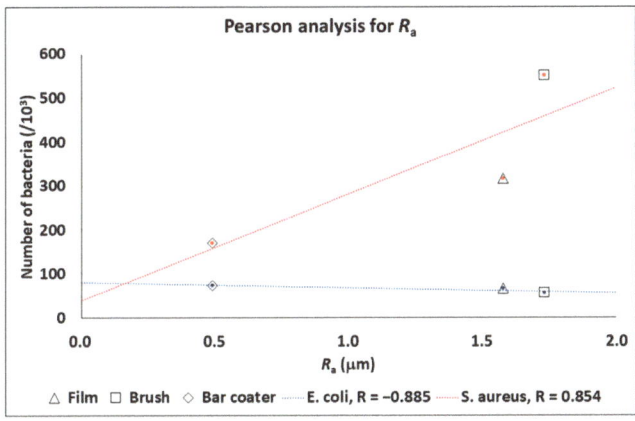

Figure 4. Pearson analysis for rugosity R_a.

3.4. Effect of TPU Surfaces on Bacterial Biofilms

After the adhesion of planktonic bacteria, we have evaluated the ability of that bacteria to form biofilms on the surfaces. Figure 5 shows that the bacterial biofilms grew on all samples, although the bar coater-modified surface is able to reduce the *E. coli* biofilm viability by circa 40% (A,a) and the *S. aureus* biofilm viability by circa 80% (A,b, Table 1). The film surface can reduce the *E. coli* biofilm by circa 20% and the staphylococcal one by circa 50%. The brush-modified surface, instead, showed the same percentage of reduction (circa 30%) for both bacterial biofilms (A, Table 1). Panel B shows the SEM images of the bacterial biofilms.

As reported in numerous papers in the literature [13,42,43], the surface roughness is often correlated with high levels of biofilm formation as it increases the surface area available for bacterial attachment. This helps to explain why, particularly on the TPU Brush samples (which had the highest roughness compared to the Film and Bar Coater samples), the biofilm viability of *S. aureus* was higher.

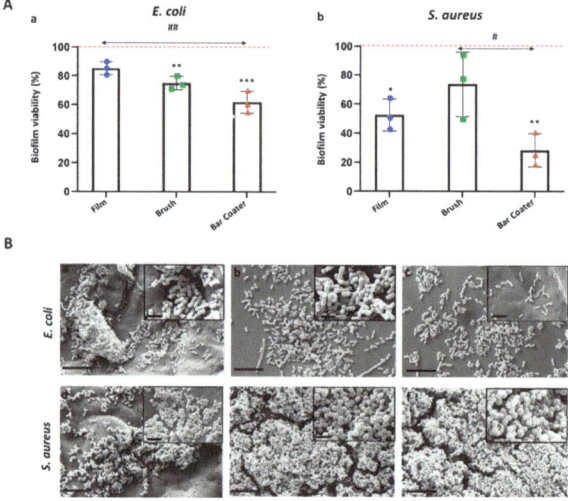

Figure 5. Bacterial biofilm on TPUs. *E. coli* (**A**, **a**; **B**, **a–c**) and *S. aureus* (**A**, **b**; **B**, **d–f**) were incubated in biofilm conditions on TPU Film, Brush, and Bar Coater for 24 h at 37 °C. After removal of supernatant, viability of biofilms was determined through MTT (**A**). Biofilm viabilities (%) were reported with respect to the TCP control, represented by biofilm grown in medium and set as 100% (red line). Data are represented as the mean values of the replicates ($n = 3$) ± the standard deviation (SD), represented by the error bars. Statistical analysis (*, #) indicates the analysis vs. TCP: $p < 0.001$ (***), $p < 0.01$ (**), $p < 0.05$ (*). One-way analysis of variance (ANOVA), followed by Bonferroni's test between samples (#) within bacterium, was performed: $p < 0.05$ (#) and $p < 0.01$ (##). SEM images (**B**) of *E. coli* (**a–c**) and *S. aureus* (**d–f**) biofilms on Film (**a,d**), Brush (**b,e**), and Bar Coater (**c,f**) were acquired at 6k× magnification (scale bar 8 µm), and insets at 30k× (scale bar 2 µm).

3.5. Evaluation of TPU Surface Effect on Platelets, Fibrinogen, and Cells Adhesion

To further characterize the biological properties of the TPU surfaces, the adhesion of platelets, fibrinogen [44,45], and eukaryotic cells was evaluated [46].

Figure 6 shows data regarding platelets seeded for 1 h at 37 °C on the TPU Film, Brush, and Bar Coater compared to the TCP control, represented by platelets adhered on a well (red line). The data demonstrate that there is no significant difference between samples and all three surfaces did not allow platelets to adhere (A) (<0.5% adhesion vs. TCP). The results were due to the hydrophobicity of TPU, already reported by Villani et al. [34], and our findings are in accordance with the literature [44,45]. Quantitative data are supported by SEM images (B). No activation of platelets was observed on either the control or samples, since no bulbous and pseudopodia were present on the adhered platelet's surface [46–48].

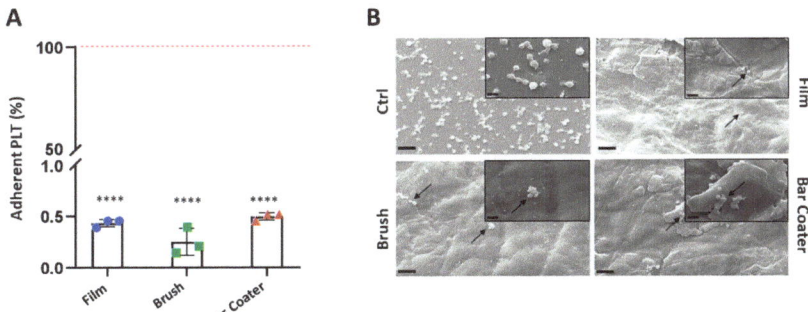

Figure 6. Platelets adhesion. Platelets (PLT) were incubated for 1 h at 37 °C + 5% CO_2 on TPU samples: Film, Brush, and Bar Coater. Viability has been determined through LDH assay on supernatant (**A**). Data are represented as percentage of adherent platelets on TPUs with respect to the TCP control, denoted by the platelets seeded in a well and set as 100% (red line). Data are shown as the mean values of the replicates (n = 3) ± the standard deviation (SD), represented by the error bars. Statistically significant differences of samples vs. TCP were reported: $p < 0.0001$ (****). One-way analysis of variance (ANOVA), followed by Bonferroni's test between samples, showed no significant difference between samples. After removal of supernatant, the adherent platelets on TPU surfaces and on control glass were fixed and the SEM images (**B**) were acquired at 3k× magnification (scale bar 20 µm), and insets at 10k× (scale bar 2 µm). Platelets are indicated by arrows on the TPU samples. No pseudopodia, characteristics of activated PLTs, were observed on either the control or the samples.

Furthermore, the capacity of fibrinogen to adhere on modified TPU surfaces was evaluated, since the importance for platelets adhesion. The results, shown in Figure 7 and Table 1, confirmed that a low percentage, with respect to the TCP control, could bind to the surface [44]. There is no significant difference between film and brush, whose surfaces displayed circa 15% of fibrinogen adhesion. The Bar Coater surface, on the contrary, demonstrated an ability to bind circa 20% of the protein compared to TCP control.

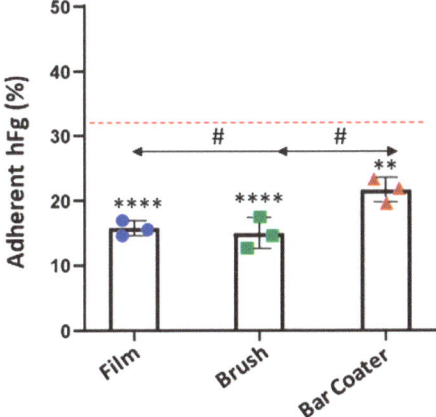

Figure 7. Fibrinogen quantification. Human fibrinogen (hFg) was incubated, overnight at 4 °C, on TPU Film, Brush, and Bar Coater. The adherent protein on TPU was detected through an anti-fibrinogen HRP-conjugated antibody and quantified via ELISA assay. Data are represented as

percentage of adherent hFg on TPU materials with respect to the TCP control (red line). Data are shown as the mean values of the replicates ($n = 3$) ± the standard deviation (SD), represented by the error bars. Statistically significant differences of samples vs. TCP were reported: $p < 0.0001$ (****), $p < 0.01$ (**). One-way analysis of variance (ANOVA), followed by Bonferroni's test between samples (#), was performed: $p < 0.05$.

Finally, the biocompatibility and the adhesive properties of TPU vs. NIH-3T3 fibroblasts were assessed [49,50] and are shown in Figure 8 and summarized in Table 1. Panel A reports data obtained from the indirect cytotoxicity assay, where the content of TPU, released overnight in the cell medium, was tested on cells. As shown in the figure, only the undiluted solutions, recovered from Film and Bar Coater, reduced the fibroblast viability of circa 20% with respect to the TCP control (red line), represented by cells grown in a well. On the other hand, the more diluted solutions were not toxic for the cells, as illustrated in the figure. No significant differences between samples were observed. Finally, panel B reports the percentage and the SEM images of NIH-3T3 cells' adhesion onto the three surfaces. Fibroblasts' adhesion on all surfaces was <2.5% with respect to TCP control. Significant differences were observed with respect to the TCP. The very low fibroblast adhesion was due to the hydrophobic nature of the TPU [35], which led to a reduction in protein adsorption (Figure 7) and, consequently, to low cell adhesion [51].

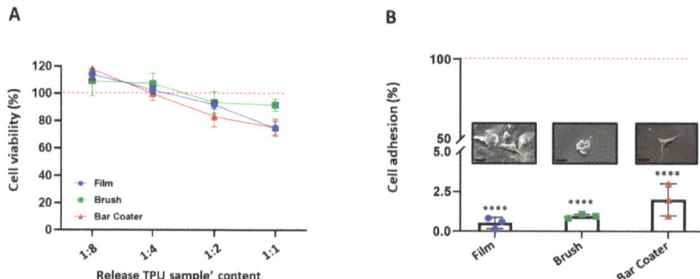

Figure 8. Cell viability (A) and adhesion (B). NIH-3T3 cell medium was incubated with TPU samples overnight at 37 °C + 5% CO_2. The released content of polymer from the samples was 2-fold diluted and incubated with NIH-3T3 cells for 24 h. The viability was evaluated through MTT colorimetric test (A). Data are shown as percentage of cell viability with respect to TCP control (red line) represented by cells grown in a well. Statistical analysis reported no significant differences ($p > 0.05$) with respect to TCP control and between samples. Cells were seeded on TPU samples for 24 h at 37 °C + 5% CO_2 (B). The viability of adherent cells was evaluated through MTT. Data are shown as percentage of cell adhesion with respect to TCP control (red line). Data are represented as the mean values of the replicates ($n = 3$) ± the standard deviation (SD), denoted by the error bars. Statistics indicates the analysis vs. TCP: $p < 0.0001$ (****). ANOVA analysis was performed, and no significant differences ($p > 0.05$) were observed. SEM images of the cell adhesion on TPU surfaces were acquired at 3k× (scale bar 20 µm).

4. Discussion

The development of biomaterials with specific characteristics is crucial for their application in medicine and in tissue engineering. Surface topography as well as wettability [13] play an important role in prokaryotic and eukaryotic cells' adhesion.

In this work, we studied whether the different deposition methods of a TPU solution, distributed by brush and bar coater applicators on TPU substrates (TPU film) [35], would have altered the TPU-modified surfaces' topography and would have affected their anti-adhesive and biological properties.

In this study, the texture analysis of three surfaces has been performed by AFM, which provided information regarding the TPU-modified surfaces' roughness, compared to the un-modified one (TPU Film). The roughness parameters [13,52], which measure the different height between areas of a surface [53], are important for evaluating prokaryotic and eukaryotic cells-biomaterial interaction.

The obtained AFM topography data confirmed that no characteristic traits were present on the surfaces. They were smooth, but the bar coater-modified surface was flatter than the others, probably due to the type of TPU deposition [35]. What further bolstered our findings was the fact that the bar coater sample displayed a notably narrower dispersion of results when compared to Brush and Film. As reported by the literature [2,54] the different type of deposition methods can vary the roughness of the surface and, consequently, the interaction with cells. The anti-adhesive effect of the modified surfaces was evaluated against planktonic cultures of Gram-negative *E. coli* and Gram-positive *S. aureus*. Briefly, the viability of planktonic adherent bacteria was assessed after 6 h vs. the TCP control, represented by bacteria grown in a well. The obtained data demonstrated the anti-adhesive effect of Film, Brush and Bar Coater surfaces against *E. coli*. Staphylococcal cells, instead, displayed major adhesion on the brush-modified surface and minor adhesion on the Bar Coater's. As known in the literature, the surface characteristics such as roughness, wettability (hydrophilicity and hydrophobicity), play a fundamental role for cell adhesion [13,52]. A better adhesion of prokaryotic and eukaryotic cells, indeed, is observable both on rough surfaces, since they present more areas to let cells anchor [55], and on hydrophilic surfaces [13]. For this reason, we explain why the higher staphylococcal adhesion is observable on the brush-modified surface [2]. However, the opposite bacterial behavior, displayed by planktonic *E. coli* and *S. aureus* bacteria, could be explained by their different characteristics mainly in the cell wall and motility [56–58] since they belong to Gram-negative and Gram-positive strain, respectively. Interestingly, we performed Pearson's R coefficient analysis, which showed that both R_a roughness and Haralick correlation feature [59–61], were trend predictors for the adhesion of planktonic bacterial cells.

We evaluated the ability of adherent bacteria to form biofilms, which are complex microbial communities protected by a self-produced polysaccharide matrix [2,62,63]. The obtained data showed that the brush-modified surface favored, as supported by the literature [2], the formation of both biofilms, whereas the bar coater's smooth surface reduced them. The surfaces, since they did not contain antibacterial agents, were not able to inhibit the formation of both biofilms, as reported in the literature [64].

Furthermore, we evaluated the platelets' adhesion and the fibrinogen adsorption on brush- and bar coater-modified surfaces, and their biocompatibility for a potential use as coatings in cardiovascular devices. Our findings showed that both surfaces, compared to the TPU Film, did not release any toxic compound for cells [28]. Moreover, from platelets' adhesion and fibrinogen adsorption analyses [27–29], important for a preliminary evaluation of the hemocompatibility [65], and from the assessment of fibroblasts' adhesion, we confirmed the anti-adhesive effect of TPU and of its brush- and bar coater-modified surfaces. These results are supported by the hydrophobic nature of the TPU [34], which causes proteins to be adsorbed onto the surface in a denatured state [13], not allowing platelets [27–29] and fibroblasts to adhere [66].

5. Conclusions

In this study, a brush and bar coater, both interesting for the deposition of polymer solutions on TPU films, were able to modify the surface topography of the TPU material by changing the surface roughness. However, these changes did not significantly alter the anti-adhesive properties of the TPU-modified surfaces, as well as their ability to hinder human fibrinogen adsorption, human platelets', and fibroblasts' adhesion. However, further analyses, both in vitro and in vivo, will be required to confirm all this experimental evidence. Finally, using Pearson's analysis to correlate the bacterial adhesion with roughness data and with Haralick's correlation feature, we confirmed how important it is to have a good characterization of the surface as a predictor of the cell–material interaction.

Author Contributions: Conceptualization, E.R., N.B., L.F. and L.V.; investigation, E.R., E.P., N.B., G.L.B., G.B. and M.G.; formal analysis, software, L.F.; writing—original draft preparation, E.R.; writing—review and editing, E.R., E.P., N.B., G.L.B., G.B., M.G., R.R., L.F. and L.V.; supervision, R.R. and L.V.; funding acquisition, L.V. All authors have read and agreed to the published version of the manuscript.

Funding: This research was funded by a grant of the Italian Ministry of University and Research (MUR) to the Department of Molecular Medicine of the University of Pavia under the initiative "Dipartimenti di Eccellenza (2018–2022) and (2023–2027)".

Data Availability Statement: The data presented in this study are available on request from the corresponding author.

Acknowledgments: The authors thank Maurizio Villani for having provided the TPU samples, Roberta Migliavacca (Department of Clinical, Surgical, Diagnostic and Pediatric Sciences, University of Pavia, Italy) for providing bacterial strains and Centro Lavorazione e Validazione, Servizio di Immunoematologia e Medicina Trasfusionale, Fondazione IRCCS Policlinico San Matteo, Pavia for PRP samples. G.B. acknowledges the support from the Italian Ministry of University and Research (MUR) and the University of Pavia through the program "Dipartimenti di Eccellenza 2023–2027". The authors thank Bianca Abbadessa (IULM University, Milan, Italy) for linguistic proofreading.

Conflicts of Interest: The authors declare no conflicts of interest. The funders had no role in the design of the study; in the collection, analyses, or interpretation of data; in the writing of the manuscript; or in the decision to publish the results.

References

1. Xu, L.C.; Siedlecki, C.A. Submicron topography design for controlling staphylococcal bacterial adhesion and biofilm formation. *J. Biomed. Mater. Res. A* **2022**, *110*, 1238–1250. [CrossRef]
2. Muszanska, A.K.; Rochford, E.T.J.; Gruszka, A.; Bastian, A.A.; Busscher, H.J.; Norde, W.; Van Der Mei, H.C.; Herrmann, A. Antiadhesive polymer brush coating functionalized with antimicrobial and RGD peptides to reduce biofilm formation and enhance tissue integration. *Biomacromolecules* **2014**, *15*, 2019–2026. [CrossRef] [PubMed]
3. Skovdal, S.M.; Jørgensen, N.P.; Petersen, E.; Jensen-Fangel, S.; Ogaki, R.; Zeng, G.; Johansen, M.I.; Wang, M.; Rohde, H.; Meyer, R.L. Ultra-dense polymer brush coating reduces Staphylococcus epidermidis biofilms on medical implants and improves antibiotic treatment outcome. *Acta Biomater.* **2018**, *76*, 46–55. [CrossRef] [PubMed]
4. Ramasamy, M.; Lee, J. Recent nanotechnology approaches for prevention and treatment of biofilm-associated infections on medical devices. *Biomed. Res. Int.* **2016**, *2016*, 1–18. [CrossRef] [PubMed]
5. Stewart, P.S.; Bjarnsholt, T. Risk factors for chronic biofilm-related infection associated with implanted medical devices. *Clin. Microbiol. Infect.* **2020**, *26*, 1034–1038. [CrossRef]
6. Uddin, T.M.; Chakraborty, A.J.; Khusro, A.; Zidan, B.R.M.; Mitra, S.; Emran, T.B.; Dhama, K.; Ripon, M.K.H.; Gajdács, M.; Sahibzada, M.U.K.; et al. Antibiotic resistance in microbes: History, mechanisms, therapeutic strategies and future prospects. *J. Infect. Public Health* **2021**, *14*, 1750–1766. [CrossRef] [PubMed]
7. O'Neill, J. Tackling drug resistant infections globally: Final report and recommendations. *Rev. Antimicrob. Resist.* **2016**, 1–84. Available online: https://amr-review.org/sites/default/files/160518_Final%20paper_with%20cover.pdf (accessed on 11 January 2024).
8. Wang, C.G.; Surat'man, N.E.B.; Mah, J.J.Q.; Qu, C.; Li, Z. Surface antimicrobial functionalization with polymers: Fabrication, mechanisms and applications. *J. Mater. Chem. B* **2022**, *10*, 9349–9368. [CrossRef]
9. Nhu Hieu, V.; Thanh Van, T.T.; Hang, C.T.T.; Mischenko, N.P.; Sergey, A.F.; Truong, H. Polyhydroxynaphthoquinone Pigment from Vietnam Sea Urchins as a Potential Bioactive Ingredient in Cosmeceuticals. *Nat. Prod. Commun.* **2020**, *15*, 1–8. [CrossRef]
10. Zayed, N.; Munjaković, H.; Aktan, M.K.; Simoens, K.; Bernaerts, K.; Boon, N.; Braem, A.; Pamuk, F.; Saghi, M.; Van Holm, W.; et al. Electrolyzed Saline Targets Biofilm Periodontal Pathogens In Vitro. *J. Dent. Res.* **2024**, 1–10. [CrossRef]
11. Káčerová, S.; Muchová, M.; Doudová, H.; Münster, L.; Hanulíková, B.; Valášková, K.; Kašpárková, V.; Kuřitka, I.; Humpolíček, P.; Víchová, Z.; et al. Chitosan/dialdehyde cellulose hydrogels with covalently anchored polypyrrole: Novel conductive, antibacterial, antioxidant, immunomodulatory, and anti-inflammatory materials. *Carbohydr. Polym.* **2024**, *327*, 121640. [CrossRef]
12. Restivo, E.; Pugliese, D.; Gallichi-Nottiani, D.; Sammartino, J.C.; Bloise, N.; Peluso, E.; Percivalle, E.; Janner, D.; Milanese, D.; Visai, L. Effect of Low Copper Doping on the Optical, Cytocompatible, Antibacterial, and SARS-CoV-2 Trapping Properties of Calcium Phosphate Glasses. *ACS Omega* **2023**, *8*, 42264–42274. [CrossRef]
13. Cai, S.; Wu, C.; Yang, W.; Liang, W.; Yu, H.; Liu, L. Recent advance in surface modification for regulating cell adhesion and behaviors. *Nanotechnol. Rev.* **2020**, *9*, 971–989. [CrossRef]
14. Tudureanu, R.; Handrea-Dragan, I.M.; Boca, S.; Botiz, I. Insight and Recent Advances into the Role of Topography on the Cell Differentiation and Proliferation on Biopolymeric Surfaces. *Int. J. Mol. Sci.* **2022**, *23*, 7731. [CrossRef]
15. Clarke, D.E.; Mccullen, S.D.; Chow, A.; Stevens, M.M. 5.02 Functional Biomaterials. In *Comprehensive Biotechnology*, 2nd ed.; Pergamon: Oxford, UK, 2011; pp. 3–10.

16. Kulangara, K.; Leong, K.W. Substrate topography shapes cell function. *Soft Matter* **2009**, *5*, 4072–4076. [CrossRef]
17. Yu, H.; Xu, Y.; Zhang, M.; Zhang, L.; Wu, W.; Huang, K. Magnetically-separable cobalt catalyst embedded in metal nitrate-promoted hierarchically porous N-doped carbon nanospheres for hydrodeoxygenation of lignin-derived species. *Fuel* **2023**, *331*, 125917. [CrossRef]
18. Yu, H.; Xu, Y.; Havener, K.; Zhang, L.; Wu, W.; Liao, X.; Huang, K. Efficient catalysis using honeycomb-like N-doped porous carbon supported Pt nanoparticles for the hydrogenation of cinnamaldehyde in water. *Mol. Catal.* **2022**, *525*, 112343. [CrossRef]
19. Vishnoi, M.; Kumar, P.; Murtaza, Q. Surface texturing techniques to enhance tribological performance: A review. *Surf. Interfaces* **2021**, *27*, 101463. [CrossRef]
20. Haralick, R.; Shanmugam, K.; Dinstein, I. Textural Features for Image Classification. *IEEE Trans. Syst. Man. Cybern.* **1973**, *3*, 610–621. [CrossRef]
21. Brynolfsson, P.; Nilsson, D.; Torheim, T.; Asklund, T.; Karlsson, C.T.; Trygg, J.; Nyholm, T.; Garpebring, A. Haralick texture features from apparent diffusion coefficient (ADC) MRI images depend on imaging and pre-processing parameters. *Sci. Rep.* **2017**, *7*, 4041. [CrossRef]
22. Vrbik, I.; Van Nest, S.J.; Meksiarun, P.; Loeppky, J.; Brolo, A.; Lum, J.J.; Jirasek, A. Haralick texture feature analysis for quantifying radiation response heterogeneity in murine models observed using Raman spectroscopic mapping. *PLoS ONE* **2019**, *14*, e0212225. [CrossRef]
23. Das, A.; Mahanwar, P. A brief discussion on advances in polyurethane applications. *Adv. Ind. Eng. Polym. Res.* **2020**, *3*, 93–101. [CrossRef]
24. Maestri, C.; Plancher, L.; Duthoit, A.; Hébert, R.L.; Di Martino, P. Fungal Biodegradation of Polyurethanes. *J. Fungi* **2023**, *9*, 760. [CrossRef]
25. Borcan, F.; Vlase, T.; Vlase, G.; Popescu, R.; Soica, C.M. The Influence of an Isocyanate Structure on a Polyurethane Delivery System for 2′-Deoxycytidine-5′-monophosphate. *J. Funct. Biomater.* **2023**, *14*, 526. [CrossRef]
26. Wang, J.; Dai, D.; Xie, H.; Li, D.; Xiong, G.; Zhang, C. Biological Effects, Applications and Design Strategies of Medical Polyurethanes Modified by Nanomaterials. *Int. J. Nanomed.* **2022**, *17*, 6791–6819. [CrossRef]
27. Cortella, L.R.X.; Cestari, I.A.; Guenther, D.; Lasagni, A.F.; Cestari, I.N. Endothelial cell responses to castor oil-based polyurethane substrates functionalized by direct laser ablation. *Biomed. Mater.* **2017**, *12*, 065010. [CrossRef] [PubMed]
28. Navas-Gómez, K.; Valero, M.F. Why polyurethanes have been used in the manufacture and design of cardiovascular devices: A systematic review. *Materials* **2020**, *13*, 3250. [CrossRef] [PubMed]
29. Fernandes, K.R.; Zhang, Y.; Magri, A.M.P.; Renno, A.C.M.; Van Den Beucken, J.J.J.P. Biomaterial Property Effects on Platelets and Macrophages: An in vitro Study. *ACS Biomater. Sci. Eng.* **2017**, *3*, 3318–3327. [CrossRef]
30. Pavithra, D.; Doble, M. Biofilm formation, bacterial adhesion and host response on polymeric implants—Issues and prevention. *Biomed. Mater.* **2008**, *3*, 034003. [CrossRef] [PubMed]
31. Ekonomou, S.; Soe, S.; Stratakos, A.C. An explorative study on the antimicrobial effects and mechanical properties of 3D printed PLA and TPU surfaces loaded with Ag and Cu against nosocomial and foodborne pathogens. *J. Mech. Behav. Biomed. Mater.* **2023**, *137*, 105536. [CrossRef]
32. Feng, Q.; Fan, B.; He, Y.-C.; Ma, C. Antibacterial, antioxidant and fruit packaging ability of biochar-based silver nanoparticles-polyvinyl alcohol-chitosan composite film. *Int. J. Biol. Macromol.* **2023**, *256*, 128297. [CrossRef]
33. Fu, Y.; Dudley, E.G. Antimicrobial-coated films as food packaging: A review. *Compr. Rev. Food Sci. Food Saf.* **2021**, *20*, 3404–3437. [CrossRef]
34. Villani, M.; Consonni, R.; Canetti, M.; Bertoglio, F.; Iervese, S.; Bruni, G.; Visai, L.; Iannace, S.; Bertini, F. Polyurethane-based composites: Effects of antibacterial fillers on the physical-mechanical behavior of thermoplastic polyurethanes. *Polymers* **2020**, *12*, 362. [CrossRef] [PubMed]
35. Villani, M.; Bertoglio, F.; Restivo, E.; Bruni, G.; Iervese, S.; Arciola, C.R.; Carulli, F.; Iannace, S.; Bertini, F.; Visai, L. Polyurethane-based coatings with promising antibacterial properties. *Materials* **2020**, *13*, 4296. [CrossRef] [PubMed]
36. Sader, J.E.; Chon, J.W.M.; Mulvaney, P. Calibration of rectangular atomic force microscope cantilevers. *Rev. Sci. Instrum.* **1999**, *70*, 3967–3969. [CrossRef]
37. Trespidi, G.; Scoffone, V.C.; Barbieri, G.; Marchesini, F.; Abualsha'ar, A.; Coenye, T.; Ungaro, F.; Makarov, V.; Migliavacca, R.; De Rossi, E.; et al. Antistaphylococcal activity of the FtsZ inhibitor C109. *Pathogens* **2021**, *10*, 886. [CrossRef]
38. Pallavicini, P.; Arciola, C.R.; Bertoglio, F.; Curtosi, S.; Dacarro, G.; D'Agostino, A.; Ferrari, F.; Merli, D.; Milanese, C.; Rossi, S.; et al. Silver nanoparticles synthesized and coated with pectin: An ideal compromise for anti-bacterial and anti-biofilm action combined with wound-healing properties. *J. Colloid Interface Sci.* **2017**, *498*, 271–281. [CrossRef] [PubMed]
39. Bloise, N.; Fassina, L.; Focarete, M.L.; Lotti, N.; Visai, L. Haralick's texture analysis to predict cellular proliferation on randomly oriented electrospun nanomaterials. *Nanoscale Adv.* **2022**, *4*, 1330–1335. [CrossRef]
40. Guerra-Flórez, D.Y.; Valencia-Osorio, L.M.; Zapata-González, A.F.; Álvarez-Láinez, M.L.; Cadavid-Torres, E.; Meneses-Ramírez, E.A.; Torres-Osorio, V.; Botero-Valencia, J.S.; Pareja-López, A. In vitro toxicity of fine and coarse particulate matter on the skin, ocular and lung microphysiological cell-culture systems. *Toxicology* **2023**, *500*, 153685. [CrossRef] [PubMed]
41. Gatto, M.L.; Furlani, M.; Giuliani, A.; Cabibbo, M.; Bloise, N.; Fassina, L.; Petruczuk, M.; Visai, L.; Mengucci, P. Combined Effects of HA Concentration and Unit Cell Geometry on the Biomechanical Behavior of PCL/HA Scaffold for Tissue Engineering Applications Produced by LPBF. *Materials* **2023**, *16*, 4950. [CrossRef] [PubMed]

42. Zhang, X.; Wang, L.; Levänen, E. Superhydrophobic surfaces for the reduction of bacterial adhesion. *RSC Adv.* **2013**, *3*, 12003–12020. [CrossRef]
43. Sharma, S.; Jaimes-Lizcano, Y.A.; McLay, R.B.; Cirino, P.C.; Conrad, J.C. Subnanometric Roughness Affects the Deposition and Mobile Adhesion of Escherichia coli on Silanized Glass Surfaces. *Langmuir* **2016**, *32*, 5422–5433. [CrossRef]
44. Wu, X.; Jia, H.; Fu, W.; Li, M.; Pan, Y. Enhanced Tensile Properties, Biostability, and Biocompatibility of Siloxane–Cross-Linked Polyurethane Containing Ordered Hard Segments for Durable Implant Application. *Molecules* **2023**, *28*, 2464. [CrossRef] [PubMed]
45. Lee, J.H.; Ju, Y.M.; Kim, D.M. Platelet adhesion onto segmented polyurethane film surfaces modified by addition and crosslinking of PEO-containing block copolymers. *Biomaterials* **2000**, *21*, 683–691. [CrossRef]
46. Shin, E.K.; Park, H.; Noh, J.Y.; Lim, K.M.; Chung, J.H. Platelet shape changes and cytoskeleton dynamics as novel therapeutic targets for anti-thrombotic drugs. *Biomol. Ther.* **2017**, *25*, 223–230. [CrossRef]
47. Cho, J.; Kim, H.; Song, J.; Cheong, J.W.; Shin, J.W.; Yang, W.I.; Kim, H.O. Platelet storage induces accelerated desialylation of platelets and increases hepatic thrombopoietin production. *J. Transl. Med.* **2018**, *16*, 1–9. [CrossRef] [PubMed]
48. Apte, G.; Börke, J.; Rothe, H.; Liefeith, K.; Nguyen, T.H. Modulation of Platelet-Surface Activation: Current State and Future Perspectives. *ACS Appl. Bio. Mater.* **2020**, *3*, 5574–5589. [CrossRef] [PubMed]
49. Al Nakib, R.; Toncheva, A.; Fontaine, V.; Vanheuverzwijn, J.; Raquez, J.M.; Meyer, F. Design of Thermoplastic Polyurethanes with Conferred Antibacterial, Mechanical, and Cytotoxic Properties for Catheter Application. *ACS Appl. Bio. Mater.* **2022**, *5*, 5532–5544. [CrossRef]
50. Ensoylu, M.; Deliormanlı, A.M.; Atmaca, H. Preparation, Characterization, and Drug Delivery of Hexagonal Boron Nitride-Borate Bioactive Glass Biomimetic Scaffolds for Bone Tissue Engineering. *Biomimetics* **2023**, *8*, 10. [CrossRef]
51. Gautrot, J.E.; Trappmann, B.; Oceguera-Yanez, F.; Connelly, J.; He, X.; Watt, F.M.; Huck, W.T.S. Exploiting the superior protein resistance of polymer brushes to control single cell adhesion and polarisation at the micron scale. *Biomaterials* **2010**, *31*, 5030–5041. [CrossRef]
52. Robotti, F.; Bottan, S.; Fraschetti, F.; Mallone, A.; Pellegrini, G.; Lindenblatt, N.; Starck, C.; Falk, V.; Poulikakos, D.; Ferrari, A. A micron-scale surface topography design reducing cell adhesion to implanted materials. *Sci. Rep.* **2018**, *8*, 10887. [CrossRef]
53. Gorji Kandi, S.; Panahi, B.; Zoghi, N. Impact of surface texture from fine to coarse on perceptual and instrumental gloss. *Prog. Org. Coat.* **2022**, *171*, 107028. [CrossRef]
54. Rastogi, V.K.; Samyn, P. Bio-based coatings for paper applications. *Coatings* **2015**, *5*, 887–930. [CrossRef]
55. Crawford, R.J.; Webb, H.K.; Truong, V.K.; Hasan, J.; Ivanova, E.P. Surface topographical factors influencing bacterial attachment. *Adv. Colloid Interface Sci.* **2012**, *179–182*, 142–149. [CrossRef] [PubMed]
56. Wu, S.; Zhang, B.; Liu, Y.; Suo, X.; Li, H. Influence of surface topography on bacterial adhesion: A review (Review). *Biointerphases* **2018**, *13*, 60801. [CrossRef] [PubMed]
57. Silhavy, T.J.; Kahne, D.; Walker, S. The bacterial cell envelope. *Cold Spring Harb. Perspect. Biol.* **2010**, *2*, a000414. [CrossRef]
58. Zheng, S.; Bawazir, M.; Dhall, A.; Kim, H.E.; He, L.; Heo, J.; Hwang, G. Implication of Surface Properties, Bacterial Motility, and Hydrodynamic Conditions on Bacterial Surface Sensing and Their Initial Adhesion. *Front. Bioeng. Biotechnol.* **2021**, *9*, 643722. [CrossRef]
59. Xu, L.; Dara, Y.; Magar, S.; Badughaish, A.; Xiao, F. Morphological and rheological investigation of emulsified asphalt/polymer composite based on gray-level co-occurrence matrix. *Int. J. Transp. Sci. Technol.* **2023**, 1–18. [CrossRef]
60. Liang, Y.; Kou, W.; Lai, H.; Wang, J.; Wang, Q.; Xu, W.; Wang, H.; Lu, N. Improved estimation of aboveground biomass in rubber plantations by fusing spectral and textural information from UAV-based RGB imagery. *Ecol. Indic.* **2022**, *142*, 109286. [CrossRef]
61. Mansour, I.R.; Thomson, R.M. Haralick texture feature analysis for characterization of specific energy and absorbed dose distributions across cellular to patient length scales. *Phys. Med. Biol.* **2023**, *68*, 075006. [CrossRef]
62. Pathak, R.; Bierman, S.F.; D'arnaud, P. Inhibition of bacterial attachment and biofilm formation by a novel intravenous catheter material using an in vitro percutaneous catheter insertion model. *Med. Devices Evid. Res.* **2018**, *11*, 427–432. [CrossRef]
63. Schelin, J.; Wallin-Carlquist, N.; Cohn, M.T.; Lindqvist, R.; Barker, G.C.; Rådström, P. The formation of Staphylococcus aureus enterotoxin in food environments and advances in risk assessment. *Virulence* **2011**, *2*, 580–592. [CrossRef] [PubMed]
64. Uneputty, A.; Dávila-Lezama, A.; Garibo, D.; Oknianska, A.; Bogdanchikova, N.; Hernández-Sánchez, J.F.; Susarrey-Arce, A. Strategies applied to modify structured and smooth surfaces: A step closer to reduce bacterial adhesion and biofilm formation. *Colloids Interface Sci. Commun.* **2022**, *46*, 100560. [CrossRef]
65. Weber, M.; Steinle, H.; Golombek, S.; Hann, L.; Schlensak, C.; Wendel, H.P.; Avci-Adali, M. Blood-Contacting Biomaterials: In Vitro Evaluation of the Hemocompatibility. *Front. Bioeng. Biotechnol.* **2018**, *6*, 99. [CrossRef] [PubMed]
66. Khorasani, M.T.; MoemenBellah, S.; Mirzadeh, H.; Sadatnia, B. Effect of surface charge and hydrophobicity of polyurethanes and silicone rubbers on L929 cells response. *Colloids Surf. B Biointerfaces* **2006**, *51*, 112–119. [CrossRef]

Disclaimer/Publisher's Note: The statements, opinions and data contained in all publications are solely those of the individual author(s) and contributor(s) and not of MDPI and/or the editor(s). MDPI and/or the editor(s) disclaim responsibility for any injury to people or property resulting from any ideas, methods, instructions or products referred to in the content.

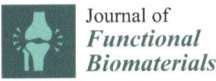

Article

Toxicological Evaluation toward Refined Montmorillonite with Human Colon Associated Cells and Human Skin Associated Cells

Zhou Wang [†], Yibei Jiang [†], Guangjian Tian, Chuyu Zhu * and Yi Zhang *

Department of Inorganic Materials, School of Minerals Processing and Bioengineering, Central South University, Changsha 410083, China; zhouwang@csu.edu.cn (Z.W.); 215611016@csu.edu.cn (Y.J.); 215613081@csu.edu.cn (G.T.)
* Correspondence: 220133@csu.edu.cn (C.Z.); yee_z10@csu.edu.cn (Y.Z.)
[†] These authors contributed equally to this work.

Abstract: Montmorillonite has been refined to overcome uncertainties originating from different sources, which offers opportunities for addressing various health issues, e.g., cosmetics, wound dressings, and antidiarrheal medicines. Herein, three commercial montmorillonite samples were obtained from different sources and labeled M1, M2, and M3 for Ca-montmorillonite, magnesium-enriched Ca-montmorillonite, and silicon-enriched Na-montmorillonite, respectively. Commercial montmorillonite was refined via ultrasonic scission-differential centrifugation and labeled S, M, or L according to the particle sizes (small, medium, or large, respectively). The size distribution decreased from 2000 nm to 250 nm with increasing centrifugation rates from 3000 rpm to 12,000 rpm. Toxicological evaluations with human colon-associated cells and human skin-associated cells indicated that side effects were correlated with excess dosages and silica sand. These side effects were more obvious with human colon-associated cells. The microscopic interactions between micro/nanosized montmorillonite and human colon-associated cells or human skin-associated cells indicated that those interactions were correlated with the size distributions. The interactions of the M1 series with the human cells were attributed to size effects because montmorillonite with a broad size distribution was stored in the M1 series. The M2 series interactions with human cells did not seem to be correlated with size effects because large montmorillonite particles were retained after refining. The M3 series interactions with human cells were attributed to size effects because small montmorillonite particles were retained after refining. This illustrates that toxicological evaluations with refined montmorillonite must be performed in accordance with clinical medical practices.

Keywords: refine; montmorillonite; toxicological evaluation; microscopic interaction; clinical medical orientation

1. Introduction

Montmorillonite (MMT) is obtained from natural bentonite and used in various fields because of its natural abundance, cost-effectiveness, and nontoxic nature [1–3]. MMT has the chemical formula $(Na, Ca)_{0.33}(Al, Mg, Fe)_2[(Si, Al)_4O_{10}](OH)_2 \cdot 4H_2O$, containing one Al-octahedral sheet and two Si-tetrahedral sheets. These elements, such as Si, Al, Fe, Ti, and Mn, could cause side effects in clinical medical studies, which might be due to silicon-containing minerals, iron-containing minerals, and titanium-containing minerals [4]. Several treatments and chemical methods have been used to refine MMT in laboratories and industry, such as sieving, sonication, sedimentation or centrifugation, and even long-term sedimentation combined with sonication and/or centrifugation [5,6]. In addition, selective dissolution under acidic or alkaline conditions was used to remove soluble salts, carbonates, organics, and toxic elements.

Refined MMT has been studied for various common health applications, such as cosmetics [7,8], wound dressings [9–13], and anti-diarrhea medicines [14], owing to the uniform bidimensional particle shapes, high length-to-height ratios, inherent stiffness, dual charge distribution, chemical inertness, biocompatibility, and active sites on the surface [15–18]. The results of these studies have attracted the interest of scientists and biotechnologists since micro/nanosized materials might also exhibit the same micro/nano biological interactions because one functional dimension is outside the nanoscale range of 1 nm to 100 nm, whereas organ-modified micro/nanosized materials might have uncertain effects on micro/nanobiological interactions [19–22]. The material parameters included size, shape, surface chemical characteristics, and surface topological structure, whereas the biological information included signaling molecule transmission, cell internalization, tissue distribution, and organ filtration [23–26]. Therefore, the refinement of MMT with a controllable length–radius and toxicological evaluation of refined MMT must be carried out in accordance with clinical methods, which will enable standardized evaluation in micro/nanobiological studies. Overall, the factors influencing MMT material information and cell biological information, such as the toxicological effects on human-derived cell lines and MMT–cell interactions, should be considered.

As shown in this manuscript, MMT refining for medical use required evaluation of trace impurities and size distribution, which were neglected in traditional MMT refining, i.e., the MMT content was the main criterion. Toxicological evaluations of refined MMT with human colon-associated cells and human skin-associated cells have been performed because oral administration and external use of MMT are the main medical utilization directions. Three commercial MMTs were described according to their sources, i.e., Ca-MMT (M1), magnesium-enriched Ca-MMT (M2), and silicon-enriched Na-MMT (M3). Commercial MMTs were refined through ultrasonic scission-differential centrifugation and divided into three categories. The material characteristics of the commercial MMT and the refined MMT were measured via X-ray fluorescence (XRF), X-ray diffraction (XRD), Fourier transform infrared (FTIR), differential scanning calorimetry (DSC-TG), scanning electron microscopy (SEM), and DSL. In addition, micro/nano MMT–human cell line interactions were investigated.

2. Materials and Methods

2.1. Materials

MMTs were obtained from Sand Technology Co., Ltd. (Ezhou, China) and labeled M1, M2, and M3 for Ca-MMT, magnesium-enriched Ca-MMT, and silicon-enriched Na-MMT. Human umbilical vein endothelial cells (HUVECs), human intestinal epithelial cells (HIEC6), and human colonic epithelial cells (NCM460) were obtained from the American Type Culture Collection (ATCC) (Manassas, VA, USA). Human immortalized keratinocytes (HaCaT) were obtained from Changsha Abiowell Biotechnology Co., Ltd. (Changsha, China). A Cell Counting Kit-8 (CCK-8) was obtained from Beijing Lablead Biotech Co., Ltd. (Beijing, China).

2.2. Processed MMT with Ultrasonic Scission-Differential Centrifugation

The MMT was refined through ultrasonic fission-differential centrifugation. In brief, 2.5 g of MMT was mixed with 50 mL of water to form an MMT suspension and sonicated at 750 W for 10 min. Subsequently, the sonicated MMT suspension was centrifuged at 3000, 6000, and 12,000 rpm to collect the sediment. The centrifuged supernatant was reserved for subsequent centrifugation. The Ca-MMT, magnesium-enriched Ca-MMT, and silicon-enriched Na-MMT were labeled M1, M2, and M3, respectively. Sonicated M1, M2, and M3 were centrifuged at 3000 rpm for 10 min to collect M(1,2,3)-L with large particles. Subsequently, the supernatant was recentrifuged at 6000 rpm for 10 min to collect the medium M(1,2,3)-M particles. The supernatant was recentrifuged at 12,000 rpm for 10 min to collect small M(1,2,3)-S particles. All sediments were cleaned with deionized water 1–3 times and then dried overnight at 60 °C.

2.3. Characterization

Scanning electron microscopy (SEM) images were recorded using an MIRA3 LMU scanning electron microscope from Tescan (Brno, Czech Republic). The vacuum pressure was 5×10^{-3} Pa, and the accelerating voltage was 20 kV. All samples were suspended in deionized water at a concentration of 1 mg/mL, and then the solutions were dripped onto silicon slices and freeze-dried for 2 h. The X-ray diffraction (XRD) data were recorded using a TD-3500 instrument from Dandong Tongda Science & Technology Co., Ltd. (Dandong, China). The wavelength of the copper anode was $\lambda(K\alpha) = 0.15406$ nm. Fourier transform infrared (FTIR) spectra were recorded using a TENSOR II instrument from Bruker (Berlin, Germany). The spectra were scanned over the range of 400 to 4000 cm^{-1}. X-ray fluorescence (XRF) data were recorded using an Axios mAX wavelength dispersive XRF spectrometer from PANalytical B.V. (Almelo, The Netherlands).

2.4. Toxicological Evaluation and Interaction Observation

Cell culture. Human skin-associated cell lines were incubated at 37 °C with 5% CO_2 in DMEM containing 10% FBS and 1% Pen/Strep, i.e., the HUVEC line and HaCaT cell line. Human colon-associated cells were incubated at 37 °C with 5% CO_2 in RPMI 1640 medium supplemented with 10% FBS and 1% Pen/Strep, i.e., the HIEC6 cell line and the NCM460 cell line. Single cells were isolated from 0.25% trypsin-EDTA solutions and cultured in the medium.

Toxicological evaluation. The cell lines were incubated for 12–24 h in 96-well cell culture plates (2×10^3 cells/well) with different culture media and then incubated for 24 h in fresh culture media supplemented with MMT solutions at concentrations ranging from 0 to 300 µg/mL. CCK-8 was used to evaluate the cell survival rate by detecting formazan (450 nm) produced by the reduction of dehydrogenase in living cells. Cell viability was calculated as follows:

$$\text{Cell viability} = (\text{OD}_{experiment})/(\text{OD}_{Control}) \times 100\%$$

Interaction observations. The cell lines were incubated for 12–24 h in 12-well cell culture plates (1×10^4 cells/well) with different culture media and then incubated for 24 h in a fresh culture medium containing 200 µg/mL MMT solution. The treated cell lines were fixed for 24 h in 2.5% glutaraldehyde and then dehydrated in a graded ethanol series for SEM observation.

2.5. Statistical Analyses

The mean and standard deviation (S.D.) were calculated from the original data. All studies were conducted with three independent biological replicates. Statistical analyses were conducted with ANOVA and subsequent Student's t tests. p-values less than 0.05, 0.005, and 0.0005 were considered significant at the *, **, and *** levels, respectively.

3. Results and Discussion

3.1. Material Characterization and Toxicological Evaluation of MMT

The XRF results for the MMTs from different sources are shown in Table 1. Ca-MMT and Na-MMT had different Ca and Na contents. The chemical contents in M1 decreased in the order Si, Al, Mg, Ca, Fe, F, Na, K, Ti, etc. The high Si content in M1 was attributed to silicon-containing minerals. The chemical element contents in M2 decreased in the order Si, Mg, Al, Fe, Ca, Na, F, K, Cl, Ti, etc. The high Mg content and Si content in M2 were attributed to magnesium-containing minerals and silicon-containing minerals. The element contents in M3 decreased in the order Si, Al, Mg, Fe, Na, Ca, Ti, F, K, S, etc. The high Si content and Fe content in M3 were attributed to silicon-containing minerals and iron-containing minerals. Metal ions such as Ca, Fe, and Zn are essential trace elements associated with human health. Ca intake, according to the WHO recommendation, should be 1000–1200 mg/d; the blood Ca concentration in adults is approximately 2.25–2.75 mmol/L; the total Ca content in adults is 850–1200 kg; and excess calcium intake or overload of Ca stores could induce diseases due to broken ion homeostasis. According to the WHO recommendations, the Fe intake should be 8–10 mg/d, the blood Fe concentration in adults is approximately 1.1–1.6 mol/L, the total Fe content in adults is 4–5 g, and excess Fe intake or overload of iron stores could induce diseases due to reactive •OH radicals. The Zn intake, according to the WHO recommendation, should be 8–11 mg/d; the blood Zn concentration in adults is approximately 11–18 μmol/L; the total Zn content in adults is 2–3 g; and excess Zn intake or overload of Zn stores could induce diseases due to disrupted ion homeostasis and impaired immune function. In addition, metal ions with different hemostatic mechanisms are used in wound healing; for example, Ca accelerates thrombosis by facilitating the conversion of prothrombin to thrombin, Fe stabilizes thrombin and plays a role in accelerating blood coagulation, and Zn is involved in all stages of wound healing.

Table 1. Characterization evaluation of MMT via XRF.

Sample	Oxide Contents by Analysis, wt %												
	SiO_2	Al_2O_3	MgO	Na_2O	Fe_2O_3	CaO	TiO_2	MnO	K_2O	ZrO_2	SO_3	Cl	F
M1-RAW	65.554	20.309	7.400	0.568	2.001	2.575	0.156	0.071	0.286	0.014	0.034	0.027	0.955
M2-RAW	55.685	14.886	23.884	0.630	1.787	1.609	0.134	0.031	0.290	0.012	0.092	0.302	0.613
M3-RAW	61.369	20.793	4.860	3.757	3.940	2.493	1.410	0.010	0.228	0.025	0.371	0.059	0.535

The XRD patterns of the MMT samples from different sources are shown in Figure 1A. According to the M1 XRD results in Supplementary Materials Table S1, reflections were observed at 19.79°, 35.17°, 53.98°, and 61.88°, which were consistent with the Ca-MMT standard card (JCPDS Card No. 00-058-2007). The strongest reflection was located in the 4–8° range, which was ascribed to the 001 plane in MMT, and the basal spacing, d_{001}, was calculated as approximately 1.48 nm. These reflections were observed at 21.86°, 22.75°, 27.97°, and 73.02°, which were consistent with the standard card for cristobalite (JCPDS Card No. 00-039-1425), the standard card for quartz (JCPDS Card No. 01-070-2537), the standard card for albite (JCPDS Card No. 00-010-0393), and the standard card for illite (JCPDS Card No. 00-029-1496). According to the M2 XRD results in Table S2, reflections were observed at 19.79°, 35.08°, 53.95°, and 62.09°, which were consistent with the Ca-MMT standard card (JCPDS Card No. 00-058-2007). The strongest reflection was located in the 4–8° range, which was ascribed to the 001 plane in MMT, and the basal spacing, d_{001}, was approximately 1.49 nm. These reflections were observed at 18.61°, 38.00°, 50.82°, 58.66°, and 68.35°, which were consistent with the standard card for brucite (JCPDS Card No. 00-007-0239). These reflections were observed at 21.97°, 26.68°, 29.51°, and 73.02°, which were consistent with the standard card for cristobalite (JCPDS Card No. 00-039-1425), the standard card for quartz (JCPDS Card No. 00-033-1161), the standard card for calcite (JCPDS Card No. 00-047-1743), and the standard card for illite (JCPDS Card No. 00-029-1496). According to the M3 XRD results in Table S3, reflections were observed at 19.86°, 34.85°, 54.08°, and 62.01°, which were consistent with the Na-MMT standard card (JCPDS Card No. 00-029-1498). The strongest reflection was located in the 4–8° range, which was ascribed to the 001 plane in MMT, and the basal spacing, d_{001}, was approximately 1.37 nm. These reflections were observed at 26.74°, 28.07°, and 73.04°, which were consistent with the quartz standard card (JCPDS Card No. 01-070-2537), albite standard card (JCPDS Card No. 00-010-0393), and illite standard card (JCPDS Card No. 00-029-1496), respectively. Therefore, these XRD patterns indicated that MMT was the dominant mineral. The impurities include brucite, quartz, cristobalite, calcite, albite, illite, etc., which can cause side effects in humans. For example, quartz enhances the production of reactive oxygen species and results in oxidative damage [27–29].

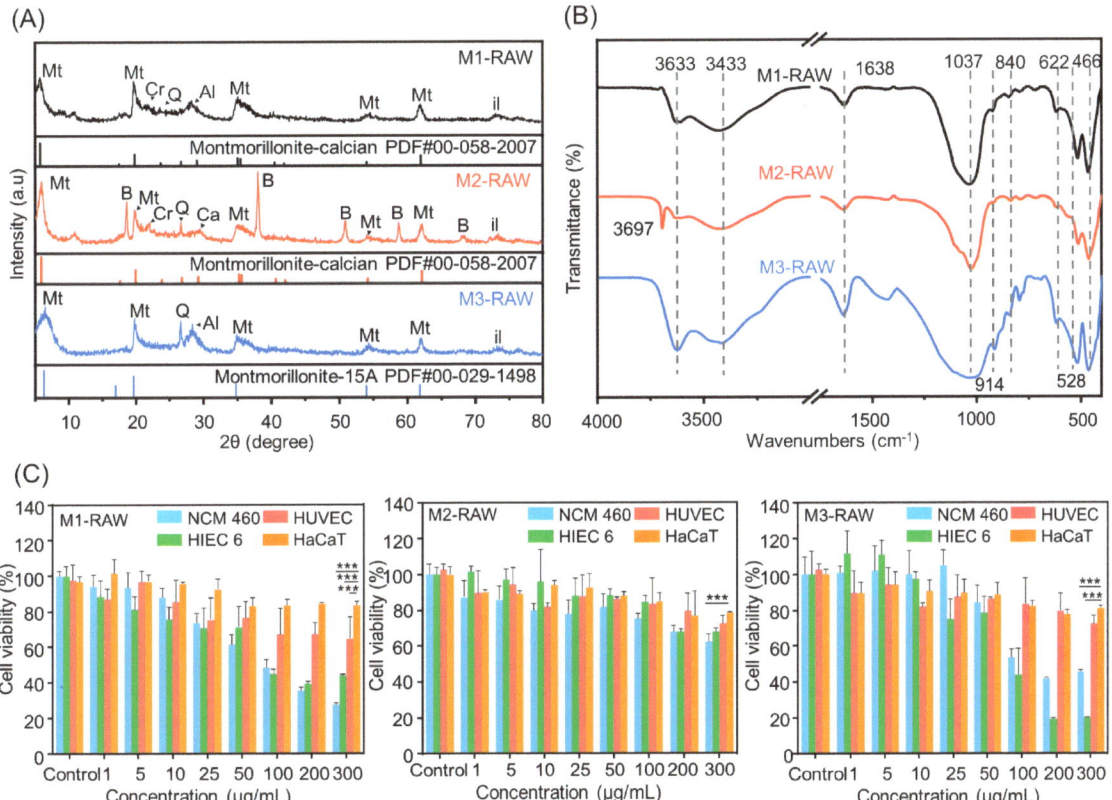

Figure 1. Characterization and toxicological evaluation of MMT via (**A**) XRD, (**B**) FTIR, and (**C**) CCK-8. M1-RAW: unrefined Ca-MMT; M2-RAW: unrefined magnesium-enriched Ca-MMT; M3-RAW: unrefined silicon-enriched Na-MMT. The P value was determined by ANOVA and Student's t tests. *** $p < 0.0005$.

The FTIR spectra of MMT from different sources are shown in Figure 1B. The structural O–H stretching vibration of alumina was located at approximately 3633 cm^{-1}, the O–H stretching vibration of water was located at approximately 3433 cm^{-1}, the O–H deformation vibration of water was located at approximately 1638 cm^{-1}, and the O–H deformation vibration at approximately 1638 cm^{-1} was correlated with the water content in MMT, indicating a high water content in M3. For the Si–O bonds in MMT, the Si–O–Si stretching vibration was located at approximately 1037 cm^{-1}, the Si–O–Si stretching vibration was located at approximately 622 cm^{-1}, the Si–O–Al deformation vibration was located at approximately 523 cm^{-1}, and the Si–O–Si deformation vibration was located at approximately 466 cm^{-1}. For the Al–O bonds in MMT, the Al–Al–OH deformation vibration band was located at approximately 914 cm^{-1}, the Al–Fe–OH deformation vibration band was located at approximately 840 cm^{-1}, and the strength of the Al–Fe–OH deformation vibration band was correlated with the Fe content in MMT, indicating a high Fe content in M3. In addition, the Si–O stretching vibration was located at approximately 840 cm^{-1} and attributed to silica sand, and the Mg–OH stretching vibration was located at approximately 3697 cm^{-1} and attributed to brucite, which was observed in M2. Therefore, the FTIR data indicated that MMT contained Si–OH and Al–OH, and Si–OH or Al–OH at the structural or basal sites would cause constant charges, while surface -OH at edge sites would cause variable charges. Additionally, the net negative charge could facilitate MMT interactions with cationic molecules, and contact with opposite charges could facilitate MMT–cell interactions.

Toxicological evaluations of MMT from different sources with human colon-associated cells and human skin-associated cells are shown in Figure 1C. For M1, the cell survival rate of the HaCaT cell line was above 80% until the maximum amount was added; the cell survival rate of the HUVEC line was close to 80% with 50 µg/mL M1 treatment and decreased at a constant rate until the maximum addition, whereas the survival rates of the NCM460 cell line and HIEC-6 cell line were close to 80% after 25 µg/mL M1 treatment and decreased rapidly until the maximum addition. For M2, the survival rates of HaCaT cells and HUVECs were greater than 80% until maximum addition, and the survival rates of NCM460 cells and HIEC-6 cells were greater than 80% before treatment with 200 µg/mL M2. For M3, the survival rates of HaCaT cells and HUVECs were greater than 80% until the maximum addition, whereas the survival rates of the NCM460 cells and HIEC-6 cells were approximately 80% after treatment with 50 µg/mL M3, followed by a sudden decrease after treatment with 100 µg/mL M3. These results indicated that the side effects seem to correlate with excess dosages and the amounts of silica sand, and they were much more obvious in human colon-associated cells than in human skin-associated cells. In addition, MMT and brucite were harmless to human colon-associated cells and human skin-associated cells. Therefore, MMT refining must be carried out in accordance with clinical practices, which would overcome the uncertainties originating from different sources.

3.2. Material Characterization of Refined MMT

SEM images of MMTs from different sources are shown in Figures 2A, S1 and S2. The MMT aggregates with multilateral rhombus shapes formed inhomogeneous MMT sheets. Refined MMTs with homogeneous shapes and controllable sizes were obtained through ultrasonic fission-differential centrifugation, and the large MMT sheets were still aggregated and had thick laminated structures. Medium-sized MMT sheets were scattered and had a thin laminated structure. Small MMT sheets were exfoliated and had an ultrathin laminated structure. In addition, the average thickness of the MMT sheets decreased with an increasing centrifugation rate from 3000 rpm to 12,000 rpm.

The size distributions of the refined MMT prepared with centrifugation rates ranging from 3000 rpm to 12,000 rpm are shown in Figure 2B. For the M1 series, the centric size distribution ranged from 0.1 to 5.0 µm, and the average size was close to 1300 nm. The average size of refined M1 decreased from 500 nm to 250 nm with an increasing centrifugation rate. In addition, the centric size distributions of the widths and heights seemed almost the same in the M1 series. For the M2 series, the centric size distribution ranged from 1.0 to 5.0 µm, and the average size was close to 2000 nm. The average size of refined M2 decreased from 2300 nm to 1100 nm with an increasing centrifugation rate. In addition, the centric size distribution narrowed with decreasing average size. For the M3 series, the tricentric size distribution for M3 ranged from 0.2 nm to 9.0 µm, the tricentric size distribution for M3-L ranged from 0.1 nm to 7.0 µm, the centric size distribution for refined M3-M ranged from 0.1 nm to 5.0 µm with an average size close to 350 nm, and the centric size distribution for refined M3-S ranged from 0.1 nm to 1.0 µm with an average size close to 250 nm. In addition, the centric size distributions narrowed with decreasing average sizes. These results indicated that the size distributions decreased with increasing centrifugation rates from 3000 rpm to 12,000 rpm, and MMT was refined to give different size distributions through ultrasonic fission-differential centrifugation.

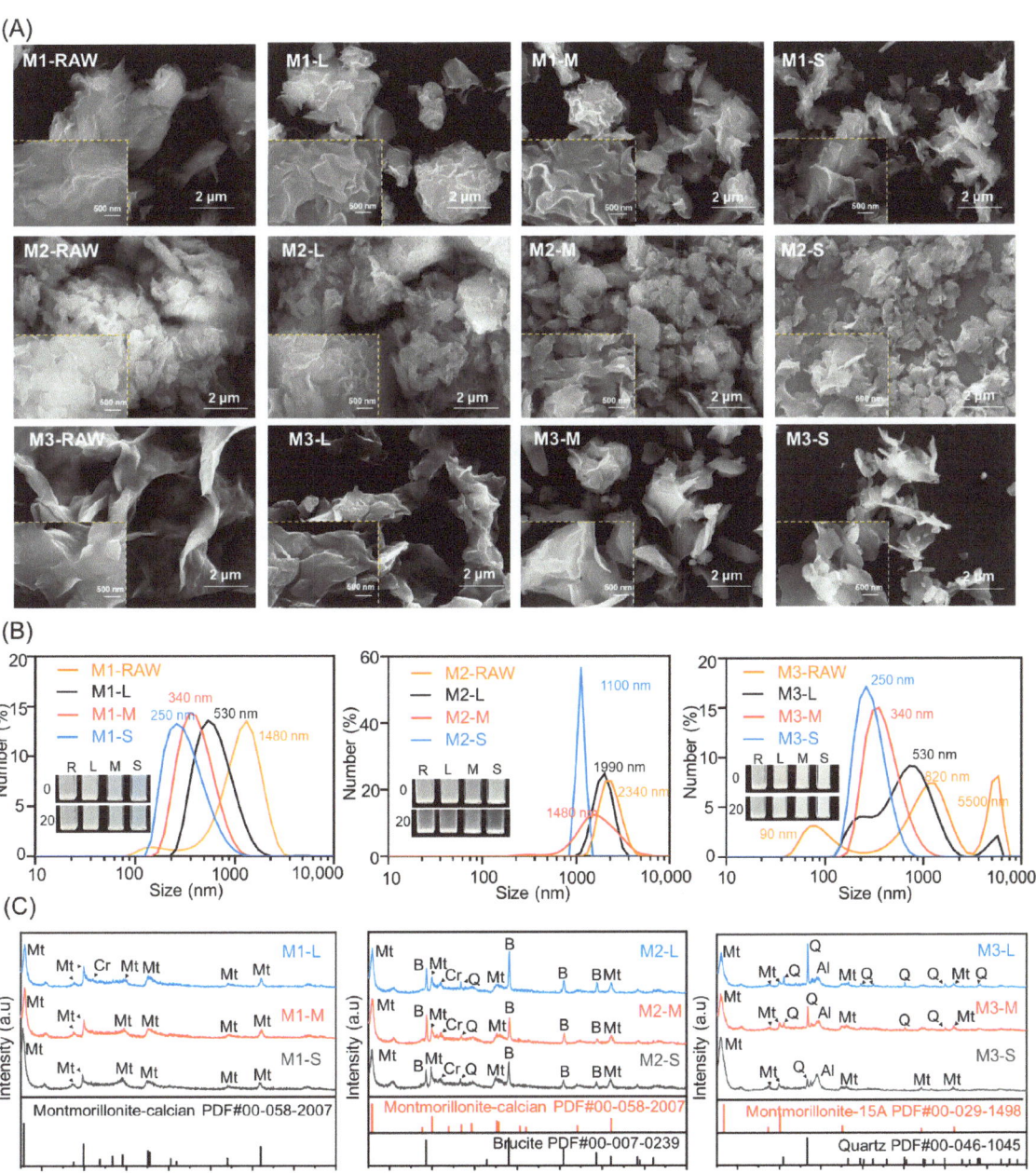

Figure 2. Characterization of refined MMT via (**A**) SEM, (**B**) DSL, and (**C**) XRD. The refined MMTs with small, medium, and large particle sizes were labeled S, M, and L, respectively.

The XRD patterns of the refined MMT are shown in Figure 2C. For the M1 series, reflections for Ca-MMT, cristobalite, and albite were observed in the XRD patterns. The (003) reflection of Ca-MMT was visible in the M1 series, which was attributed to its content and instrumental characteristics. The (101) reflection of cristobalite was almost indiscernible with a decreasing size distribution, which was attributed to its content. The (002) reflection for albite broadened with decreasing size distribution, which was attributed to structural defects. The (117) reflection of illite was almost indiscernible in the M1 series, which was attributed to the content and instrumental characteristics. For the M2 series, reflections for Ca-MMT, brucite, cristobalite, quartz, and calcite were observed in the XRD patterns. The (100) peak for the Ca-MMT increased with decreasing size distribution, which was attributed to the presence of an intact structure. The (101) reflection of cristobalite broadened with decreasing size distribution, which was attributed to structural defects. The intensities of these brucite reflections increased with decreasing size distribution, which was attributed to the brucite content and particle sizes. The (117) reflection of illite was almost indiscernible in the M2 series, which was attributed to its content and instrumental characteristics. For the M3 series, the reflections of Na-MMT, quartz, and albite were observed in the XRD patterns. The (001) peak for Na-MMT increased with decreasing size distribution, which was attributed to an intact structure. The intensities of the reflections for the quartz grains increased with decreasing size distribution, which was attributed to the quartz content and particle sizes. The (002) reflection for albite increased with decreasing size distribution, which was attributed to the intact structure. The (117) reflection of illite was almost indiscernible in the M1 series, which was attributed to the content and instrumental characteristics. Therefore, the XRD results indicated that some impurities were difficult to remove from the refined MMT, and these impurities did not seem to correlate with the size distribution. In addition, selective dissolution under acidic or alkaline conditions was used to remove soluble salts, carbonates, organics, and toxic elements.

3.3. Toxicological Evaluation of the Refined MMT

Toxicological evaluations of refined MMT with human colon-associated cells and human skin-associated cells are shown in Figure 3. For human colon-associated cells, the cell survival rate with the refined M1 series was close to 80% with 50 µg/mL refined M1 and then decreased at a flat rate until maximum addition. The cell survival rate with the refined M2 series was close to 80% with the 100 µg/mL treatment, and the cell survival rate for the refined M2-S was above 80% until maximum addition. The cell survival rate for the refined M3 series was close to 80% with the 50 µg/mL treatment and then decreased rapidly until the maximum addition. For human skin-associated cells, the cell survival rate with the refined M1 series was greater than 80% until maximum addition, the cell survival rate with the refined M2 series was greater than 80% until maximum addition, and the cell survival rate with the refined M3 series was greater than 80% until maximum addition, but we excluded the HUVEC line with the 200 µg/mL M3 series treatment. These results indicated that the impurities were correlated with excess dosages and the amount of silica sand, and they were much more obvious in the human colon-associated cells than the human skin-associated cells. In addition, MMT and brucite are harmless to human colon-associated cells and human skin-associated cells.

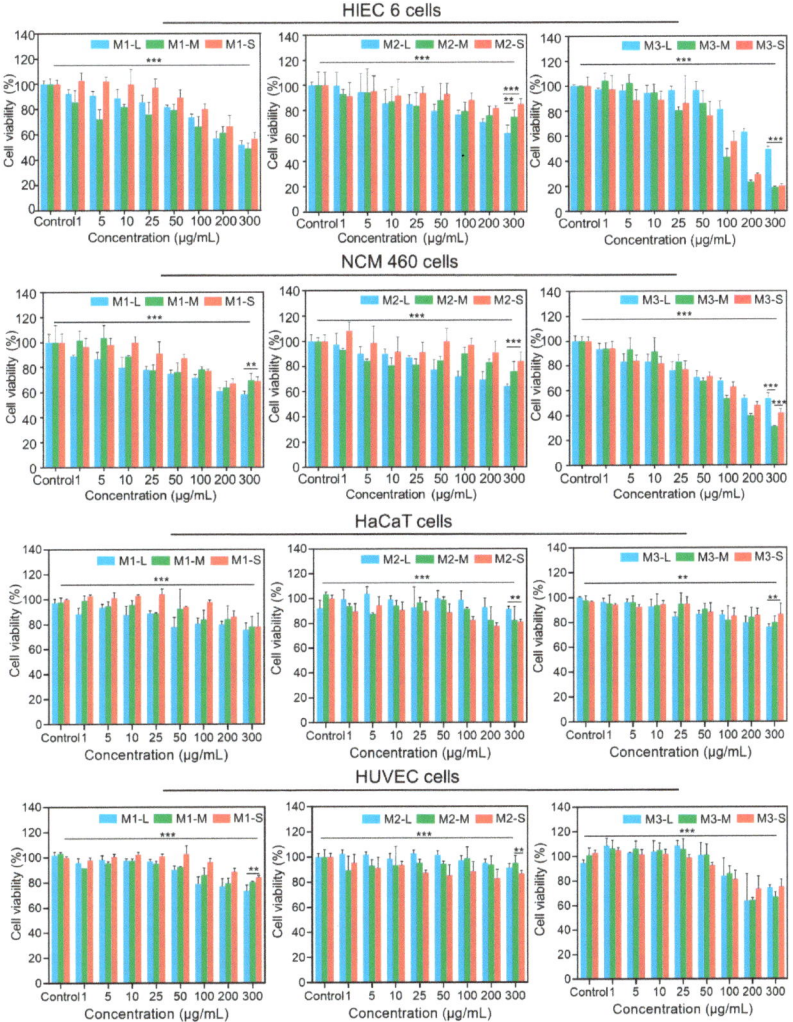

Figure 3. Toxicological effects of refined MMT on human colon-associated cells (HIEC 6 and NCM460) and human skin-associated cells (HaCaT and HUVECs). The p value was determined by ANOVA and Student's t tests. ** $p < 0.005$, *** $p < 0.0005$.

3.4. MMT–Human Cell Interactions

SEM images of MMT–human cell interactions are shown in Figure 4. In the literature, the cellular morphologies in SEM images were described as round and slender. The cell surface exhibited a negative electrostatic charge attributed to the presence of glycoproteins on the membrane. Upon stimulation, the cell surface underwent a transition from smooth to rough and experienced a reduction in mucus secretion [30,31]. The microscopic interactions between micro/nanosized MMT and human colon-associated cells or human skin-associated cells indicated that these side effects were correlated with the size distribution. Notably, MMT-RAW was internalized with an undispersed agglomerated morphology, which caused an increase in the MMT particle sizes. This interaction may have caused the aggregation of MMT-RAW into larger particles, resulting in increased cytotoxicity. The human cells interacted with M1 more than with M1-S, which was attributed to the broader size distribution and smaller sizes. In addition, mucus secretion resulting from mechanical stimuli was observed in the M1 series–human skin-associated cell interactions. For M2 and M2-S, human colon-associated cells seemed to have no response to the M2 series, which was attributed to large particle sizes, whereas human skin-associated cells interacted with the M2 series due to mechanical stimulus-induced mucus secretion. In addition, microscopic interactions with M2 featuring a small size distribution were more obvious and more uniform with human skin-associated cells. For M3 and M3-S, the human cells interacted with M3 more than with M3-S, which was attributed to more small MMT particles stored in M3. Therefore, the M1 series–human cell interactions were attributed to size effects because MMTs with broader size distributions were stored in the M1 series, and the M2 series–human cell interactions did not seem to correlate with size effects because large MMTs were stored in the M2 series. The M3 series–human cell interactions were attributed to size effects because small MMTs were stored in the M3 series.

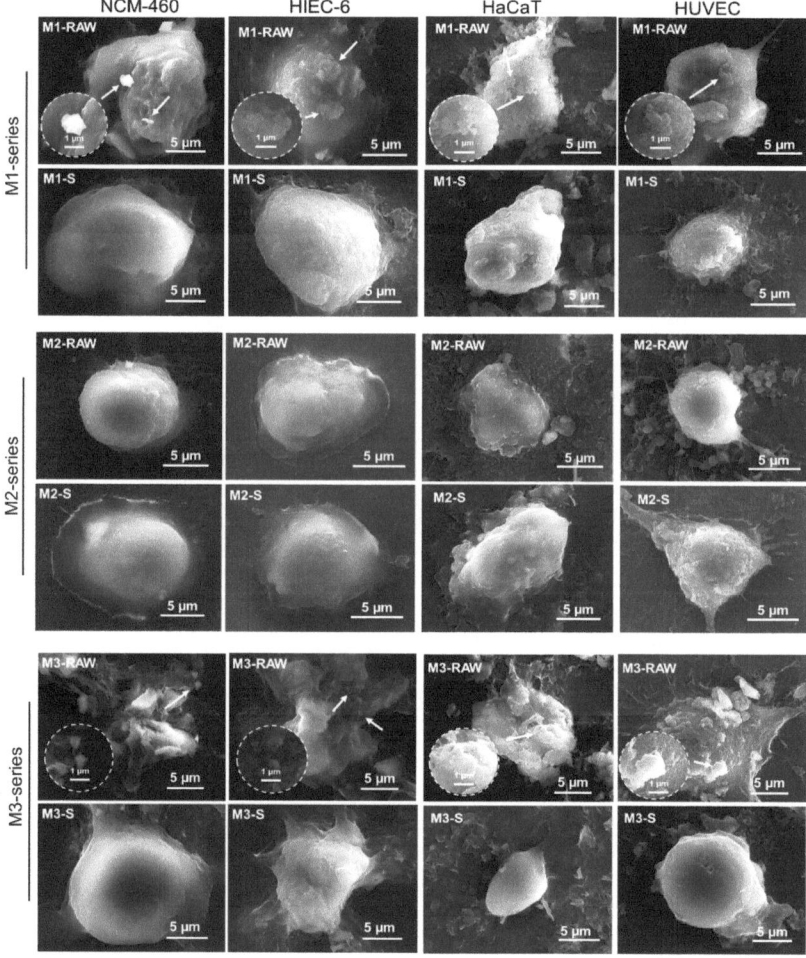

Figure 4. SEM images of MMT–human cell interactions. Unrefined Ca-MMT was labeled M1-RAW, and refined M1-RAW with small particle sizes was labeled M1-S. Unrefined magnesium-enriched Ca-MMT was labeled M2-RAW, and refined M2-RAW with small particle sizes was labeled M2-S. Unrefined silicon-enriched Na-MMT was labeled M3-RAW, and refined M3-RAW with small particle sizes was labeled M3-S. The thumbnail showed an enlarged image featuring a white arrow indicating the presence of MMT.

4. Conclusions

Refinement of MMT has been used to overcome uncertainties originating from different sources and offers opportunities for addressing various common health issues. Refined MMT with different particle size distributions was obtained through ultrasonic scission-differential centrifugation, and some harmful chemical elements were difficult to remove from the refined MMT. The characterization data indicated that the size distribution decreased with increasing centrifugation rate, while the structural morphology changed from aggregates with a thick laminated structure to an exfoliated ultrathin laminated structure. Toxicological evaluations with human colon-associated cells and human skin-associated cells indicated that the cell survival rates with MMT were not correlated with the size distribution, whereas side effects were correlated with excess dosages and silica sand. Instead, the microscopic interactions between micro/nanosized MMT and human colon-associated cells or human skin-associated cells indicated that those interactions were correlated with the size distributions. Therefore, refinement of MMT must be carried out in accordance with clinical medical practices, i.e., those for cosmetics, wound dressings, and anti-diarrhea medicines, to overcome the uncertainties originating from different sources.

Supplementary Materials: The following supporting information can be downloaded at https://www.mdpi.com/article/10.3390/jfb15030075/s1, Figure S1: SEM images of refined MMT at 50 k× and 100 k× magnification. Figure S2: SEM images of refined MMT at magnifications of 2 k× and 20 k×. Table S1: XRD data for M1. Table S2: XRD data for M2. Table S3: XRD data for M3.

Author Contributions: Z.W.: data curation, formal analysis, investigation, and writing—original draft; Y.J.: data curation, formal analysis, and investigation; G.T.: data curation and investigation; C.Z.: conceptualization, supervision, and writing—review and editing; Y.Z.: conceptualization, supervision, and writing—review and editing. All authors have read and agreed to the published version of the manuscript.

Funding: This work was supported by the National Natural Science Foundation of China (52374289) and the Central South University Innovation-Driven Research Programme (2023CXQD041). The Graduate Independent Exploration and Innovation Project of Central South University (2024ZZTS0409).

Data Availability Statement: The original contributions presented in the study are included in the article/supplementary material, further inquiries can be directed to the corresponding authors.

Conflicts of Interest: The authors declare no conflicts of interest.

References

1. Murugesan, S.; Scheibel, T. Copolymer/clay nanocomposites for biomedical applications. *Adv. Funct. Mater.* **2020**, *30*, 1908101. [CrossRef]
2. Liu, J.; Cai, W.; Khatoon, N.; Yu, W.; Zhou, C. On how montmorillonite as an ingredient in animal feed functions. *Appl. Clay Sci.* **2021**, *202*, 105963. [CrossRef]
3. Khachani, M.; Stealey, S.; Dharmesh, E.; Kader, M.; Buckner, S.; Jelliss, P.; Zustiak, S. Silicate clay-hydrogel nanoscale composites for sustained delivery of small molecules. *ACS Appl. Nano Mater.* **2022**, *5*, 18940–18954. [CrossRef]
4. Zhang, J.; Pan, Y.; Dong, S.; Yang, M.; Huang, Z.; Yan, C.; Gao, Y. Montmorillonite/agarose three-dimensional network gel sponge for wound healing with hemostatic and durable antibacterial properties. *ACS Appl. Nano Mater.* **2023**, *6*, 17263–17275. [CrossRef]
5. Rong, R.; Xu, X.; Zhu, S.; Li, B.; Wang, X.; Tang, K. Facile preparation of homogeneous and length controllable halloysite nanotubes by ultrasonic scission and uniform viscosity centrifugation. *Chem. Eng. J.* **2016**, *291*, 20–29. [CrossRef]
6. Qiao, Z.; Liu, Z.; Zhang, S.; Yang, Y.; Wu, Y.; Liu, L.; Liu, Q. Purification of montmorillonite and the influence of the purification method on textural properties. *Appl. Clay Sci.* **2020**, *187*, 105491. [CrossRef]
7. Wang, M.; Phillips, T. Inclusion of montmorillonite clays in environmental barrier formulations to reduce skin exposure to water-soluble chemicals from polluted water. *ACS Appl. Mater. Interfaces* **2022**, *14*, 23232–23244. [CrossRef]
8. Wang, M.; Phillips, T. Lecithin-amended montmorillonite clays enhance the antibacterial effect of barrier creams. *Colloid Surf. B—Biointerfaces* **2023**, *229*, 113450. [CrossRef]
9. Li, G.; Quan, K.; Liang, Y.; Li, T.; Yuan, Q.; Tao, L.; Xie, Q.; Wang, X. Graphene-montmorillonite composite sponge for safe and effective hemostasis. *ACS Appl. Mater. Interfaces* **2016**, *8*, 35071–35080. [CrossRef]
10. Ma, P.; Wang, Z.; Jiang, Y.; Huang, Z.; Xia, L.; Jiang, J.; Yuan, F.; Xia, H.; Zhang, Y. Clay-based nanocomposite hydrogels with microstructures and sustained ozone release for antibacterial activity. *Colloid Surf. A—Physicochem. Eng. Asp.* **2022**, *641*, 128497. [CrossRef]

11. Gil-Korilis, A.; Cojocaru, M.; Berzosa, M.; Gamazo, C.; Andrade, N.; Ciuffi, K. Comparison of antibacterial activity and cytotoxicity of silver nanoparticles and silver-loaded montmorillonite and saponite. *Appl. Clay Sci.* **2023**, *240*, 106968. [CrossRef]
12. Liang, H.; Wang, H.; Sun, X.; Xu, W.; Meng, N.; Zhou, N. Development of ZnO/Ag nanoparticles supported polydopamine-modified montmorillonite nanocomposites with synergistic antibacterial performance. *Appl. Clay Sci.* **2023**, *244*, 107112. [CrossRef]
13. Qin, X.; Wu, Z.; Fang, J.; Li, S.; Tang, S.; Wang, X. MXene-intercalated montmorillonite nanocomposites for long-acting antibacterial. *Appl. Clay Sci.* **2023**, *616*, 156521. [CrossRef]
14. Zhao, H.; Ye, H.; Zhou, J.; Tang, G.; Hou, Z.; Bai, H. Montmorillonite-enveloped zeolitic imidazolate framework as a nourishing oral nano-platform for gastrointestinal drug delivery. *ACS Appl. Mater. Interfaces.* **2020**, *12*, 49431–49441. [CrossRef]
15. Dening, T.; Thomas, N.; Rao, S.; Looveren, C.; Cuyckens, F.; Holm, R.; Prestidge, C. Montmorillonite and laponite clay materials for the solidification of lipid-based formulations for the basic drug blonanserin: In Vitro and in vivo investigations. *Mol. Pharm.* **2018**, *15*, 4148–4160. [CrossRef]
16. Rebitski, E.; Aranda, P.; Darder, M.; Carraro, R.; Ruiz-Hitzky, E. Intercalation of metformin into montmorillonite. *Dalton Trans.* **2018**, *9*, 3185–3192. [CrossRef]
17. Cui, Z.; Kim, S.; Baljon, J.; Wu, B.; Aghaloo, T.; Lee, M. Microporous methacrylated glycol chitosan-montmorillonite nanocomposite hydrogel for bone tissue engineering. *Nat. Commun.* **2019**, *10*, 3523. [CrossRef]
18. Zuo, Z.; Zhang, X.; Li, S.; Zhang, Y.; Liang, J.; Li, C.; Zheng, S.; Sun, Z. Synergistic promotion system of montmorillonite with Cu^{2+} and benzalkonium chloride for efficient and broad-spectrum antibacterial activity. *ACS Appl. Bio Mater.* **2023**, *6*, 4961–4971. [CrossRef]
19. Malvar, J.; Martín, J.; Orta, M.; Medina-Carrasco, S.; Santos, J.; Aparicio, I.; Alonso, E. Simultaneous and individual adsorption of ibuprofen metabolites by a modified montmorillonite. *Appl. Clay Sci.* **2020**, *189*, 105529. [CrossRef]
20. Yan, H.; Zhang, P.; Chen, X.; Bao, C.; Zhao, R.; Hu, J.; Liu, C.; Lin, Q. Preparation and characterization of octyl phenyl polyoxyethylene ether modified organo-montmorillonite for ibuprofen controlled release. *Appl. Clay Sci.* **2020**, *189*, 105519. [CrossRef]
21. Xu, W.; Qin, H.; Zhu, J.; Johnson, T.; Tan, D.; Liu, C.; Takahashi, Y. Selenium isotope fractionation during adsorption onto montmorillonite and kaolinite. *Appl. Clay Sci.* **2021**, *211*, 106189. [CrossRef]
22. Huang, X.; Ge, M.; Wang, H.; Liang, H.; Meng, N.; Zhou, N. Functional modification of polydimethylsiloxane nanocomposite with silver nanoparticles-based montmorillonite for antibacterial applications. *Colloid Surf. A—Physicochem. Eng. Asp.* **2022**, *642*, 128666. [CrossRef]
23. Feng, Y.; Luo, X.; Li, Z.; Fan, X.; Wang, Y.; He, R.; Liu, M. A ferroptosis-targeting ceria anchored halloysite as orally drug delivery system for radiation colitis therapy. *Nat. Commun.* **2023**, *14*, 5083. [CrossRef]
24. Long, Z.; Wu, Y.; Gao, H.; Zhang, J.; Ou, X.; He, R.; Liu, M. In vitro and in vivo toxicity evaluation of halloysite nanotubes. *J. Mater. Chem. B* **2018**, *6*, 7204–7216. [CrossRef]
25. Sabzevari, A.; Sabahi, H.; Nikbakht, M. Montmorillonite, a natural biocompatible nanosheet with intrinsic antitumor activity. *Colloid Surf. B—Biointerfaces* **2020**, *190*, 110884. [CrossRef]
26. Rozhina, E.; Batasheva, S.; Miftakhova, R.; Yan, X.; Vikulina, A.; Volodkin, D.; Fakhrullin, R. Comparative cytotoxicity of kaolinite, halloysite, multiwalled carbon nanotubes and graphene oxide. *Appl. Clay Sci.* **2021**, *205*, 106041. [CrossRef]
27. Sushma; Kumar, H.; Ahmad, I.; Dutta, P. In-vitro toxicity induced by quartz nanoparticles: Role of ER stress. *Toxicology* **2018**, *404*, 1–9. [CrossRef]
28. Leinardi, R.; Pavan, C.; Yedavally, H.; Tomatis, M.; Salvati, A.; Turci, F. Cytotoxicity of fractured quartz on THP-1 human macrophages: Role of the membranolytic activity of quartz and phagolysosome destabilization. *Arch. Toxicol.* **2020**, *94*, 2981–2995. [CrossRef]
29. Nattrass, C.; Horwell, C.; Damby, D.; Brown, D.; Stone, V. The effect of aluminium and sodium impurities on the in vitro toxicity and pro-inflammatory potential of cristobalite. *Environ. Res.* **2017**, *159*, 164–175. [CrossRef]
30. Takahashi, C.; Umemura, Y.; Naka, A.; Yamamoto, H. SEM imaging of the stimulatory response of RAW264.7 cells against Porphyromonas gingivalis using a simple technique employing new conductive materials. *J. Biomed. Mater. Res.* **2018**, *106*, 1280–1285. [CrossRef]
31. Goldstein, A.; Soroka, Y.; Frusic-zlotkin, M.; Popov, I.; Kohen, R. High resolution SEM imaging of gold nanoparticles in cells and tissues. *J. Microsc.* **2014**, *256*, 237–247. [CrossRef]

Disclaimer/Publisher's Note: The statements, opinions and data contained in all publications are solely those of the individual author(s) and contributor(s) and not of MDPI and/or the editor(s). MDPI and/or the editor(s) disclaim responsibility for any injury to people or property resulting from any ideas, methods, instructions or products referred to in the content.

MDPI AG
Grosspeteranlage 5
4052 Basel
Switzerland
Tel.: +41 61 683 77 34

Journal of Functional Biomaterials Editorial Office
E-mail: jfb@mdpi.com
www.mdpi.com/journal/jfb

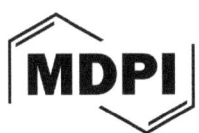

Disclaimer/Publisher's Note: The title and front matter of this reprint are at the discretion of the Guest Editor. The publisher is not responsible for their content or any associated concerns. The statements, opinions and data contained in all individual articles are solely those of the individual Editor and contributors and not of MDPI. MDPI disclaims responsibility for any injury to people or property resulting from any ideas, methods, instructions or products referred to in the content.